Make All of the Right Moves

Make All

of the

Right

Moves

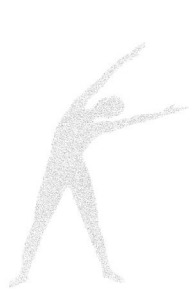

BRIAN P. LAMBERT, PT

B.L. Enterprises, LLC
Charlottesville, Virginia

Cover design by Jane Hagaman
Cover art by istockphoto.com/thenys
Photos by Rhonda Roebuck
Anatomy illustrations by Ann Lambert
Distress and smoke images by Corel and istockphoto, respectively
Text design by Jane Hagaman

The material presented in this book is not intended to be a substitute for direct and personal, professional medical care and opinion. To reduce the risk of injury, none of the exercises or activities mentioned in this book should be performed without clearance from your physician.

Exercise is not without its risks, and the exercises contained in this book, or other exercises, may result in injury.

The information in this book is in no way intended to replace or to be construed as medical advice and is offered for informational purposes only. As with any exercise, if you begin to feel faint, dizzy, or have physical discomfort, you should stop immediately and consult a physician. The information should not be considered complete, nor should it be relied on to suggest a course of treatment for a particular individual. It should not be used in place of a visit, call, consultation, or the advice of your physician or other qualified health-care provider. Should you have any health-care-related questions, call or see your physician or other qualified health-care provider promptly.

Reliance by you on any information contained in this book is solely at your own risk, and the author assumes no liability or responsibility for damage or injury to persons or property arising from your use of any information, idea, or instruction contained in this book.

Library of Congress Control Number: 2013955458

ISBN: 978-0-9748092-2-9

10 9 8 7 6 5 4 3 2 1

Printed on acid-free paper in the United States

Table of Contents

Acknowledgments

I wish to acknowledge the assistance of my family, friends, and colleagues who helped make this book possible. A special thanks to my wife, Ann, for her love, support, and artwork.

Thanks to Rhonda Roebuck for pictures, Don Fry for editing, Katherine Garstang for her assistance, Jane Hagaman for the cover, and Sara Sgarlat for advice.

Many people have shaped my views on the musculoskeletal system. Mark Bookout, Edward Isaacs, Philip Greenman, Florence Kendall, and David Butler are just a few who have had the greatest influence.

I wish to acknowledge all of my special patients (and you know who you are) who provide me with challenge and encouragement on a daily basis.

Dedication

This book is dedicated to the memory of my mom and dad. They raised their four boys to be honest and hardworking men. Mom and dad had nine grandsons, all of whom were involved in various sports. Dad would always tell his grandsons to "make all of the right moves" both on and off the field. So far it seems to be working.

Introduction

During my 30 years treating musculoskeletal problems, I have identified four to five deficits that usually result in pain in the spine and/or extremities. This pain usually results from a portion of the musculoskeletal system doing more work than it was designed to do.

Our bodies are efficiently designed as hunting and gathering machines. People who still hunt and gather don't have the problems with their neck, back, and extremities that we face in a modern society. These people use the body as it was designed to be used. In the last one to two hundred years, we have become a more sedentary society. With increased education, computers, automobiles, and video games, we spend much more time sitting. Sitting is a negative exercise. It is worse than no exercise at all, because it creates most of the problems that lead to abnormal mechanics and subtle improper movement patterns suffered by people today.

The musculoskeletal system must be viewed as an integrated system. All of the components depend on one another. Any component that is not being used optimally shifts work to another area. When four or five components are not optimally used, a great deal of work gets shifted elsewhere.

Chronic musculoskeletal problems probably start developing the first day we enter kindergarten. At that time, we begin using our largest muscles as seat cushions, and we begin slumping forward. This combination leads to many problems. With proper reprogramming of the musculoskeletal system, many of these problems can be alleviated. This book contains the exercises I use on a daily basis with my patients. Most of them experience a significant degree of improvement just by doing the exercises alone. Manual therapy by a qualified professional will help optimize motion in restricted joints and accelerate recovery from a musculoskeletal problem.

The exercises in this book derive from many sources. Many of them were designed in response to the needs of a specific patient. When they worked well, they were then tried with other patients. If an exercise worked well enough, often enough, it was incorporated into an exercise program.

Much of my physical therapy training involved learning the principles of exercise for both orthopedic and neurological rehabilitation. In continuing-education programs, the faculty of Michigan State University's School of Osteopathic Medicine emphasizes combining the principles of each area for musculoskeletal problems. There are exercises in this book taken directly from their course work. There are other exercises, whose sources I cannot recall, that are neither original nor from Michigan State Programs. I hope you can use these exercises to stay pain free and functional throughout your lifetime.

This is almost the same introduction that I used in my first book; *Precision Exercises*. I still firmly believe in the rationale outlined above. Based on client feedback, I have eliminated exercises that were not particularly helpful, added a few, and tried to explain better how to do the ones that were kept. I know that some of the exercises seem complicated and difficult, but keep in mind that you are going to try to learn something new while simultaneously unlearning something old. Old bad habits can be hard to break, and new good ones hard to learn. If you are patient and mindful, you should be able to do the exercises that you need. If you have problems, ask for help. Find a physical therapist, trainer, or friend who can help you figure things out. You will be glad you did!

Anatomy

This book deals mainly with the spine, pelvis, knees, and shoulders. Place your hands over your waist. Your hands come into contact with the pelvic bones. A little below that, we have the hip bones. Inside the hip bones are the ball and socket that make up the hip joint. The socket is part of the pelvis. The top of the thigh bone or femur is made up of the hip bone and the ball portion of the hip joint. The bottom of the femur is the top half of the knee. There is a wedge-shaped bone between the pelvic bones called the

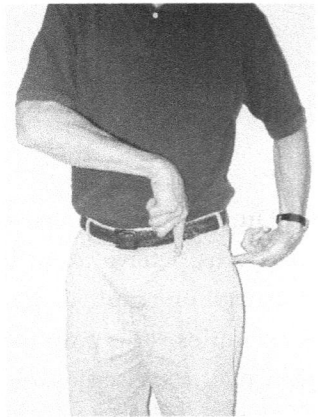

Hip Joint

sacrum. The sacrum is composed of five fused vertebrae. They generally fuse from individual vertebrae by the time we reach our late teens. The sacrum is connected to the pelvic bone by sacroiliac joints. These joints are tied to the pelvis by very strong ligaments from the front and the back. The pelvic bones are joined in the front at the pubic symphysis, which is also tied together with ligaments.

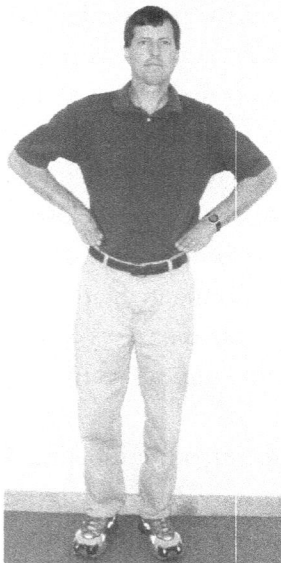

Pelvic Bones

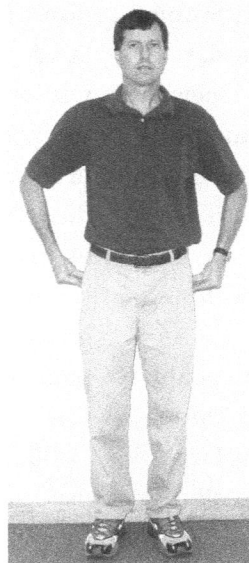

Hip Bones

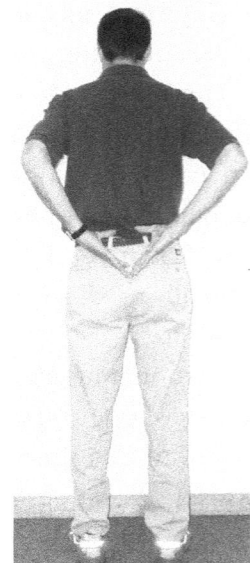

The Sacrum is between the pelvic bones

Neck or
Cervical
spine

Cervical
curve

Upper
back or
Thoracic
spine
where
the ribs
attach

Thoracic
curve

Low
back or
Lumbar
spine

Lumbar
curve

Sacrum

Sacral
curve

Tailbone
or
Coccyx

Spine from rear

Spine from left side

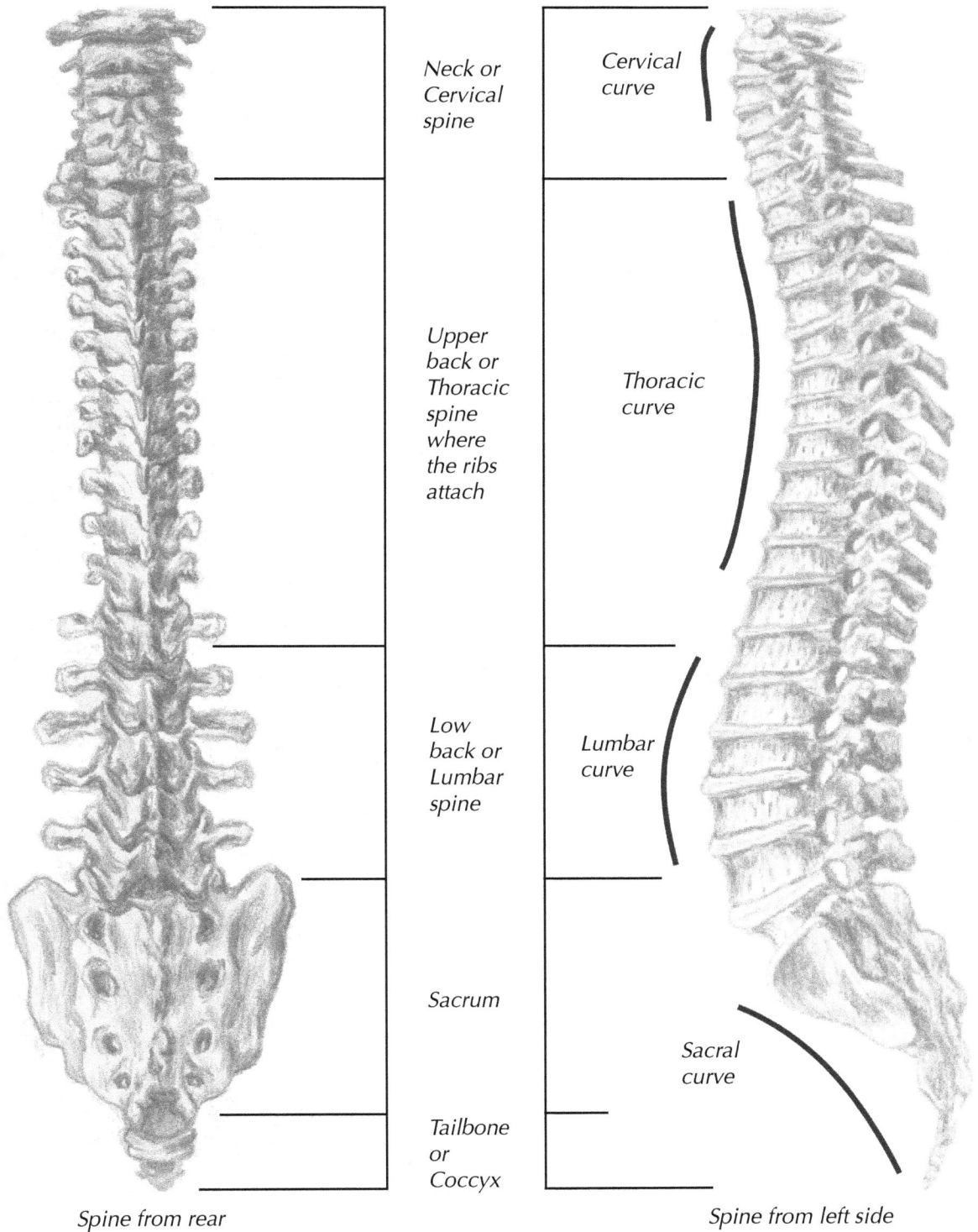

Bones of the Back

The spine is composed of individual bones called vertebra. Just above the sacrum, the bottom five vertebrae make up the lumbar spine. The ribs join the thoracic spine. Our twelve ribs attach to the twelve thoracic vertebrae. The seven cervical vertebrae are located between the base of the skull and the top of the thoracic spine.

The blocks of bone that make up the front of most vertebrae are called vertebral bodies. The vertebral bodies are separated by discs. The discs are very much like high- performance jelly doughnuts. The inside of the disc is called a nucleus and, in adults, has the consistency of crabmeat. The outside of the disc is called

Nucleus

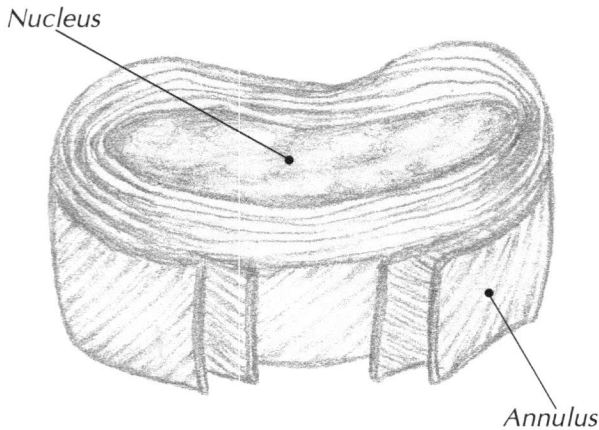

Annulus

Disc cross section

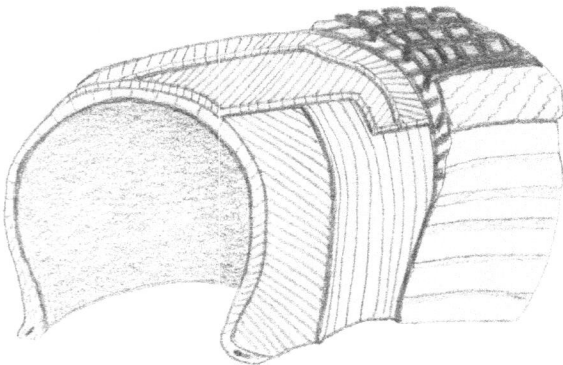

Tire cross section

the annulus, and is very much like automobile tire material. The annulus is very strong, but, over time, it can be worn down and ruptured if subjected to chronic overload. The discs are basically joints that provide multi-directional movement in the spine. They are not designed to act as shock absorbers.

On the back of the spine, there are a pair of joints. These "facet joints" link each of the vertebrae together. The surfaces of the facet joints are lined with cartilage. A joint capsule that surrounds them has an inner lining, the synovial membrane, that secretes synovial fluid into the joint. As the surface of one facet moves over the surface of another, the synovial fluid provides nutrition and lubrication to the cartilage. The facet joints stand at different angles in different parts of the spine. The orientation of the facet joints will determine how a given section of the spine can move. The thoracic spine also has attachment points for the rib cage. Problems with movement in the rib cage will influence the thoracic spine and vice versa.

The whole spinal column is bound with strong ligaments that hold it together, but are loose enough to allow movement. Bone spurs may occur where the ligaments attach to the bone as a result of continuous stress on that attachment.

Mechanical Considerations

One of the first things to observe in the spine, pelvis, and rib cage is how well everything moves. Motion in any direction should be uniform from the bottom of the sacrum to the top of the neck. All of the vertebrae should move like links in a chain. Since life's activities tend to bend us forward, the thoracic spine and sacrum become stuck in some degree of forward bending or "flexion." To achieve upright posture, we tend to overextend and overuse the low back and the middle of the neck. Localized overuse is partially responsible for arthritis or other signs of degeneration commonly seen in the low back and in the middle of the neck.

The facet joints influence how a given section of the spine will move. When viewing the lumbar spine from the back, the facet surfaces are oriented vertically. Place your hands in front of your face in a "prayer position" to illustrate the orientation of the lumbar facet joints. This allows forward bending, backward bending, and side bending, but restricts twisting. Excessive twisting in the low back jams the facet surfaces together and causes a shearing force across the disc.

In the thoracic spine, the facet pairs are almost vertical when viewed from the side. This configuration would allow movement in almost all directions, but the ribcage adds complexity to this part of the spine.

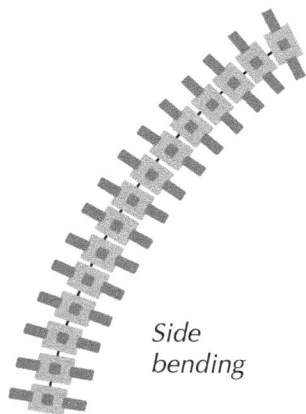

There are small joints called "demi-facets" where the ribs attach to the transverse processes (the boney struts that poke out from the sides of the vertebrae) and vertebral bodies. The bumps that you can feel on the back of your spine are called a spinous processes, and the vertebral body is the block of bone on the front of the vertebrae.

Ideally, the ribcage must move with movement of the thoracic spine. With forward bending of the thoracic spine, the back of the vertebrae with the transverse processes moves vertically because of the vertical orientation of the facet joints. Because the ribs are attached to the transverse processes, they also move vertically. Twisting in the thoracic spine pushes one rib and pulls the opposite rib. If ribs and spine move freely, life is good, but what is commonly seen is a thoracic spine that is stuck in a flexed or forward bent position. When the spine is stuck in this position, then, most likely, so are the ribs. Backward bending and rotation then become very limited. This is why grandpa has so much trouble backing the car out of the driveway.

In the neck, when viewed from the side, the facet joints in all but the top two vertebrae are at a 45 degree angle. This

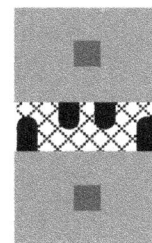

Side bending

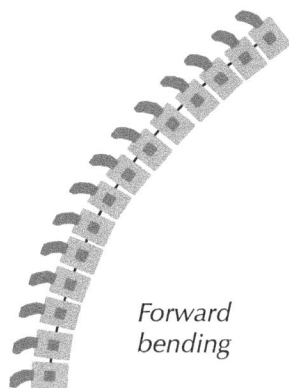

Forward bending

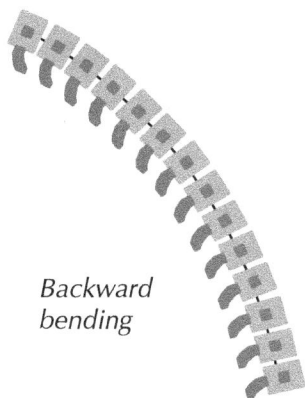

Backward bending

Lumbar facets

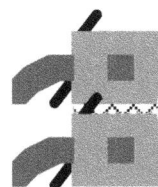

Thoracic facets

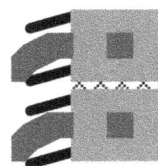

Neck facets

allows free motion in all directions. The top two vertebrae are very atypical, and, by themselves, allow your head some of its side bending and turning movements.

Mechanics of the sacrum and pelvis can be very confusing. If mechanics are good, forward bending of the trunk causes the top of the sacrum to move slightly backwards and the bottom of the sacrum to move slightly forward. The opposite motions occur with bending backward.

Imagine three cereal boxes lined up side by side. The outside boxes are the pelvic bones, and the center box is the sacrum. A fourth box on top of the center one would represent the bottom of the lumbar spine. When the top box

Sacral motion
between the pelvic bones

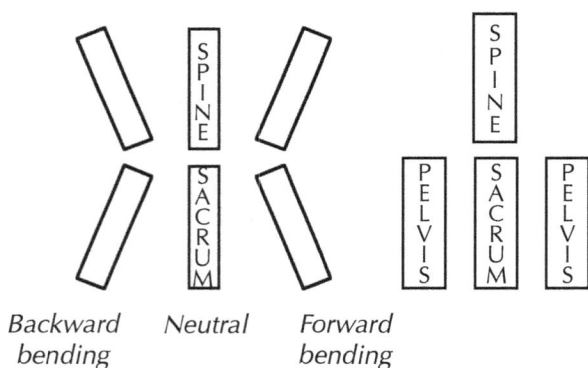

Backward   Neutral   Forward
bending   bending

is tipped forward or backwards, the bottom center box tends to tip in the opposite direction. The outside boxes are unaffected by movement of the center boxes until we connect them with "ligaments." Movement of the center box or sacral motion occurs until the slack is taken up in the ligaments, then the pelvic bones (outside boxes) move with the trunk. The first few degrees of forward or backward motion should be isolated to the spine and sacrum.

The mechanics of the pelvis and spine become more complicated when we walk or run. One side of the pelvis is rotating with the lead leg. The other side of the pelvis is rotating in the opposite direction with the trailing leg. This is generally accompanied by a slight bit of rotation and sidebending in the spine and sacrum. The spine, sacrum, and pelvic bones must move freely. One of the most common mechanical problems in the pelvis occurs when the top of the sacrum is tipped back and stuck. One side is usually worse than the other. This makes the pelvis function as one big solid bone instead of three individual bones. The lack of motion in any area of the body, including the sacroiliac joints, is called "mechanical dysfunction." Adaptation above the pelvis contributes to increased work in the low back. Since the hip socket is part of the pelvic bone, extra work may also be transmitted to the hip joint, then to the knee, then to the foot.

In the musculoskeletal system, a deficit in one area increases the workload in another area. This principle applies to the hip joints as well. Restriction of mobility in the hip joints will increase workload of the spine, pelvis, and legs. Good mobility of the hips should allow you to pull your leg towards the center of the chest to within twelve inches of your chest. A tight piriformis muscle deep in the buttock will restrict this movement.

Inward rotation of the hips should allow you to sit in a chair with your knees and thighs together and your feet 18 to 20 inches apart. Good outward rotation would allow the shin of one leg to be almost parallel to the floor when the ankle is placed on the opposite knee. Restrictions in rotation of the thighbone may be due to tightness of the muscles at the hip joint or arthritic changes in the hip joint. Hip extension is the

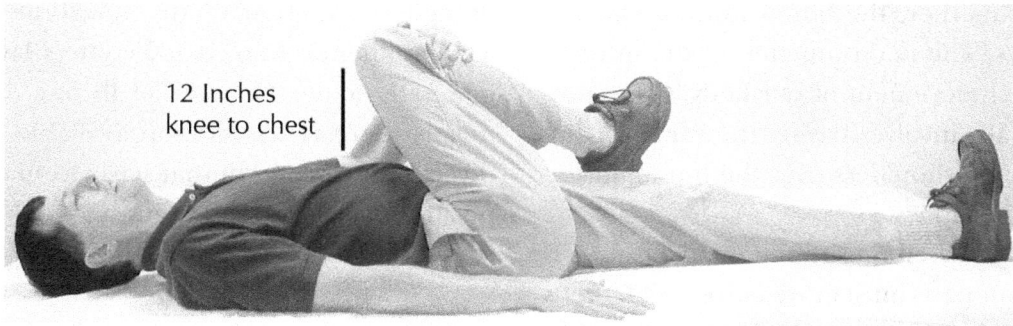

12 Inches
knee to chest

Piriformis Muscle

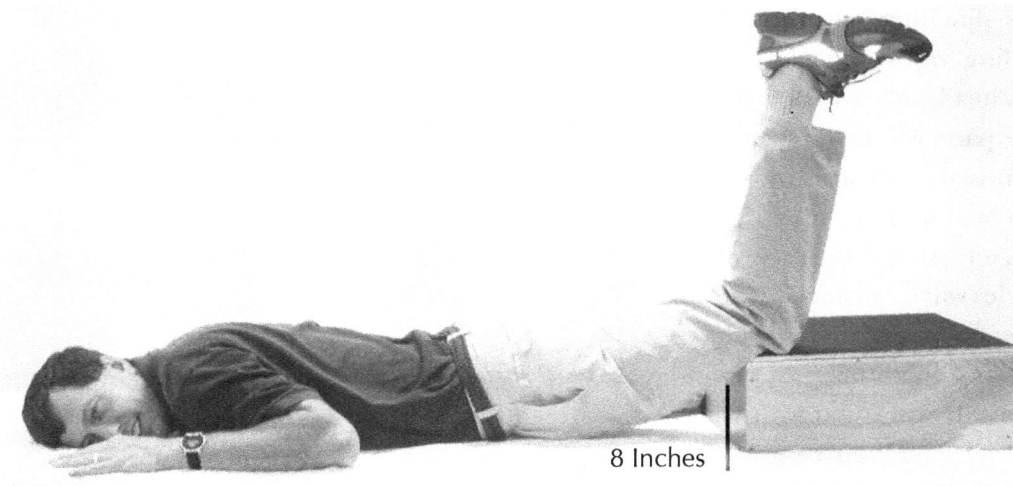

8 Inches

Hip Extension

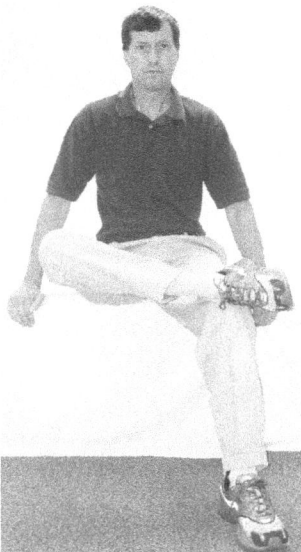

Outward Rotation of Hip

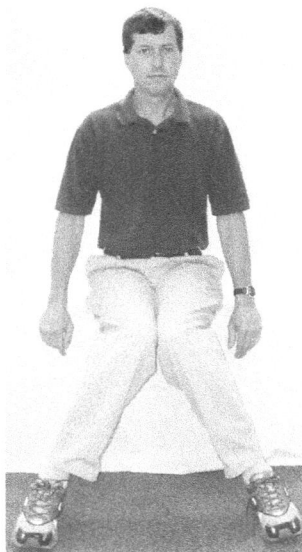

Inward Rotation of Hip

movement of the thigh behind the body when we walk and run. Good hip extension should allow you to lie face down and have someone lift your leg so that the knee is eight to twelve inches off the surface without causing movement at the pelvis. Tight hip flexors muscles can restrict this movement.

Posture

Several components must be in place for good posture. Essentially all of the parts must be stacked one on top of another, very much like a building in which all the walls are plumb. If all our components are stacked one on top of another, the bones hold us up, not the muscles. The main function of the muscles is to control movement of our body. Good posture generally involves having the ears over the shoulders, the shoulders over the hips, and the hips over the ankles.

The major prerequisite for good posture is that all of our parts must move well enough for us to easily stack things up. We should not have to force ourselves to remain upright by pinching our shoulders back, holding our stomach in, or pulling our head back over our shoulders. If the parts will easily stack up, very little muscular effort is required to remain standing. If your knees can completely straighten, then your thigh muscles will be relaxed. If your knees were to remain even slightly bent, then your thigh muscles would have to work. If you stood with your knees bent all day, then your knees and thighs would probably get very sore. Poor posture increases pressure or loading in the spine the same way bent knees increase the pressure or loading on the joint surfaces of the knee.

The benefits of good posture are many. First, all of the spinal segments are in a completely neutral position. This neutral position of the vertebrae means that the bottom surface of each vertebra is parallel to the top surface of the vertebra below it. Loading is then distributed evenly across the disc, which is sandwiched between the vertebral bodies. Another benefit

of neutral position of the vertebrae involves a phenomenon known as Fryette's law, which generally states that motion in one direction, means there is less motion available in other directions. A segment that starts from a neutral position has maximum motion available in any single direction. When you turn your head or

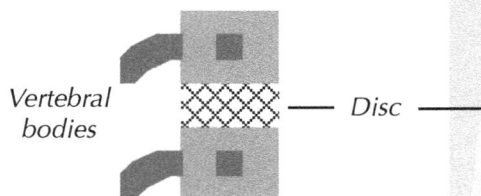

Vertebral bodies —————— *Disc* ——————

The discs are sandwiched between the vertebrae.

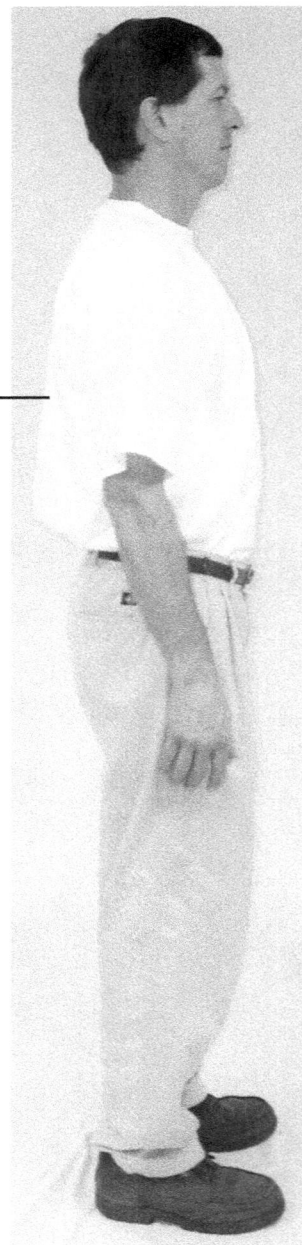

trunk, each segment should move uniformly, like links in a chain. Stress and movement will then be evenly distributed. So, if grandpa's upper back is forward bent, then his neck is probably backward bent to compensate. He then has less rotation available to look back when backing the car out of the driveway. Out-of-neutral segments create a kink in the system, and stress increases above and below the kink. An out-of-neutral segment can be stuck simply forward or backward bent but there are mechanical dysfunctions where one or more vertebrae can be stuck flexed, rotated, and sidebent or extended, rotated, and sidebent.

When walking or running, movement of the neutral spine and pelvis combines with movement of the hips, knees, ankles, and feet so that all of these joints behave like a vertical accordion. Normally, when the ends of an accordion are pressed together, all parts of the accordion should move uniformly. If three or four folds were to be blocked open, then points of high stress would be created above and below the blocked area when the accordion is compressed. With mechanical dysfunction in the spine and pelvis, we see these points of high stress in "our accordion" in the middle of the neck, lower lumbar spine, and often at the knees.

When all of the segments are in neutral positions, the spine has four primary curves. Generally there is some sway or "lordosis" to the low back and neck. There is a forward curvature or "kyphosis" through the thoracic spine as well as through the sacrum and pelvis. Like a spring, the neutral curves allow movement that will provide for shock absorption. If there is too little curve in the back, a great deal of compressive force is driven straight down, especially through the lower vertebrae. If there is too much curve, as

with a sway back, then shearing forces develop. There are many adaptations to poor posture. Some of these involve severe retraction of the head and neck, flattening of the lumbar spine, or severe forward sway to the pelvis. Too often mechanics in one area are sacrificed to compensate for problems in another. If you can't stand up straight, your muscles work too hard and cause problems.

Muscles of the Hips and Pelvis

The muscles located in your buttock area are the most important muscles in the body for control, balance, and motion. The largest muscles in your body are located there. The "tush" can be thought of as the keystone of the musculoskeletal system. It should be the main propulsion unit. It should be the foundation the spine sits on. It should be the main area for control of balance. Often it is none of the above.

The entire buttock area is a package of muscles. The largest single muscle in the body is the gluteus maximus. This muscle is a hip extensor and a hip (external) rotator. It attaches along the pelvis and sacrum and crosses the hip joint to attach to the upper portion of the thighbone. Ahead of this muscle, but behind and above the hipbone, are the gluteus medius and gluteus minimus muscles. These large muscles are commonly called hip abductors. Underneath the gluteus maximus are the smaller hip (external) rotators. These include the piriformis, the gemelli superior, gemelli inferior, quadratus femoris, obturator internus, and obturator externus (not pictured). All of these buttock muscles basically surround our body's center of gravity. The most efficient way to control an object is at its center of gravity.

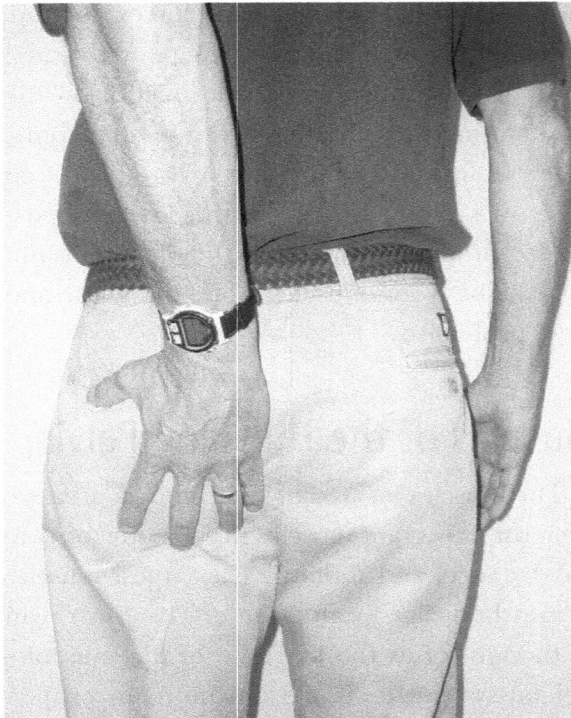

Gluteus Maximus Muscle

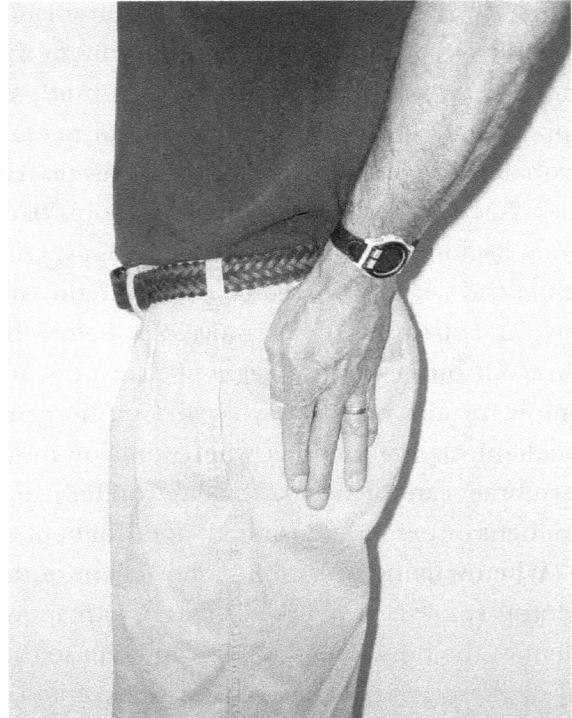

Gluteus Medius and Minimus Muscle

The buttock muscles, especially the gluteus maximus, will do multiple jobs with a single contraction. Ideally, one side of the tush muscles should be strong enough to lift and control the entire weight of the body. This should happen with every step you take. The gluteus maximus may also stabilize the sacroiliac joint (SIJ) by pulling the sacrum against the pelvic bone when the muscle contracts. Often therapists will use a belt when the SIJ seems loose or unstable. Good glute max function will stabilize the sacroiliac joints.

Good contraction of the gluteus maximus will pull the ball of the hip joint backwards and to the inside of the hip socket. Most of the wear and tear in an arthritic hip is at the top of the ball and socket. Weightbearing forces and the action of many of the hip muscles tend to push and pull the ball straight up to the top of the socket. Good

contraction of the gluteus maximus will offset this straight-up push and use more of the surface area available in the hip joint. Good gluteus activation will align the thigh bone over the lower leg for correct tracking of the knee cap and foot and ankle orientation. By extending the hip the gluteus maximus pushes us forward from directly behind our center of gravity. This uses our buttocks as our main propulsion unit. Long periods of sitting will degrade how well we can activate or recruit the gluteus maximus, medius, and minimus when we move. Because these muscles are not well recruited, they are very weak and grossly underutilized. With our body's redundant design (*i.e.* no muscle works alone), we try to shift the work to other muscle areas.

Tightness or inflexibility in muscles should be viewed as an adaptation to overuse. The spring on a garage door reduces the energy you must

Pelvic bone

Greater trochanter (hip bone)

Gluteus medius

Gluteus minimus

Piriformis

Gluteus maximus

Superior gemellus

Obturator internus

Inferior gemellus

Quadratus femoris

Ischial tuberosity
(sit bone)

Hamstrings

Calf

Back

Side

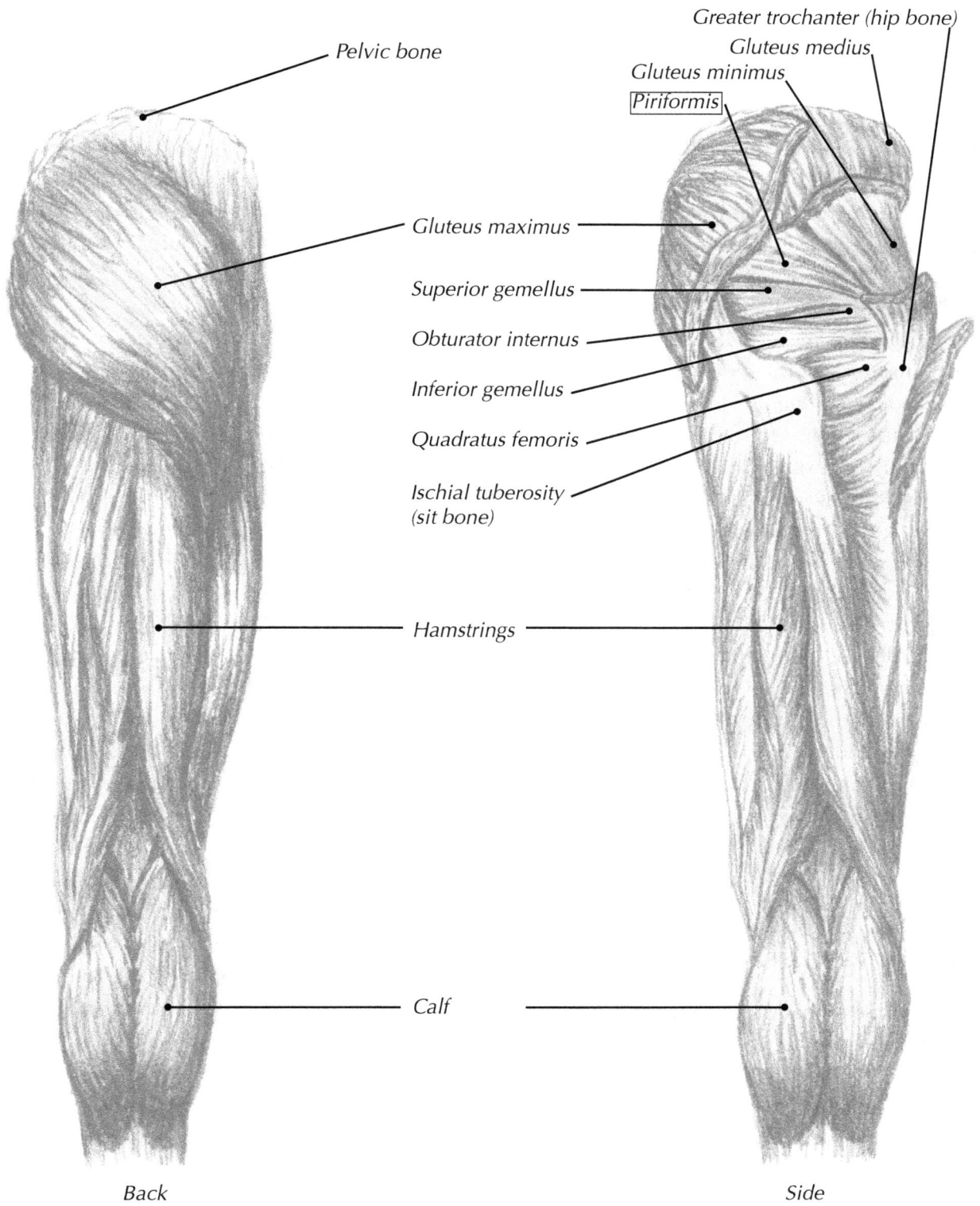

Muscles of the Right Hip and Leg

expend to open the door manually. A tight muscle is spring-loaded and becomes much more energy efficient. The same phenomenon occurs with young men who lift very heavy weights on a repetitive basis. They become "muscle bound." This term refers not only to their bulkiness, but also to their lack of mobility. If you lose too much mobility in a muscle, then the tightness itself becomes a problem. The large muscles in the hip tend to be very weak. The muscles that try to substitute for them will tend to be overused and become very tight. The hamstrings, on the back of the thigh, are secondary hip extensors but mainly control the knee. If the hamstrings have to do both jobs constantly, full-time, they will get tight. The smaller hip rotators (especially the piriformis) can substitute to some degree for the hip abductors and extensors, and will get very tight. The low back muscles can substitute to some degree for the hip abductors and extensors, and again, will get very tight if they are overused on a chronic basis. The tightness in these muscles will not be alleviated until the large muscles are not only strong, but are also activated or "recruited" appropriately when you move.

Muscles of the Cylinder/ Guy-Wire System

The muscles that wrap around the body from the rib cage down to the pelvis must work simultaneously as both a cylinder or tube system and a guy-wire system.

An upright tube or cylinder is capable of resisting compressive forces. If you take a spent toilet paper tube and stand it on a table, you could easily balance several books on its top. The weight of the books would be evenly distributed around the base of the tube. If the tube were dented or weakened on one side, then the system would collapse.

Functioning as a tube, the muscles between the rib cage and pelvis allow some of the weight of the upper torso to be carried on the upper rim of the pelvis. If functioning properly, the abdominal muscles will reduce some of the compressive forces carried by the spine. The lumbar intervertebral discs are roughly two inches in diameter. Without help from the cylinder/guy-wire system, these discs will break down because they are not large enough or strong enough to bear the entire weight of the upper torso for an entire lifetime.

An example of a guy-wire system would be the cable supports that hold up a radio antenna. The tension in these wires must balance so that the antenna is evenly supported. Obviously, the antenna must be perfectly vertical or plumb.

As we move, the muscles between the rib cage and pelvis hold the torso upright like the guy-wires holding up an antenna. In the front and sides, the muscles of the cylinder/guy-wire system include the rectus abdominis, the internal and external obliques, and the transverse abdominis. Around the back of the spine, you have the erector spinae, quadratus lumborum, and the latissimus dorsi. The layering and criss-crossing pattern of these muscles allow them to function simultaneously as a cylinder and guy-wire system.

Having poor posture is like having an antenna that is leaning over. Some of the cables will be very tight (the back muscles). Other cables will be very loose (the abdominal muscles). Having poor posture is like having a dent in the tube holding up the books. The books will fall over unless the back of the tube is reinforced. This is what our back muscles end up doing. When

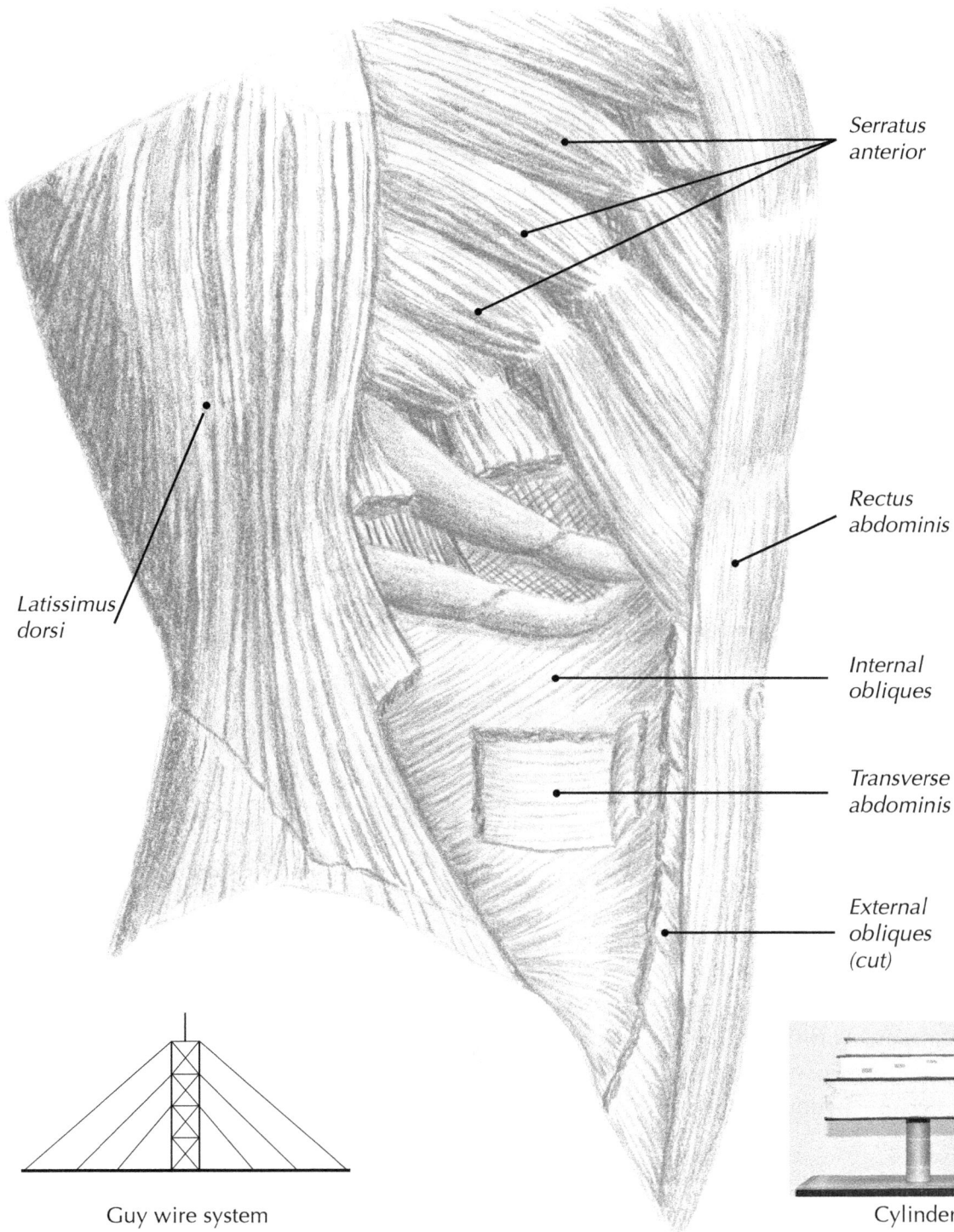

Serratus
anterior

Rectus
abdominis

Internal
obliques

Transverse
abdominis

External
obliques
(cut)

Latissimus
dorsi

Guy wire system

Cylinder

Muscles of the Cyliner/Guy-Wire System
(looking at the right side)

we are upright and moving, we need to be able to maintain some tension in all of the muscles between the rib cage and pelvis. This "co-contraction" of the muscles gives the cylinder/guy-wire system some "rigidity," and this is how we need them to work to support the back. Poor posture will under-utilize the abdominal muscles and overuse the back muscles.

Some common stomach exercises may be bad for us. The intention of crunches, sit-ups, curls, and abdominal exercise machines is to train and strengthen the abdominal muscles. Posture may worsen with these exercises by incorrectly strengthening the muscles in the front of the chest and neck, and the hip flexors when attempting to strengthen only the abdominals. The abdominal musculature is used in a sit-up motion with an activity like getting out of bed. During upright movements, these muscles should be used as a cylinder/guy-wire system.

Most people with back and leg problems have gross muscle imbalance and very poor control of the muscles of the torso. With the pelvic clock exercise (page 8), most people can selectively isolate and activate their back muscles, but, initially, they cannot selectively isolate and activate their stomach muscles. They tend to push with their legs and/or tighten their chest and neck. This pattern of muscle activation probably occurs when they are upright. Isolation and activation of opposing muscle groups in the torso should be almost as easy as using your biceps and triceps when bending and straightening your elbow.

Neck, Upper Back, and Shoulders

Most of the problems with pain in the neck and shoulders can be traced back to poor positioning and/or movement patterns. There is usually muscle imbalance in the neck, upper back, and rib cage. Forward head posture occurs when the upper back or "thoracic spine" is stuck in a flexed position. This places the head in front of the shoulders. Your head weighs as much as a bowling ball. It is easier to carry a bowling ball with one arm in an upright position, centered and balanced. If you allow the bowling ball to tip forward, more muscle effort is required to keep it in place. Forward head posture requires more effort from the muscles in the neck and upper back. These muscles should only have to work when we are moving.

Postural muscles in the front of the neck include the scalene and deep neck flexors. One end of the scalene muscles attaches along the sides of the vertebrae of the neck, and their other end attaches to the first and second ribs just behind the collarbones. The deep neck flexors attach to the front of the vertebra of the neck. Forward head posture causes overuse of the scalenes and muscles in the back of the neck and underuse of the deep neck flexors. The deep muscles along the upper back and back of the neck include the various layers of the spinal extensors or erector spinae. These muscles can attach from one vertebra to the next, from vertebra to the skull, or from rib cage to the vertebra. The shallow muscles of the back include the trapezius, levator scapulae, and rhomboids.

One end of these muscles attaches to the shoulder blade, and the other end attaches to the spine. The upper portion of the trapezius

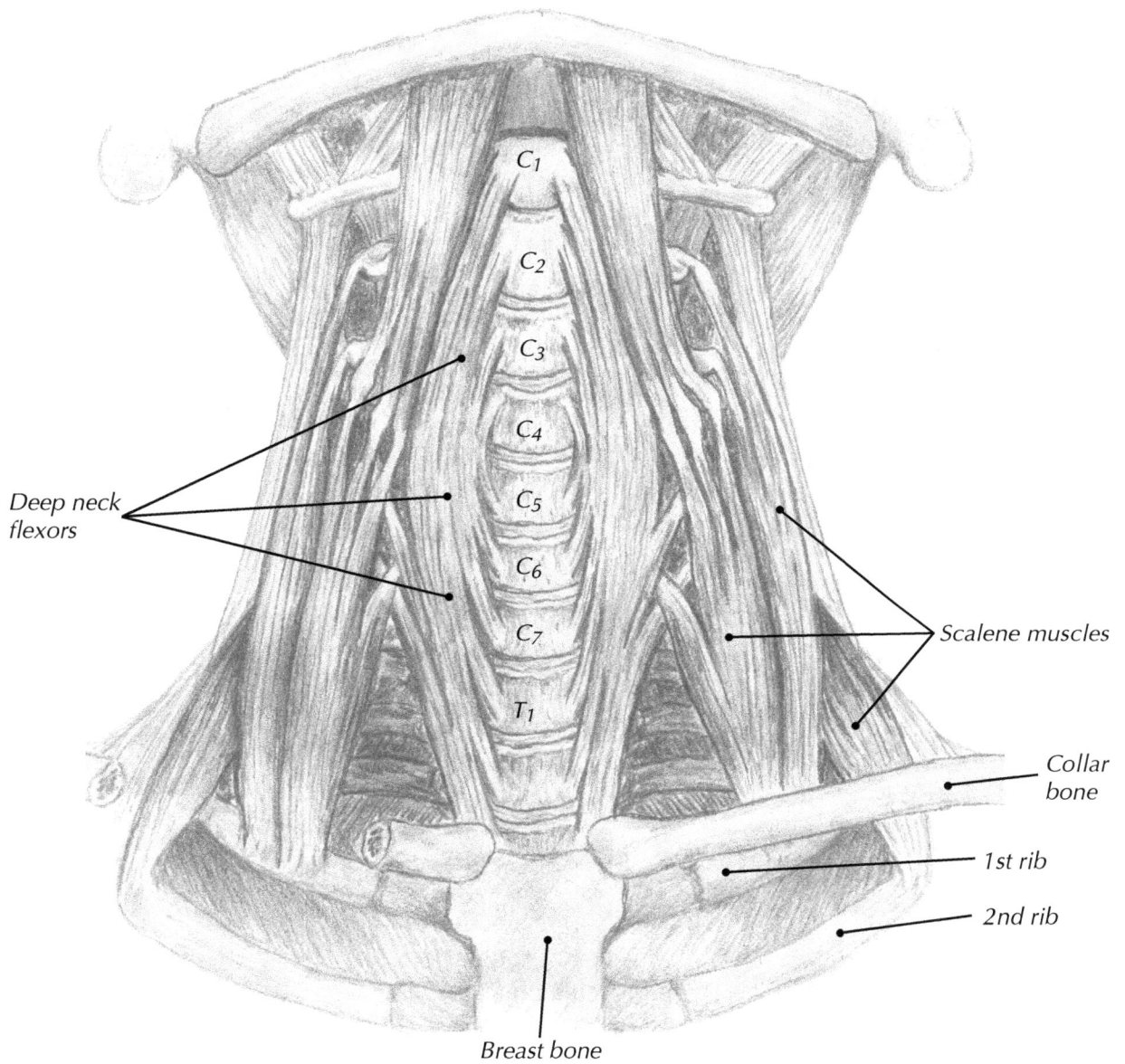

C1
C2
C3
C4
C5
C6
C7
T1

Deep neck flexors

Scalene muscles

Collar bone

1st rib

2nd rib

Breast bone

Postural Muscles in the Front of the Neck

Trapezius

Deltoid

Splenus capitus

Levator scapulae

Rhomboids

Rotator cuff

Serratus anterior

Latissimus
dorsi

Erector spinae

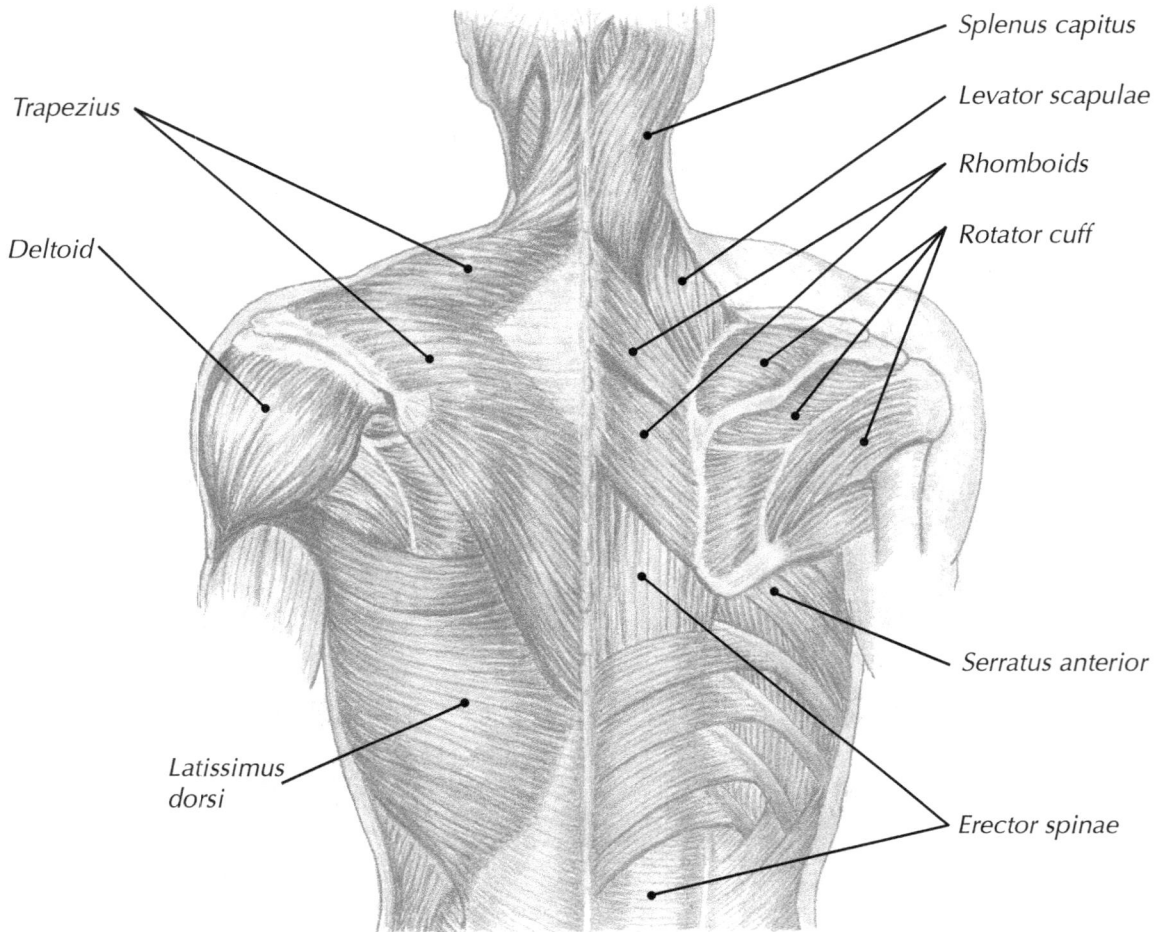

Muscles of the Back
Deep Muscles on Right Side

attaches to the back of the head. Forward head posture will cause overuse of the upper trapezius, levator scapula, and erector spinae in the neck, and underuse of the thoracic erector spinae, rhomboids, and the lower portion of the trapezius. Overused muscles will become tight and probably painful. Underused muscles will become weak and poorly recruited. Good posture involves keeping the ears over the shoul-ders, the shoulders over the hips, and the hips over the ankles. This lineup will encourage optimal usage of all of the postural musculature.

The arms attach to the spine and rib cage with a series of supportive muscles. Some of these muscles also attach to the head and neck. The only boney attachment that the arm has to the body is through the collar bone. These muscles include the trapezius, serratus anterior, rhomboids, pectoralis minor (not pictured), and levator scapula. All of these muscles attach from the spine or rib cage to the shoulder blade. The trapezius and levator musculature do double duty. One end helps support the head and neck. The other end is attached to the shoulder blade to help control and stabilize the shoulder. If posture is poor, too much of their work is devoted to controlling the head and neck, and less control is available to the shoulder. The latissimus dorsi and pectoralis or chest musculature attach to the upper arm and then to the rib cage and spine. If posture is poor, these muscles can become tight and will adversely affect shoulder function.

The rotator cuff and deltoid muscles attach to the shoulder blade and then to the upper portion of the arm. Their primary purpose is to control movement in the ball and socket that make up the shoulder or "glenohumeral joint." The socket is part of the shoulder blade, and the ball is part of the bone of the upper arm or humerus. Movement of the ball in the socket accounts for only a portion of the motion of raising your arm.

If you start with your arm at your side and raise it so your hand is straight up over your head, the total movement is usually around 180 degrees. Traditionally, it is thought that 120 degrees of movement occurs in the "shoulder joint" and the other 60 degrees is movement of the shoulder blade on the rib cage, which is a 2:1 ratio. Realistically, the ratio is closer to 1:1, where half of the arm motion of raising the arm is in the glenohumeral joint, and the other half is movement of the shoulder blade.

This one-to-one ratio can be demonstrated if your right shoulder blade is held stationary while you attempt to gently raise your right arm overhead. If you stop as soon as you feel movement of the shoulder blade, the overall

movement of right arm is usually less than 90 degrees. If you were to start with the arm 30 degrees behind your body, then the motion in the glenohumeral joint would come out to 120 degrees, but it's less than 90 degrees when the arm starts at your side.

To assess movement of the shoulder blade, hold a pen or pencil, pointed forward, on top of the flat, boney spot on top of the shoulder. With the arm beside the body, the pencil is close to horizontal. When the arm is raised to 180 degrees or straight overhead, the flat spot or "acromion process" and pencil are now close to vertical. Slight left sidebending of the upper torso helps to tilt the shoulder blade farther upward.

While these measurement techniques may not be in the most rigorous scientific method they seem to demonstrate a ratio of movement that is closer one to one (1:1) than two to one (2:1).

Ideal movement of the shoulder blade, and hence, ideal functioning of the whole shoulder complex, is dependent on the shoulder blade's ability to move on the rib cage. Poor posture and mechanical dysfunction of the rib cage will interfere with this movement. Tight pectoral, latissimus dorsi, upper trapezius, and levator scapula will interfere with this movement. Mechanical dysfunction in the rib cage usually involves the upper ribs being stuck in an elevated position which jams the ribs under the shoulder blade preventing it from moving properly when we raise our arm. The ribs are elevated by poor recruitment patterns and tightness of muscles that attach to the rib cage. These muscles include the scalenes, pectoralis minor, iliocostalis cervicis, serratus posterior superior, and levator costae. These muscles tend to be overused when posture is poor, and when our breathing pattern is more in the upper chest rather than diaphragmatic.

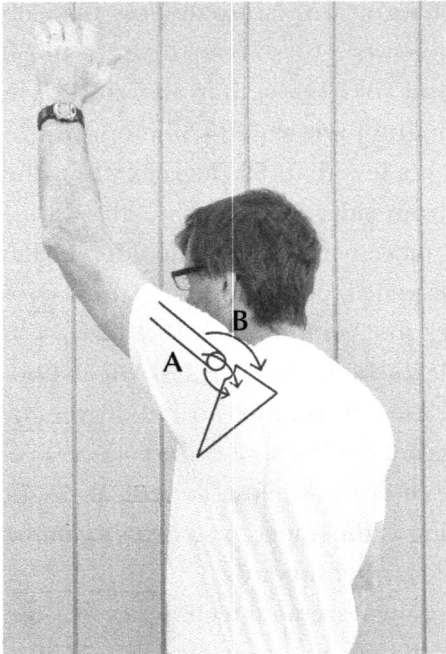

Rotator cuff (A) and deltoid (B)
muscles move the ball in the socket

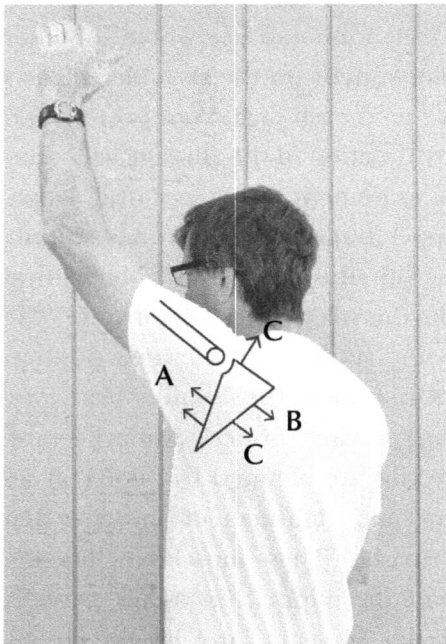

Serratus anterior (A), rhomboids (B),
trapezius (C), and other scapular
muscles move the shoulder blade on
the rib cage.

Movement issues in the upper back and rib cage can cause problems in the shoulder and neck. Rotator cuff tendonitis and bursitis may be caused if our bodies adapt to poor shoulder blade function by shifting work out to the "shoulder joint." If our bodies shift work "upward," we then have pain in the neck.

Before You Begin

Our bodies are not designed for static positioning or repetitive motion. Sitting can be viewed as a negative exercise. We were not designed for prolonged sitting because it creates tremendous pressure on the buttock muscles. This area is not designed as a seat cushion. Sitting has the same effect on the large buttock muscles as asking someone to sit on their hand for 15 or 20 minutes. The hand would not be of much use until the circulation and feeling returned. This happens to the buttock muscles every day. Theoretically, if you sat long enough, without moving, you would kill the skin and muscle tissue and subsequently develop a pressure sore. Our bodies are designed in such a redundant fashion that we can learn to do without the large muscles. Over years, the work of the gluteals is transferred up to the back, into the piriformis muscles, and down to the knees and ankles, causing problems in these areas. Not using your big muscles causes big pain elsewhere.

Sitting also increases forward bending of the upper torso, which leads to poor posture. The skeletal system out of plumb alters how the cylinder/guy-wire muscle system works. Once we have adopted abnormal movement patterns, it is difficult to unlearn them without specific exercises designed to activate or "recruit" muscles and restore movements that are no longer used on a regular basis.

Misused areas of the body will hurt, feel fatigued, feel tight, and may show increased signs of wear and tear (*i.e.* arthritis). There is usually nothing wrong with the area or part that hurts. It is just doing more work than it is meant to handle.

To illustrate: Imagine an air conditioning system for a six-story building. Our system has six units spaced evenly in the building. These units feed a central duct system. Let's say that each unit needs to run at 50 percent capacity to keep the building at 70 degrees. If, through some control malfunction, the output of unit three drops to only 20 percent, one way to compensate would be to increase the output of unit four to 70 percent. When this pattern of usage persists for a long period of time, the com-

ponents of unit four would wear out while the remaining units would appear to be working just fine. A technician could repair the worn parts in unit four but, if it continues to run at 70 percent capacity, it will again suffer a premature breakdown.

In our bodies, unit three could represent the pelvis. This would include the sacroiliac and hip joints and associated muscles. Unit four could be the low back. A poorly functioning pelvis can shift workload to the back causing premature breakdown.

We can assign the other "units" to other body parts. Unit five is the cylinder/guy-wire system. Unit six is the upper back and neck. Unit two would be our knees, and unit one would be our feet.

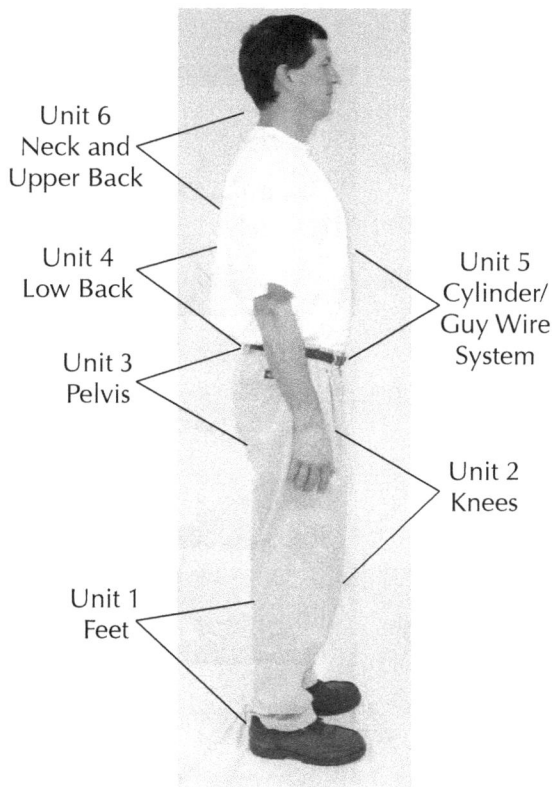

Unit 6 Neck and Upper Back

Unit 4 Low Back

Unit 3 Pelvis

Unit 1 Feet

Unit 5 Cylinder/ Guy Wire System

Unit 2 Knees

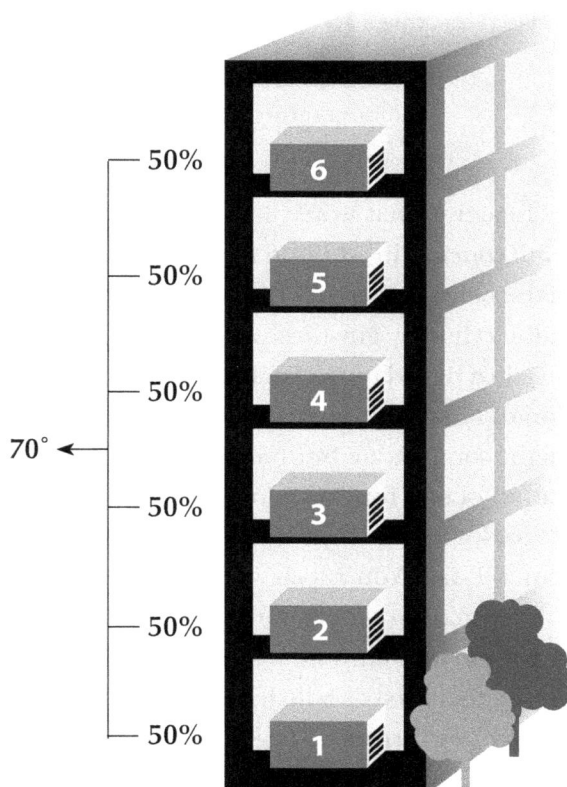

50%

50%

50%

70°

50%

50%

50%

Building with six HVAC units operating at 50% capacity

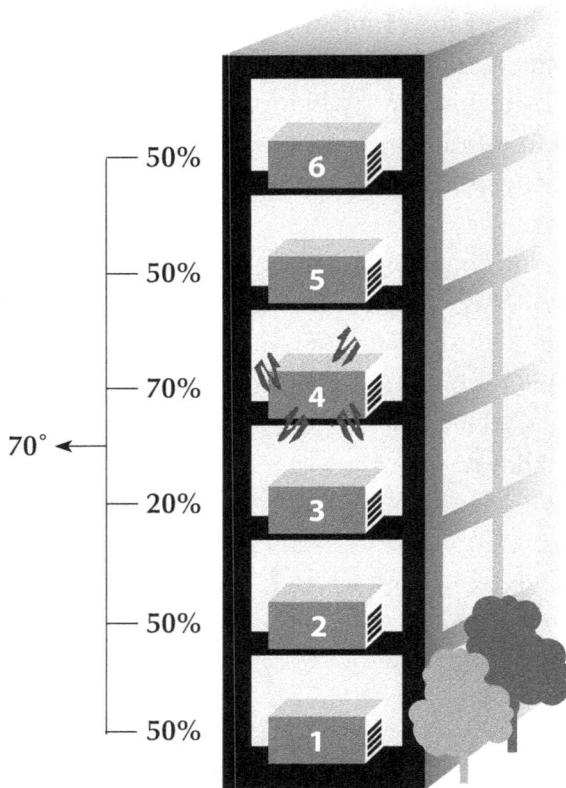

50% — 6
50% — 5
70° ← 70% — 4
20% — 3
50% — 2
50% — 1

Minor control malfunction

back, but they are not aware of the damage that is being done.

The scenario described for low back pain is not the only way the body can compensate for multiple areas of dysfunction. If you have only 30 percent function in units three, five, and six (pelvis, cylinder/guy-wire system, and upper back) but the low back function, unit 4, remains at 50 per cent, the overload might get shifted to unit two—the knees. Now unit two is routinely operating at 100 percent capacity, and we now have issues with pain and unusual wear and tear in the knees rather than the low back.

Our bodies are creative and adaptive machines. When dealing with multiple areas of dysfunction you see almost any combination of load redistribution. The overloaded area might

Imagine what would happen to the low back (unit four), if in addition to diminished function in the pelvis, we also had only 30 percent function in the cylinder/guy-wire system (unit five). Then, we add a flexed upper back which drops the function of unit six down to 30 percent. Our "system" might compensate by dramatically increasing the output of unit four. The low back now must operate under a severe overload. Sooner or later, unit four will fail. You repair it, but it will fail again. This scenario demonstrates the conditions seen in people with chronic low back pain. Some people in their sixty's will have some degenerative changes or "arthritis" (signs of overuse) in their low back and not have any back pain. These people may not be "wired" to feel pain in the same way as others. They can be overusing their low

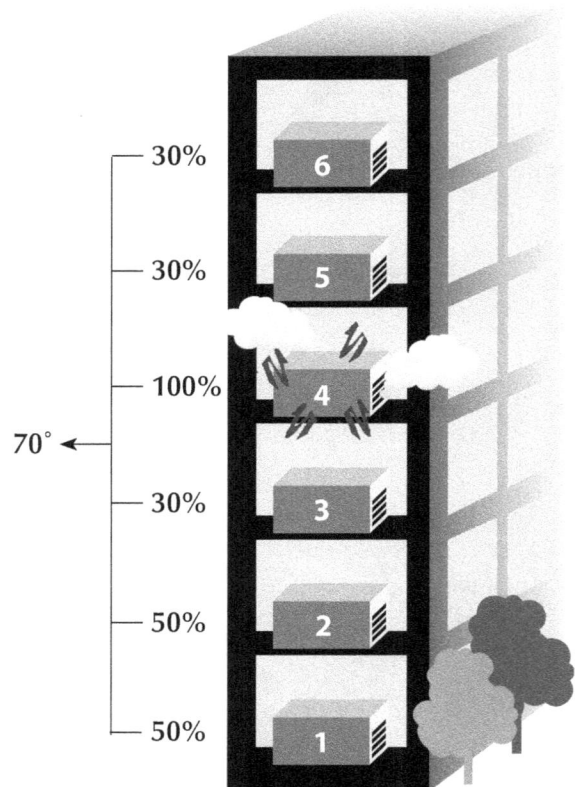

30% — 6
30% — 5
70° ← 100% — 4
30% — 3
50% — 2
50% — 1

Major control malfunction
for low back pain scenario

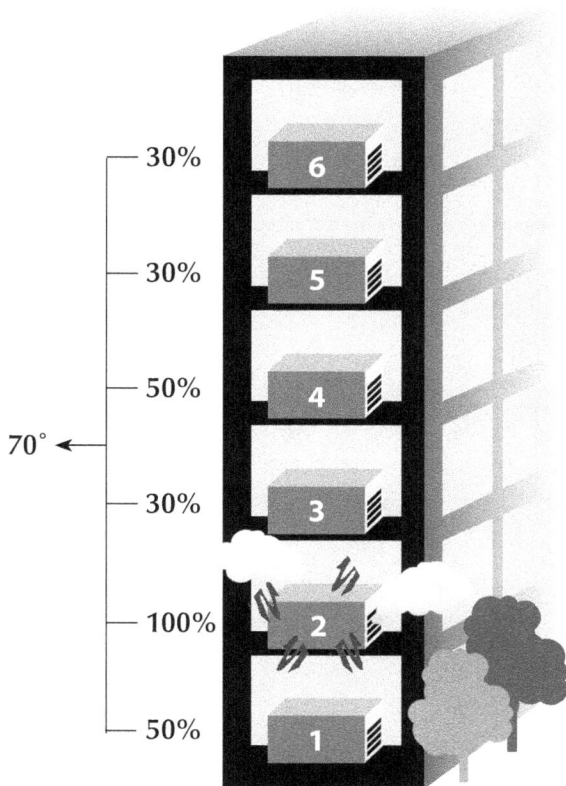

Major control malfunction for knee pain scenario

be the feet, knees, hips, back, neck, or shoulders. It all depends on our "programming."

Most of the exercises described in this book deal with reprogramming the body so that we can optimally distribute the workload of everyday life evenly over the musculoskeletal system.

All of these exercises must be done carefully with specific attention to the target of each exercise. You may consult with your physician, physical therapist, and/or trainer to be sure you can do these exercises safely and effectively. Sometimes it is helpful to have a family member observe how you are doing an exercise. They might see something that you cannot "feel" and help you do the exercise correctly.

You are not expected to do each and every exercise in this book. If you have a low back or hip problem, start with the basic low back exercises. If you have a neck or shoulder problem, start with the neck and posture exercises. For a given problem, there is no specific order in which the exercises are to be done. You can try the various stretching and foam roller exercises that might apply to your problem. A stretch that "feels good" is probably going to help you. If an exercise becomes too easy, and you are fairly certain that you are doing it correctly, try a more advanced exercise. If you master the more advanced exercise, then you may discontinue the previous one.

Avoid Pain

Pain is the body's signal that something is wrong. With the musculoskeletal system, it is often the last indicator of a problem. Dysfunction is usually present before pain. If pain seems to start gradually without a precipitating event, or if there is an injury that does not resolve, part of the body is probably working too hard. Working it harder will not fix the problem. A "no pain/no gain" approach does not work.

Exercises or other activities that cause pain are only reinforcing non-optimal muscle activation or recruitment patterns. When something hurts, you are placing strain on an area that does not need more strain. Consider a blister on the palm of your hand from too much raking or shoveling. When that area is raw and angry, the last thing you want to do is rub or irritate it in any way. Musculoskeletal pain is basically "a blister" or raw spot on the inside of the body. Causing more hurt in that area would be the same as bothering an irritated place on your palm. Don't do it: causing pain won't get rid of pain.

Many people describe a deep massage, gentle stretching, or a muscle working as "good pain."

The sensation of good pain usually dissipates when you stop doing the exercise, and you feel better. Joint pain, pinching, tingling, and numbness are "bad pain." Bad pain may linger after you stop the exercise and you don't feel any better. If you experience bad pain with a repetition of an exercise, change how you do the next repetition. Decrease the intensity or amount of movement. Stop the exercise if it cannot be done comfortably. See if there is another exercise that will "hit the target" without causing "bad pain."

1

Basic Low Back Exercises

The basic back set consists of five or six exercises. One exercise stretches the deep rotators of the hips. Two exercises are designed to reprogram the major supportive muscles in the trunk and the pelvis. The others are to improve spinal and pelvic mobility. There is no specific order in which the exercises should be done.

Each of the exercises has a purpose and a specific target. If you miss the target, the exercise is almost a waste of time. Your brain tells the body what muscles to use to make movements happen. Because the body is an adaptive, learning machine, this program can be altered. Learning a dance or other specific activity involves reprogramming or altering the body's movement program. You can start to change your motor program by doing the exercises as described.

Long periods of sitting are one of the worst positions for the body. The gluteal musculature gets smashed. The thoracic spine and sacrum get jammed into a flexed position. The abdominals are not needed. Repeated bouts of sitting (*i.e.,* K through 12) will alter our motor program into a substitution program, which ultimately becomes our standard motor program. In this substitution pattern, much of the work of balance, lift, and propulsion gets transferred away from the buttock muscles to either the lower back or the legs. The low back musculature can get grossly overused and tight, leading to increased compressive forces and increased overall work done in the lower part of the lumbar spine. If the pelvis is shifted forward, the hip flexors and thighs become involved, leading to overuse of the hips, knees, ankles, and

feet, as well as additional compressive force in the lower lumbar spine.

Runners and weekend warriors may transfer their work mostly to the legs and develop problems in those areas. Many people transfer the work to the lower back and therefore experience increased levels of low back pain.

The basic beginning exercises are the supine piriformis stretch, prone gluteal retraining, pelvic clock, sacral mobilization, and two basic foam roller exercises (pages 174 and 176). If your posture is very poor, sometimes the wall angel exercise is also needed. Substitute exercises can be done if the primary exercise does not hit the target. Do these as a group to address multiple areas of dysfunction.

The muscular retraining exercises done lying down will prepare you for doing a stand-up version of muscle re-education. Your body doesn't need supportive muscles when you lie down. You only need them when you're vertical. Complete re-integration of a muscle group into upright movement won't take place until you activate or recruit the muscle during the activity for which it is designed. The gluteal muscles need to work when the foot is on the ground, and the trunk is vertical. Good posture makes little difference when the body is horizontal, but is a big factor when you're upright.

The lie-down exercises are important to help you learn to isolate a muscle or muscle group. They teach the brain where the muscle is. The stand-up exercises teach the brain how the muscle functions, and then you can reinforce the correct motor pattern as well as strengthen the muscle.

1

Supine Piriformis Stretch

This exercise stretches the smaller hip rotators located deep in the buttock region, specifically targeting the piriformis.

Start by lying on your back with the right thigh at 90 degrees to the floor with the knee relaxed. The left leg is straight and resting on the floor. While keeping the right thigh at 90 degrees, use the right hand, bring the right knee to the midline of the body. While keeping the thigh at 90 degrees, rotate the lower portion of the leg across the body. The right heel should touch the outside of the left thigh. Keep the knee in the centerline of the body. Grab the right shin with the left hand and with the right hand, grab the outside of the right knee. Now pull equally with both hands to bring the right knee towards the center of the chest. Fine-tune by increasing the amount of rotation and/or changing the positioning of the knee by slightly moving the knee to one side or the other. You should feel a sensation of gentle stretch in the buttock area. Occasionally you may feel some of the stretch down the back of the thigh. Hold the position for at least 15 seconds, and do three repetitions on each side. If pinching occurs in the groin area, move the leg to one side or the other. Do not pull so hard that the pelvis twists or you feel pain.

For a more aggressive stretch, try the quadriped version (page 52). To work on "fibrotic" or knotted tissue, do deep massage of the piriformis (page 54).

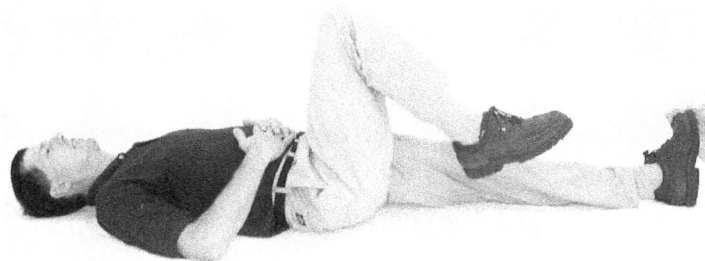

1. Lie on back. Thigh at 90° to floor.

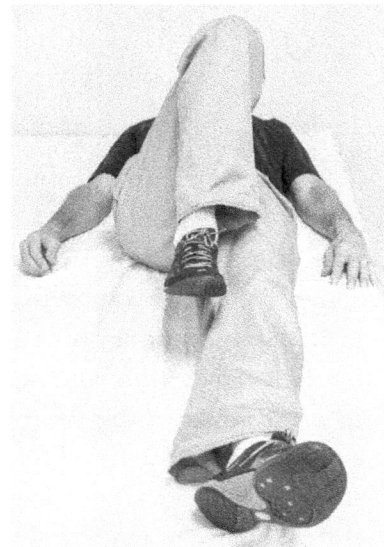

2. Maintain 90° and move knee to center of chest.

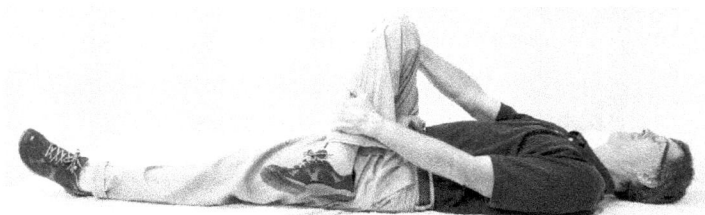

3. Maintain 90°. Rest heel on outside of opposite thigh.

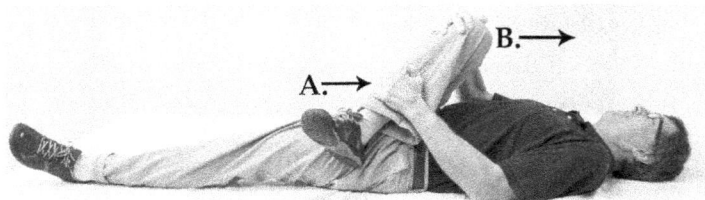

4. Pull foot toward shoulder (A) and knee toward center of chest (B) for best stretch in the buttock with least movement.

AVOID PAIN!

Prone Gluteal Retraining

The gluteus maximus (your butt muscle) is the largest muscle in the body. To begin retraining this muscle, lie on your stomach (prone) with a pillow or two under your pelvis and stomach. Put your left forearm under your forehead and, with your right hand, grab your right buttock. Bend your right ankle so the tips of the toes rest on the floor and the foot is positioned at 90 degrees to the floor. Clench the buttock muscles only and then slowly straighten the right knee. Now, "lengthen" the right side by pushing the right side of the pelvis away from the right shoulder. Maintain good right gluteal contraction, keep the knee straight then, very slowly lift the right leg only one inch. Hold the lift for about three seconds. Gently point your toe as if you were pressing on a gas pedal, and then slowly lower the leg. Relax for a moment, switch hands, and then do the same sequence on the other side. Usually ten repetitions, five on each side, are sufficient.

Keep the exercise slow and controlled. Make sure that the knee remains locked when the leg is lifted. If the knee bends, the hamstring musculature will provide too much assistance. Lifting the leg too high or too fast will over-recruit the musculature in the low back. If, because of back pain, you have trouble lying on your stomach, more pillows under the abdomen may help. If you have neck pain, the pillows can be positioned lengthwise so they are under your chest and stomach.

The work of lifting the leg should be felt mostly in the buttock muscle. If you sense that too much work is being done in other muscles (low back or leg), then don't completely lift the leg. Clench the buttock muscles, straighten the knee, lengthen, and hold this position for three to five seconds. When this gets easier, gradually progress to lifting, but never lift more than one inch.

Some people will start with the supine gluteal retraining (page 6) because, when they are on their stomachs, they can't figure out how to tighten their buttock muscles, or they are too uncomfortable on their stomachs. Tightness in the hip flexors and upper thigh muscles might make it difficult to contract the buttock muscles. You might need to stretch these muscles before good contraction of the gluteus maximus can be obtained.

If this exercise is done well, it should become very easy within five to seven days. Occasionally patients take up to three weeks before they can progress to the closed chain exercises. See Advanced Hip Exercises, page 15.

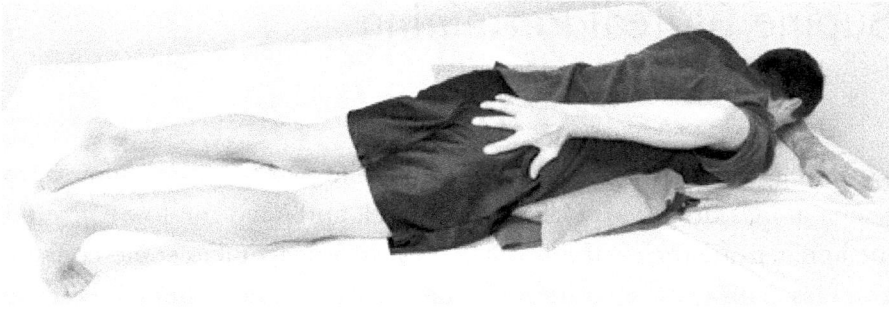

1a. Start with bent ankle.
1b. Place hand on active buttock. Clench buttock muscles ONLY.

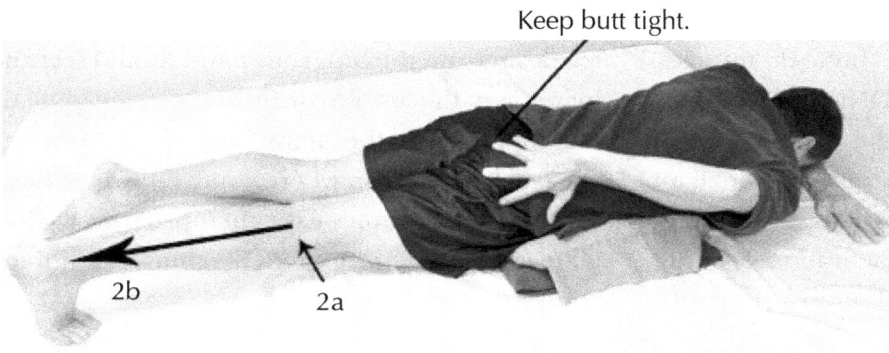

Keep butt tight.

2b   2a

2a. Straighten one knee to locked position.
2b. Then lengthen

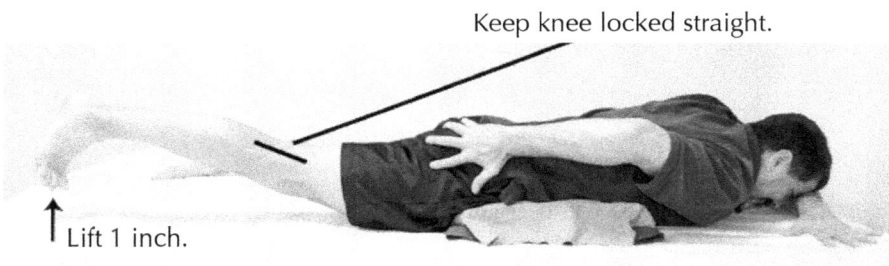

Keep knee locked straight.

Lift 1 inch.

3. Slowly lift whole leg just 1 inch. Hold 3 seconds.
4. Gently point foot, then lower slowly. Relax buttock muscles.

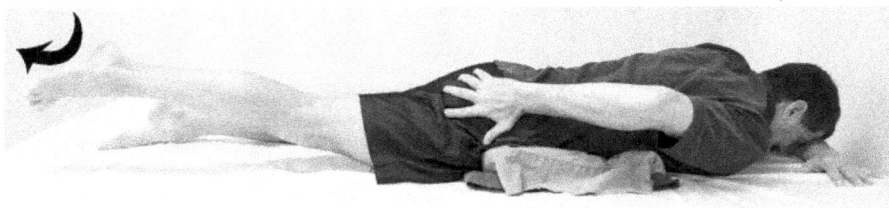

- Do 10 total.
- 5 per side.

5. Repeat sequence on other side.

AVOID PAIN!

Supine Gluteal Retraining

If the prone gluteal retraining exercise doesn't work well, the supine version may prove a better starting point to isolate and activate the gluteus maximus or buttock muscles. This exercise can be done on a bed or on the floor.

Lie on your back (supine) with two to three pillows under your knees. Cup your hands around either side of your buttock muscles. Gently contract or clench ONLY the buttock muscles! Avoid tightening the thigh and /or back muscles. It doesn't matter how small or slight the contraction of the gluteus maximus is. You do NOT want overflow activation of other muscles. Now use the buttock muscle to gently press just one knee down into the pillows. Do not raise your heel, and keep the low back and thigh relaxed. This process takes some concentration. It is almost more of a mental exercise than a physical one. Do not worry about losing contraction of the buttock of the inactive leg. Hold for five seconds. Emphasize pressing the leg down from the hip. Your hand should feel an increase in the tension or firmness in the gluteal musculature on the active side. This exercise will teach your brain where your "butt" is. When this exercise becomes easy, then progress to the prone version of the gluteus maximus retraining (previous exercise).

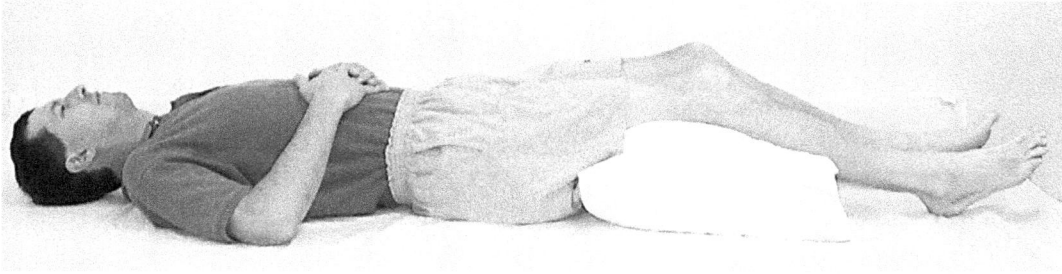

On back with pillows under knees

Keep thigh muscles relaxed.

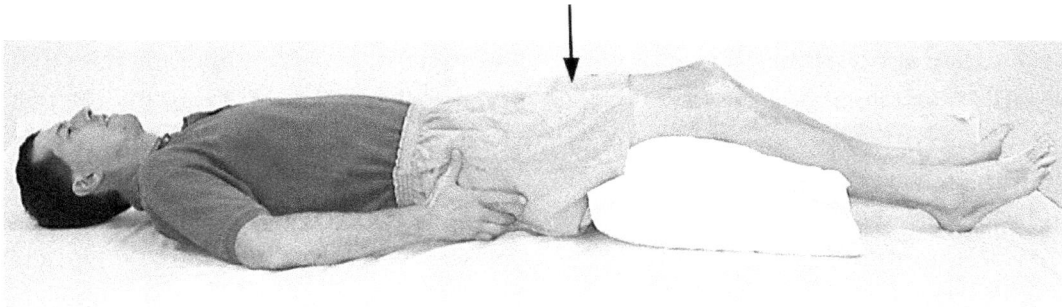

Clench buttock muscles ONLY.

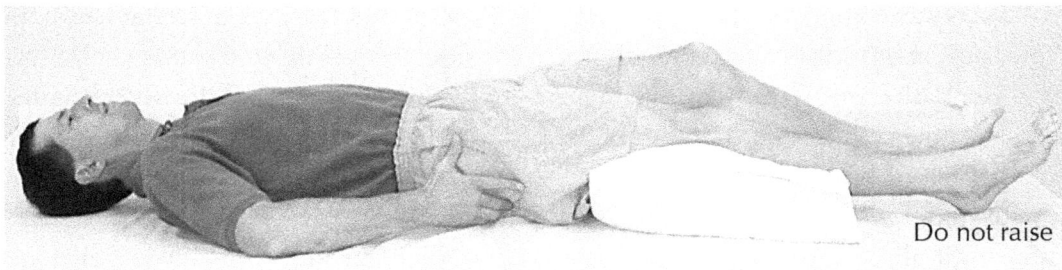

Do not raise heel.

Press ONE knee down using gluteal muscles. Hold 5 seconds. Relax, retighten buttock muscles. Press other knee down.

- Do 10 total
- 5 per side

AVOID PAIN!

Pelvic Clock

The cylinder/guy-wire system of muscles attaches from the rib cage to the pelvis, and forms a "tube" around the torso. As we move, there should be a dynamic interplay among these groups of muscles.

The pelvic clock exercise begins the process of restoring control to this area. Crunches, curls, and sit-ups will strengthen the abdominal musculature, but they also worsen posture, and do not necessarily teach good active control of the musculature. The pelvic clock is done lying on your back with your legs propped up so they can remain relaxed during the exercise. To help you feel the motion, grab the pelvis by resting the thumbs on the front of the pelvic bones, with the fingers wrapped around the hips.

Visualize a clock resting on your tummy so that 12 o'clock is up towards your head, and six o'clock is down towards your feet. When you arch just the low back, the front of the pelvis rotates in the six o'clock direction. Think of making a tunnel under your back. Keep the upper back, buttocks, and legs relaxed. If you find these areas are activated, reduce the amount of effort and motion until all of the work gets done in the low back, and the pelvis and low back are the only parts of the body that are moving. Most people can easily do a proper six o'clock tilt.

The second part, the twelve o'clock tilt, is the exact opposite motion of the six o'clock tilt. It should be done with the exact opposite muscle group: the abdominals. Most people cannot do a proper 12 o'clock tilt. They tend to use the wrong muscles. Begin the movement by pulling the belly button in and up under the rib cage. This should cause the low back to flatten against the floor and the pelvis to rotate in a posterior or 12 o'clock direction. Again make sure the thighs, buttock, shoulders, and diaphragm are quiet. These are not part of the cylinder/guy-wire system. If you have difficulty keeping other muscles relaxed, decrease the amount of pelvic movement. This is another exercise that is more mental than physical. Try doing the pelvic clock exercise in the sequence described below.

Balance the musculature by doing a six o'clock tilt first and holding for five seconds. Next, as you relax out of the six o'clock tilt, simultaneously, but gently, contract the abdominal musculature to move the pelvis to the 12 o'clock tilt and hold for five seconds. Relax for five seconds and then repeat the entire sequence. Usually a total of five repetitions are sufficient for a session. As you move towards twelve, you might help the stomach muscles work by using your hand like a claw to literally drag the belly button under your rib cage and towards your nose. Do not push your stomach towards the ceiling. You might need to use your other hand to feel the upper thigh of one leg to remind yourself to keep the legs relaxed.

The pelvic bones should move like a rolling pin when you're rolling out cookie dough. Moving smoothly six o'clock and twelve o'clock will help balance the cylinder/guy-wire muscles. Try an advanced abdominal exercise when you master the pelvic clock.

1. Start with relaxed pelvis and spine. Legs on chair or stool. Grip thigh with one hand. With other hand, make a claw. Put middle finger in the belly button.

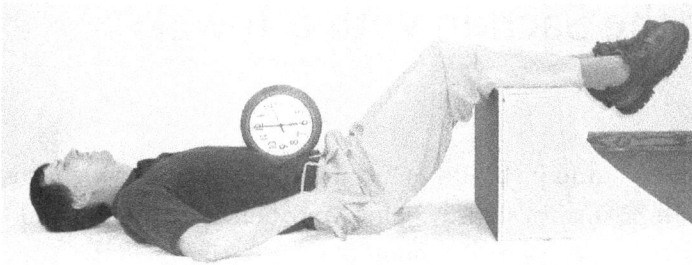

Use low back muscles ONLY.

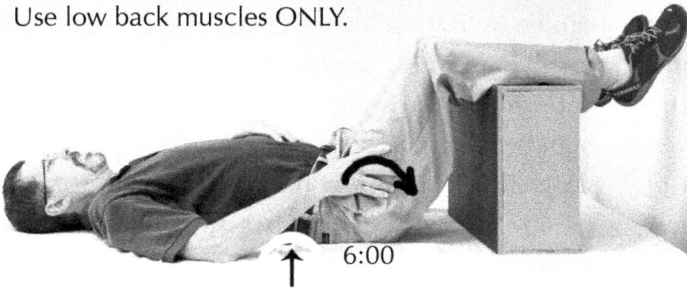

2. Gently arch into 6:00. Hold 5 seconds, then as you relax your back muscles . . .

6:00

Use low stomach muscles ONLY.

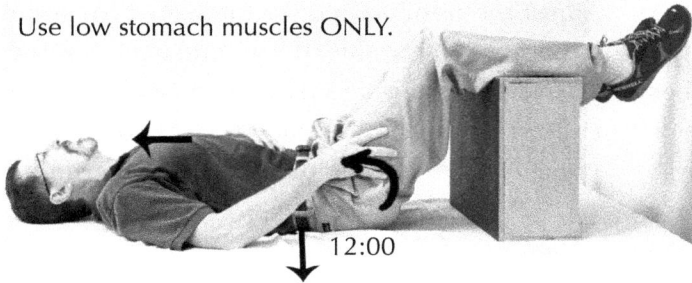

3. Gently transition to 12:00 by pulling belly button toward nose to flatten back. Hold 5 seconds.

Rest 5 seconds, then repeat sequence.

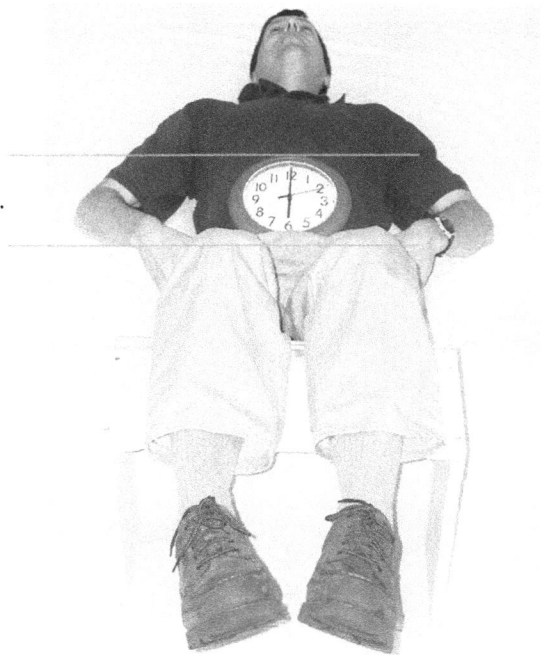

12:00

Keep chest relaxed.

Keep work between the lines.

No leg work

• Do 5 repetitions

AVOID PAIN!

Self Mobilization of the Sacrum with a Towel

The sacrum is at the bottom of your spine between the pelvic bones. It looks like an upside down triangle. Your spine sits on the top of the sacrum, and your tailbone or coccyx is at the bottom. The pelvic bones attach to either side of the sacrum to form the sacroiliac joints. To function correctly, the top of the sacrum needs to tip forward relative to the top of the pelvic bones. Sitting and bending tends to cause the top of the sacrum to be stuck, with its top tipped backwards. To help restore correct movement you can lie on a hand towel to mobilize the sacrum.

Take a 15 by 24 inch hand towel and fold it to an eight by 12 inch size. Roll it up so it is twelve inches long. Fold it in half and place a rubber band around the loose ends. Lie on the floor with the towel under the center of your pelvis. The folded end is pointed towards your head, and it should be even with the top of your pelvis or just slightly below your belt. The towel should not be in the small of your back nor under your buttocks. Keep your knees bent. A smaller towel can be used if you cannot relax. Lie on the towel for five minutes. During the first minute, alternate sliding each leg out straight, then back to bent ten times. Rest three minutes, then again, slide each leg out and back ten times in the last minute. You can gently rock your pelvis or wiggle around in the rest period.

This exercise should be very comfortable. Adjust the position and/or the size of the towel if it is not comfortable. If you want a more forceful exercise, try using a tennis ball (see next exercise). The doorframe backward bend exercise (page 36) may also help mobilize the sacrum.

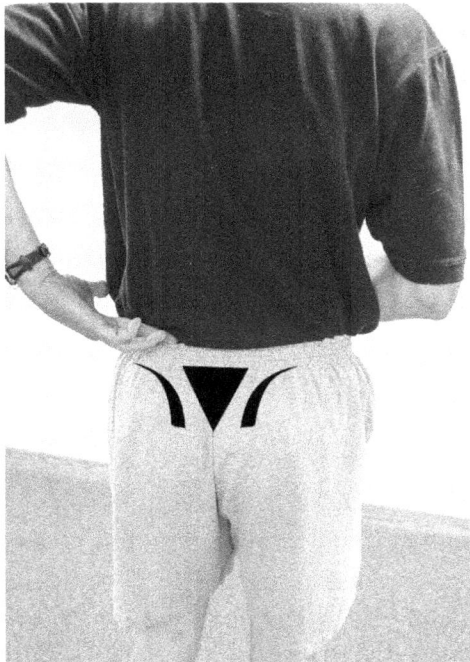

1. The sacrum is between the pelvic bones.

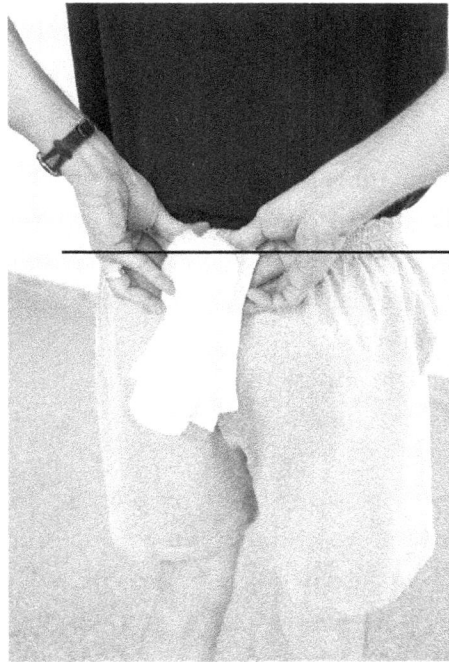

Below belt

2. Fold, roll up and bend hand towel. Place in center of sacrum, folded end toward head.

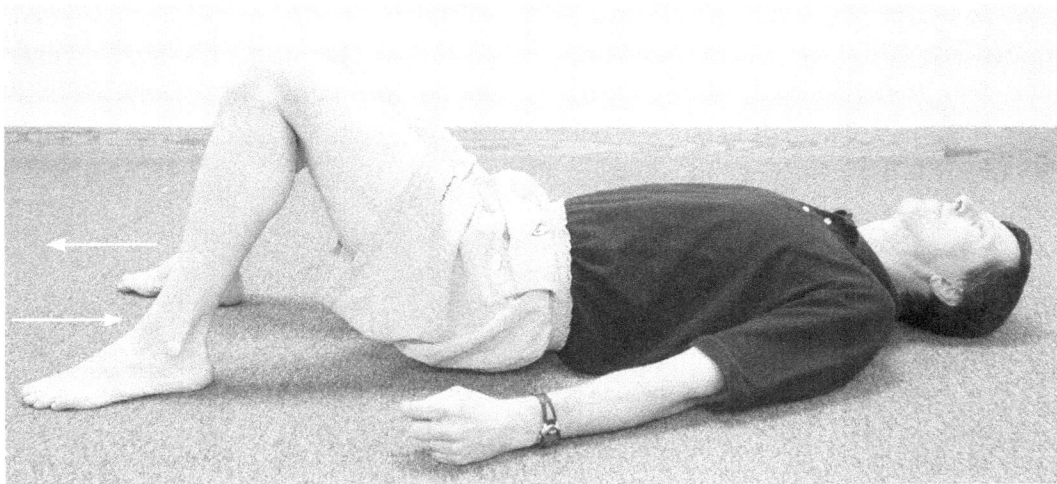

3. Lie on towel for 5 minutes. Slowly alternate sliding legs out and back.

- 10 times each leg in first minute
- Rest 3 minutes.
- 10 times each leg in last minute

AVOID PAIN!

Basic Low Back Exercises | 11

Self-Mobilization of the Sacrum with a Tennis Ball

If you need more force to mobilize the sacrum than a towel provides, then try using a tennis ball. The most difficult part of this exercise is placing the ball exactly in the sacral sulcus. The left sacral sulcus is just below your waist or belt line, at the top of the sacrum, and one quarter to one half inch to the left of the center line of the body.

To position the tennis ball correctly, lie on your back with the tennis ball under the center of the pelvis and just below your belt or waist line. Move the ball one quarter inch to the left with your hand, or by shifting your pelvis slightly to the right. The slight depression that the ball fits into is the sacral sulcus. Moving the ball too far to the left will put the ball under the left ilium or pelvic bone. The top of the sacrum is only three inches wide, and a tennis ball is two and a half inches, so the ball should feel like it is only slightly off center. Placing the ball too high means the ball will push on the lumbar spine, and too low may negate its effects.

Lie with the ball under the left sacral sulcus for at least two minutes. Alternate sliding each leg out and back ten times. Then switch the ball to the right sacral sulcus by shifting your pelvis one inch to the left. Do not move too far. Stay on this side for two minutes, and slide your legs out and back ten times again. You can repeat this sequence two or three times. If even more pressure is desired, with the ball under the left side, lift the left foot a couple of inches off the floor, and tip toe on the right side. Gently wiggle or use a slight bouncing movement for two or three minutes. For even more pressure, prop up on your forearms and lift the foot (page 14).

Sitting with good lumbar support helps keep the sacrum moving correctly. The doorframe backward bend exercise can be used as well (page 36). The towel or tennis ball exercise can be used four to five times a day for treatment or two to three times a week for maintenance.

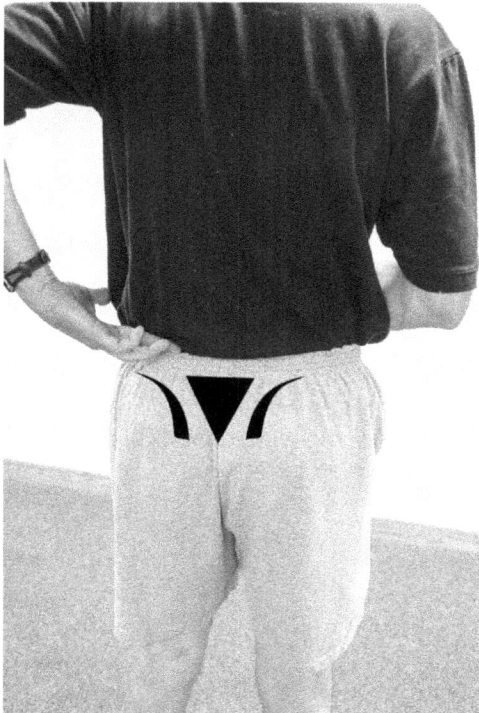

The sacrum is between the pelvic bones.

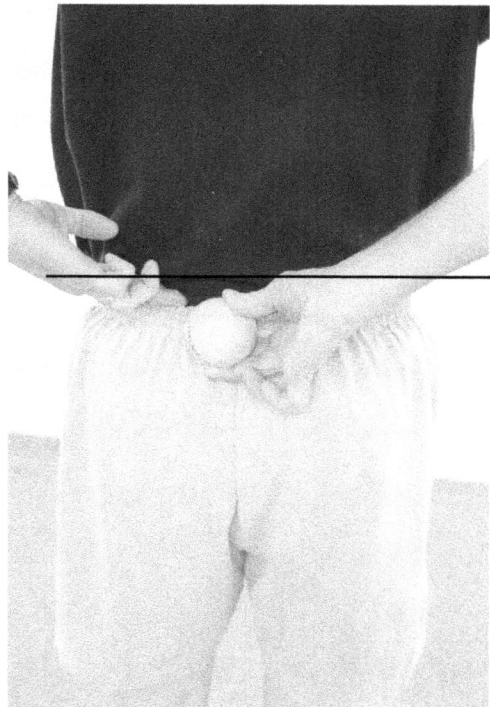

Below belt

The sacral sulcus is ¼ inch off center at the top of the sacrum.

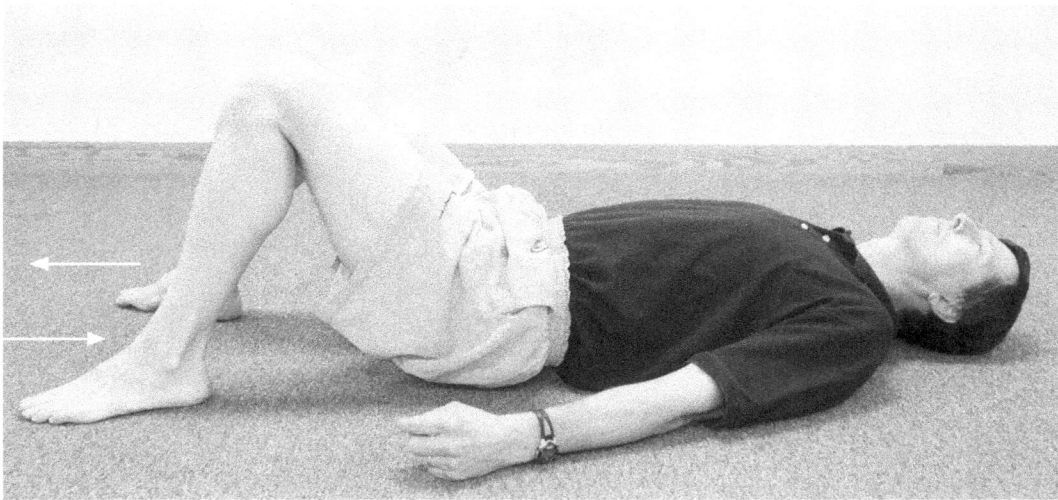

Lie on tennis ball for 2 minutes per side. Alternate sliding each leg out and back 10 times. Switch the ball to the other side and repeat.

• Do 2-3 times on each side.

AVOID PAIN!

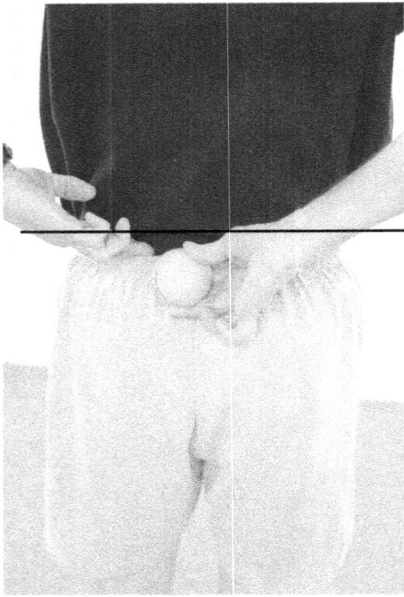

Below belt

Sacral sulcus

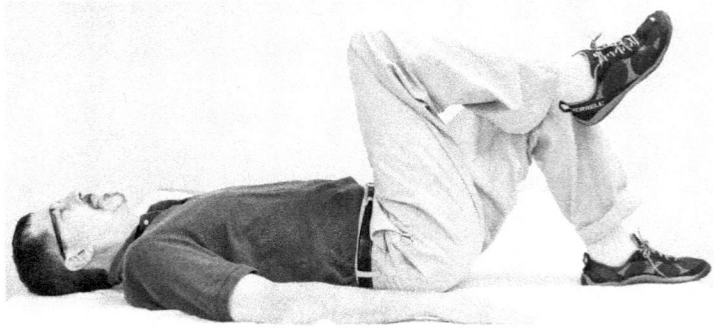

To add more pressure, lie with tennis ball in the sacral sulcus. Lift leg on that side to add pressure.

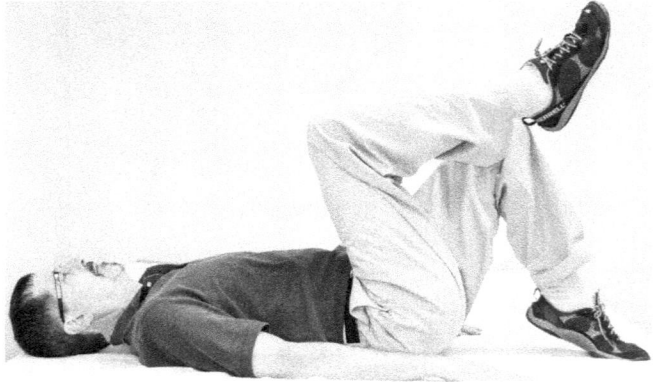

Tip toe on the other side and wiggle.

- Hold and wiggle for 20–30 seconds on "stuck" side.

AVOID PAIN!

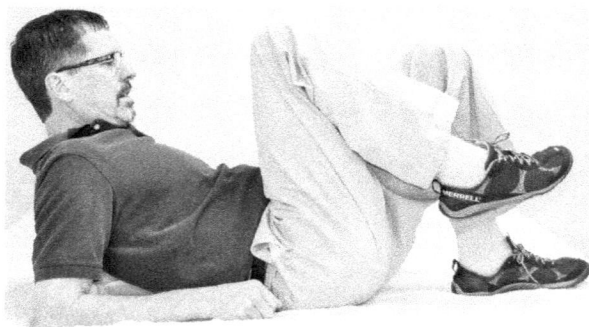

For even more pressure, prop up on the elbows, lift same leg and wiggle.

II
Advanced Hip Exercises

The preceding lying-down exercises prepare you to do the stand-up exercises. Once the lie-down exercises become easy, it's time to progress. The hip muscles are designed to work when the foot is on the ground. All of the muscles in the buttock area are needed to control the center of gravity of the body in single-leg standing and with every step you take. These muscles must keep the pelvis as level as possible. They must prevent the femur from angling and rotating inward. They also move you forward. Good contraction of the gluteous maximus will stabilize the sacroiliac joints and optimally distribute loading in the hip joint.

Walking can be broken down into several parts. The main components include heel strike, foot flat, and toe off for the leg in contact with the ground, and swing phase for the other leg. Walking differs from running in that both feet are in contact with the ground at the same time at some point. While running, only one foot at a time is in contact with the ground. If you are not over-striding, you should land a little bit flat-footed instead of directly on your heel. When the foot meets the ground, the buttock muscles control alignment. The lower extremity and the pelvis help dissipate some of the forces incurred. From landing to push off, dynamic stabilization is needed, and the gluteus maximus, acting as a hip extensor, provides propulsion to the next step.

Sloppy posture makes walking less elegant than it should be. It becomes too much of a controlled fall, with shock absorption by the thigh muscles (quadriceps, hip flexors, iliotibial band) and lumbar spine. Propulsion then shifts to the calf muscles with help from momentum of the opposite leg and forward bend of the trunk. Too much of the work of stabilization of the hip and pelvis shifts up to the low back muscles or down to the thigh and knee.

Good closed-chain functioning of the gluteal muscles is essential for unloading both the back and legs. Proper posture while walking or running allows the proper muscles to do the job nature intended.

Reverse Step Lunge

The primary stand-up or closed kinetic chain exercise for the gluteus maximus retraining is the reverse step lunge. Make sure that you can do prone gluteal retraining well before attempting this exercise. Put at least a four-inch-high platform against a doorframe or facing a post. This platform can be an aerobic step, a block of wood, a thick book, or magazines taped together. It must be stable.

Stand on the platform with your right foot. Firmly grab the doorframe, with both hands, and touch it lightly with the top of your forehead. Place the left leg off to the side and extended behind you. Pull the toes up, and turn the leg inward. The bottom of the left foot is parallel to the floor, and the heel is turned outward. Your pelvis is square and level when you are standing on both feet; keep it that way when standing on one foot. Imagine that there are headlights on the front of the pelvic bones. Keep them square and level. This is the starting position.

Holding the doorframe firmly, perform a single leg squat by arching or making your back sway to let your hips push back away from the post or doorframe. Your right knee will bend, but do not let your shin move forward. Keep the right shin stationary like a post in the ground. Most of your body weight will be on your right heel. Keep your forehead lightly touching the doorframe throughout the movement. Monitor the shin visually and by keeping your weight mostly on the heel rather than the ball of the foot. Return to the start position.

This exercise is basically a single-leg squat with emphasis on moving the buttock and the trailing leg back. If you feel too much work in the hamstrings, let your shin bone angle slightly forward. Maintain this angle throughout the movement of the lunge. If too much work is felt in the quadriceps, the shin is angled too far forward. You should be able to find the correct stationary position of the shin to keep both the quadriceps and hamstrings relatively inactive with the movement of the lunge. If you are standing on your right leg, keep your right shoulder and hip lined up over your right knee and foot. Use your grip on the post to help maintain good alignment. Keep the movement slow and controlled. Each direction should take three to four seconds.

Make sure the trailing leg stays off to one side and turned inward. The standing knee should be quiet during the entire exercise. Avoid popping or repetitive grinding in the knee. Making the motion shallower will usually relieve this problem.

If done correctly, the buttock muscles of the standing leg should do 90 percent of the work. Three sets of five repetitions once per day are usually sufficient for the first week. You may increase up to two sets of 20 repetitions as the exercise gets easier, but make sure you hit the target with each repetition of the exercise. The exercise is eventually done with only a light finger touch on the doorframe for balance.

When repetitions become easy, holding a dumbbell weight against the hip of the trailing leg will increase the resistance of the exercise. Doing wall or doorframe squats described later (pages 32 and 18 respectively) may help to perfect the technique.

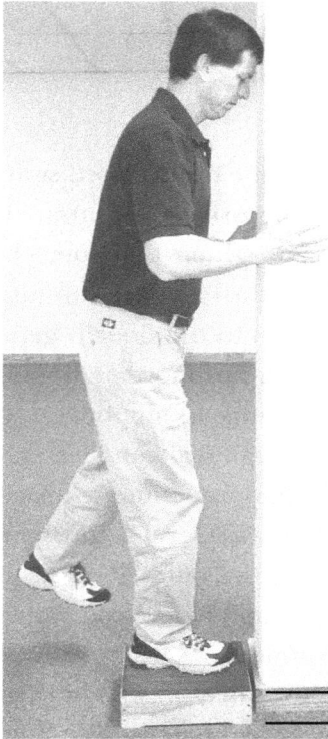

Start position

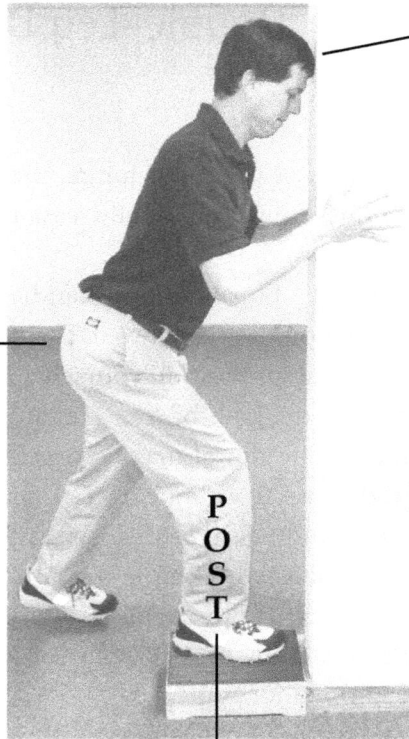

Forehead touching

Grab tight

Emphasize butt back

P O S T

Min 4 inches

- Stance leg
- Shin stationary
- Weight mostly on heel

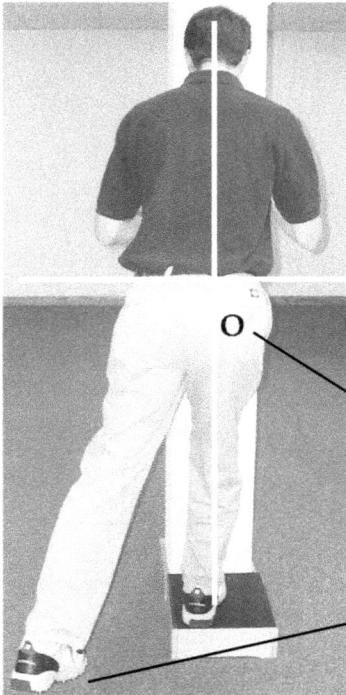

Maintain good alignment

O

Level and square pelvis

Target

- Trailing leg
- Off to side and back
- Toes up. Foot turned in.
- Knee straight

- Do in a doorframe.
- Push tush back to engage gluteal musculature.
- Slowly return to start position and repeat.
- 3 sets of 5 repetitions per side.

AVOID PAIN!

Double-Leg Doorframe Squat

An alternative to the reverse step lunge, the double-leg doorframe squat, is usually easier since both feet remain on the ground.

Place a dowel or broom/mop handle through a doorway flat on the floor two to three inches from the doorframe. Position yourself so that either your toes or the balls of your feet are resting on the dowel. The dowel may help prevent the knees and shins from moving too far forward. Your feet should be slightly wider than shoulder width and pointed straight forward. Grab the doorframe with both hands at waist level, and look down slightly. Touch your forehead lightly against the doorframe.

To squat, emphasize moving the buttock back while keeping the shins vertical. The knees are kept pushed apart as if you were sitting on a horse. You need some degree of increased sway to your spine. If too much work is concentrated in the low back, you can tighten the stomach muscles to do a slight 12 o'clock or posterior tilt. Getting your thighs parallel to the floor is generally the maximum amount of movement, but stay within a comfortable range of motion.

If you do not feel the gluteal muscles are engaged after three to four repetitions, make sure that your hands are at waist level before you start the squat. Clenching the buttock muscles at the bottom of the squat and before you come back up may help recruitment.

Avoid over-stressing the knees by monitoring sensations of strain, including noise or grinding in the knees. Three sets of five repetitions is usually a good starting point.

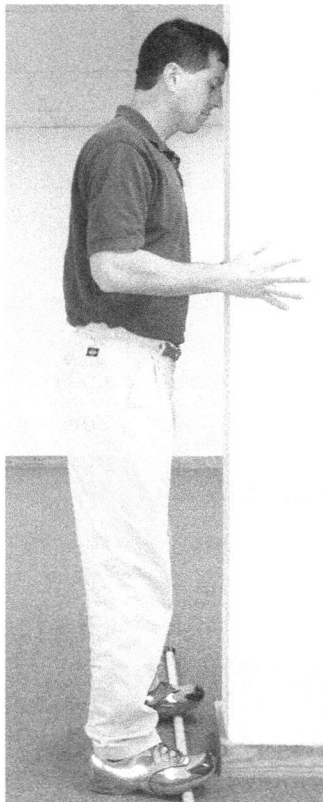

1. Forehead touching door-frame. Dowel 2–3 inches from door.

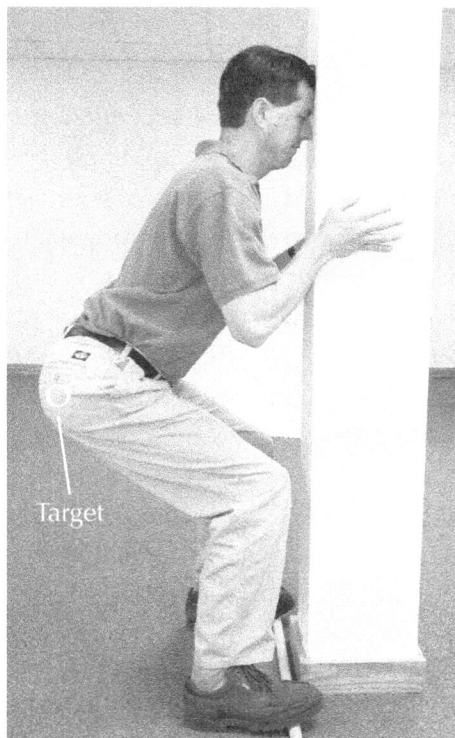

2. Point feet straight forward. Keep knees pushed apart.

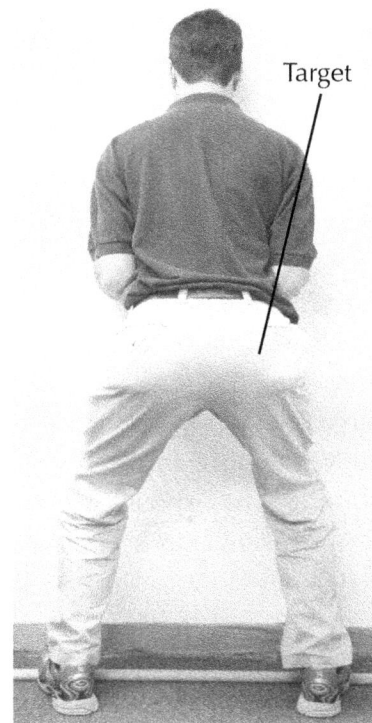

Target

Target

- Grab tight.
- Keep shins vertical.
- Chest up, butt back.
- 3 sets of 5 to start or hold for 10–15 seconds
- It can be used as an alternate to Reverse Step Lunge.

AVOID PAIN!

Side Step Lunge/Hip Wobble with a Sit

This hip wobble with a sit motion is aimed at the hip abductors. It is usually started after you master the reverse step lunge and is a closed chain upgrade for the sidelying hip abduction exercise. It is similar to the reverse step lunge: you grab the doorframe tightly, you stand on a block, your forehead touches the doorframe, and your shin remains reasonably vertical. The target is the hip abductor located behind and above the hip bone.

Begin the exercise in a doorframe, standing on a four-inch block with the inside edge of your right foot close to the side of the block. Hang your left foot in mid-air and slightly ahead of the standing leg. Move your pelvis slightly back with the left side turned slightly forward. Imaginary "headlights" on the front of the pelvis are aiming slightly to the right. Grab the doorframe firmly, and keep your forehead touching the doorframe.

Begin the motion by hiking the left hip. The left side of the pelvis should move up, and your head and shoulders should slide up the doorframe by about two inches. The area behind your hip bone should become concave. Now "un-hike" or lower the pelvis down so the hip of the stance leg is pushed slightly back and slightly to the side. This is very much like the motion people do when they wiggle their backsides. Your head and shoulders should move downward as well, and the area behind your hip bone should become convex. Make the right hip abductor muscle return you to the hip-hike position. Do not let your left side back muscle pull the left side up. Sometimes it may be helpful to rest the fingers of your right arm behind the hipbone of the standing leg to monitor the concave/convex movement. When the wobble motion works correctly, you should feel fatigue in this area. Once this motion is perfected, add a slight sit motion by bending the knee at the down portion of the wobble. If you have painful or arthritic knees, do not add the knee bend. Just move back and forth from a hip hike to the un-hike.

Remember to keep the shin of the stance leg vertical and most of your body weight on the heel. This is similar to the reverse-step lunge except that the hip is pushed to the side as well as back.

Keeping the shin stationary is often a problem in the side-step lunge. It will try to move forward when you are in the sit position, and hamstrings will try to pull it back when returning to the up position. Check it visually or have a partner lightly hold the shin just below the knee until you have reprogrammed yourself well enough to maintain good form. Keep the motion shallow in the beginning, and then increase the movement as the repetitions become easier. When correct repetitions of the exercise become easy, reduce the grip on the doorframe.

Generally start the exercise with three sets of five repetitions. Increase the repetitions as you are able. When twenty repetitions are fairly easy, add weight by holding a dumbbell weight against the hip of the hanging leg.

Forehead touching

Grab tight

Hips back

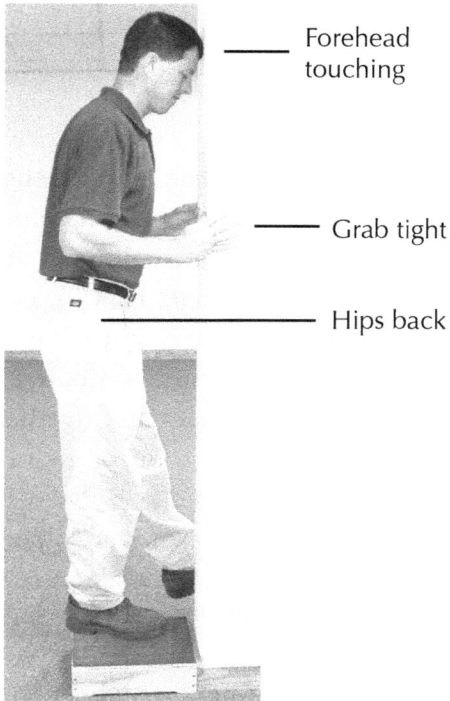

1. Hips back, weight on heel

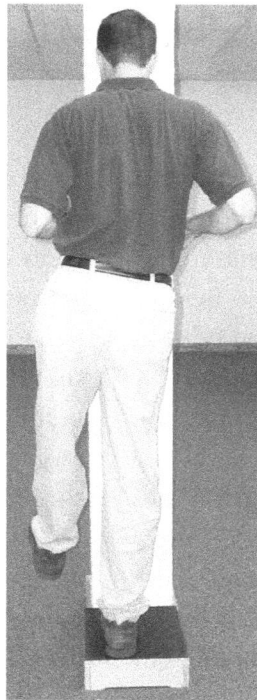

2. Hike or raise opposite hip upward.

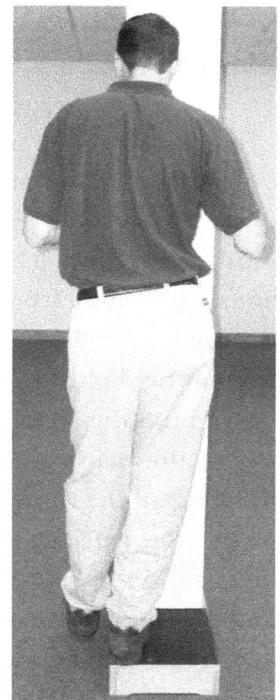

3. Lower hip down. Feel work behind hip bone on stance leg.

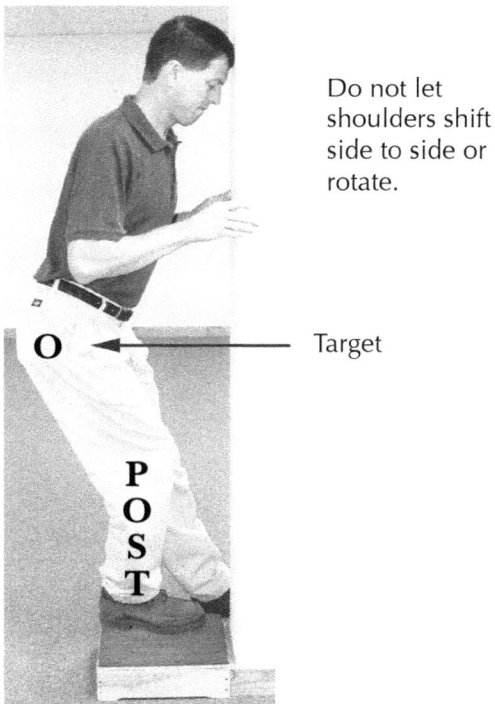

Do not let shoulders shift side to side or rotate.

O POST

Target

4. Lower further by bending knee,

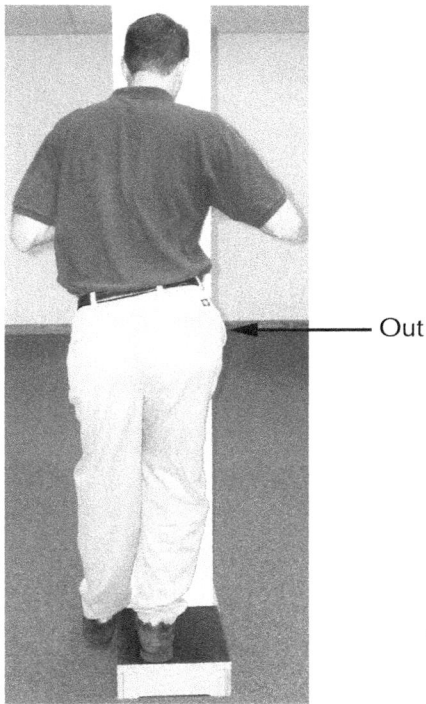

Out

5. and pushing hip out. Slowly return to hip-hike position.

• 3 sets of 5

AVOID PAIN!

Side-lying Leg Raise

Lie on your side with your back against a wall or front of a couch. Roll your pelvis slightly forward so that the top buttock cheek and shoulder are slightly away from the wall, but the heel of the top leg remains against the wall. The bottom leg may be slightly bent.

Tighten the stomach muscles, and push the top of the pelvis away from your top shoulder to elongate the top of the trunk. Point the toes of the top leg partially toward the floor. Now lift the top leg, keeping the top heel against the wall. Keep the muscles above the pelvis inactive as you raise the leg so that the foot is six to eight inches from the floor. Lower the leg slowly and repeat the leg lift. Do two to three sets of eight to ten repetitions.

This exercise attempts to isolate recruitment of the hip abductors. Sometimes it is a helpful exercise if the gluteal muscles prove difficult to activate. When doing this exercise, try to keep the top thigh relaxed and the top foot turned slightly downward. Again, if work is not felt behind the hipbone, you are not hitting the target and you may want to focus on prone or supine gluteal retraining exercises.

The "Clam" and "Hydrant" exercises are often used to attempt to strengthen the gluteal musculature, but they tend to overuse the deeper hip muscles. Use them with caution and mindfulness. Make sure that you are recruiting the appropriate muscles. If this exercise is too easy, try the "hip wobble with a sit" on the previous page.

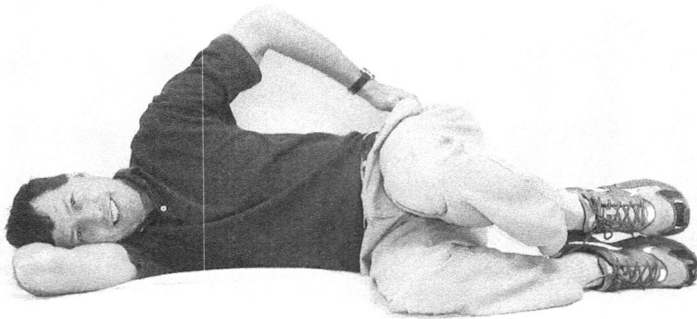

The Clam

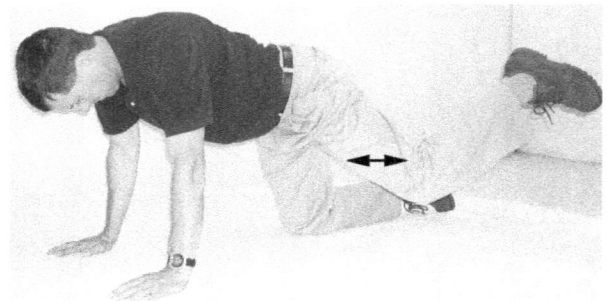

The Hydrant

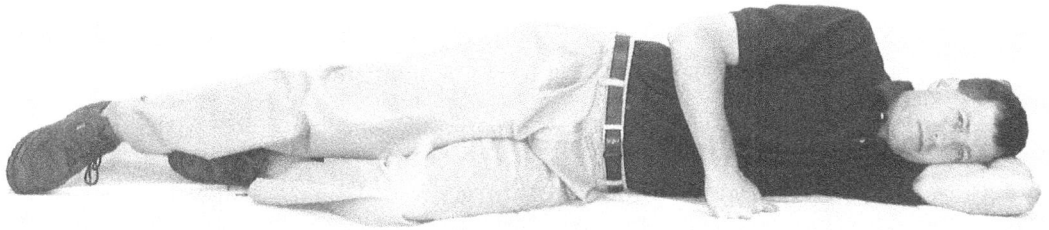

1. Lie on side, body in a straight line with back against the front of couch or wall. Bend bottom leg. Roll top butt cheek and shoulder away from couch. Top heel should touch the couch.

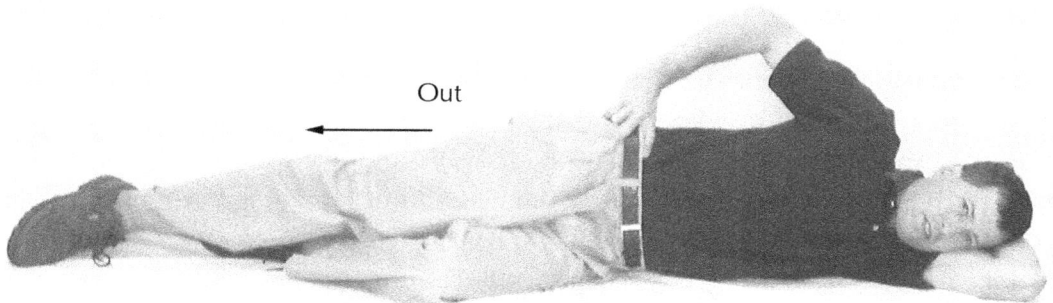

Out

2. Tighten tummy. Push the top leg straight down away from your body.

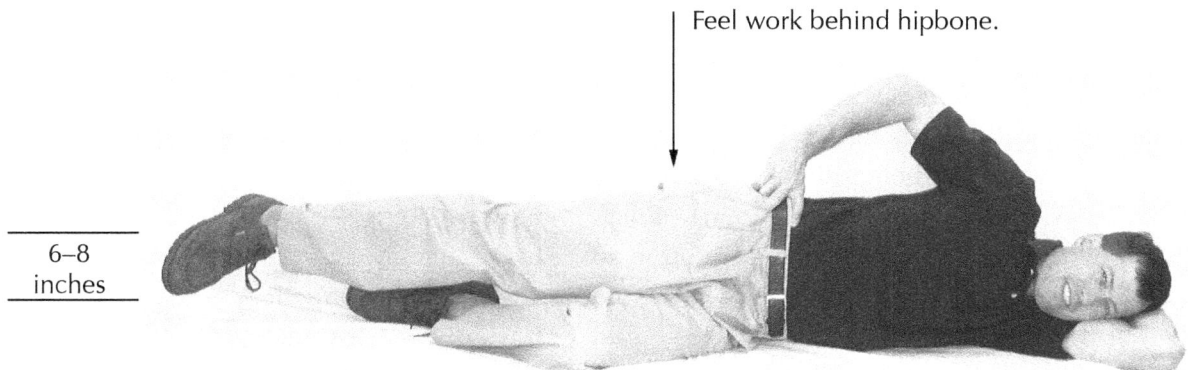

Feel work behind hipbone.

6–8
inches

3. Lift the top leg 6–8 inches. Keep the muscles above the pelvis quiet.

- 3 sets of 8–10 repetitions
- 30 second rest between sets
- Do 8–10, rest, then do other side.

AVOID PAIN!

Olympic Squat

This advanced hip exercise targets your buttock muscles. Squats may also improve posture. The weight of the bar will help push the upper rib cage downward and extend a flexed upper thoracic spine. Before attempting Olympic Squats as a strengthening exercise, you should become proficient with the wall squat exercise (page 32).

Once the wall squat has become easy, a natural progression would be to add weight to the exercise. Any squat or lift should be done as though there is a wall in front of you. Initially you can perform the wall squat with a bare bar. Doing squats in a squat rack is recommended once you are adding significant amounts of weight. You can get good activation of the gluteal and paraspinal muscles by squatting to a level where the thighs are parallel to the floor.

When squatting, keep your body weight mostly on the outside of your heels to keep your shins as vertical as possible. This should prevent too much load from being directed toward the quadriceps and knees. Make sure that you can tap your feet throughout the squat motion to help keep the shins reasonably vertical. Avoid letting the knees bow in or out. Knees should only bend in one direction like hinges, not in multiple directions like ball joints. Your body weight should be distributed evenly so that each leg is carrying 50 percent throughout the squat.

Do your squats in three sets of 12 to 15 repetitions. Do the first set as a warm-up with 50 to 70 percent of your target weight. Do the next two sets with your target weight. A safe bet for your maximum target weight would be your ideal body weight.

If you are new to squats, have an experienced helper or "spotter" available. Begin by removing the bar from the rack. Some people prefer backing up to the bar; others prefer to face it and duck under it to rest the bar on top of the shoulders. The bar should rest along the top part of the shoulder blades across the bony ridge. Add a pad or a towel around the bar for comfort. Hold the bar with your hands. Once the bar is resting comfortably on your shoulders, step away from the rack and perform the Olympic squat as though you were doing your wall squat.

Monitor knee and back positioning. Work should be felt through the buttocks, back, and to some degree, in the hamstrings. If too much work is done through the quadriceps or low back, check your form. If you are unable to isolate the gluteal muscles correctly, continue with the wall or doorframe squats, reverse step lunge, or even go back the gluteal retraining exercises.

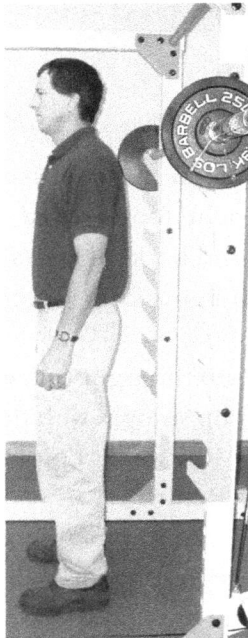

1. Squats with weights are done in a squat rack.

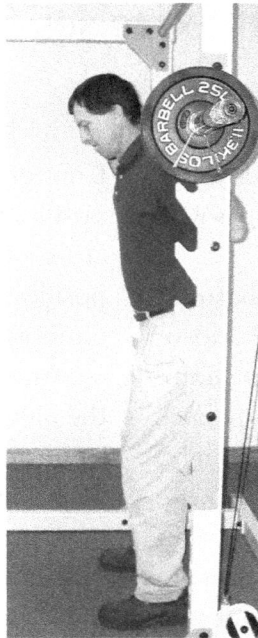

2. Back up to bar.

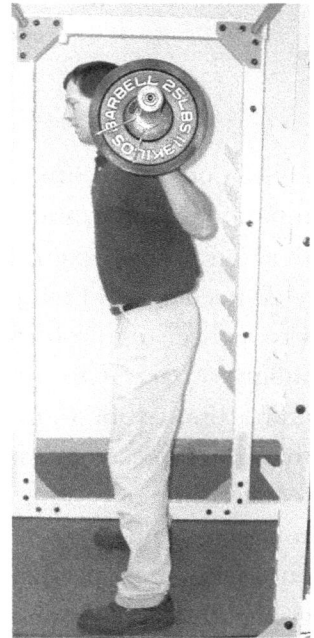

3. Step to center of rack.

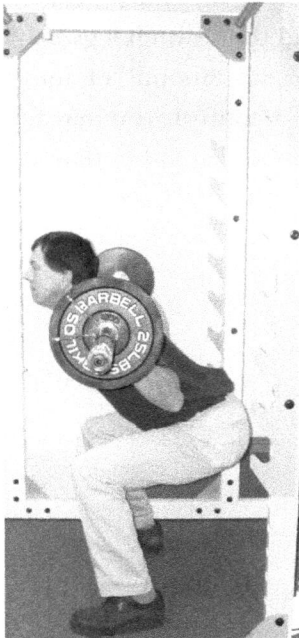

4. Squat down until thighs parallel to floor, shins vertical, chest up.

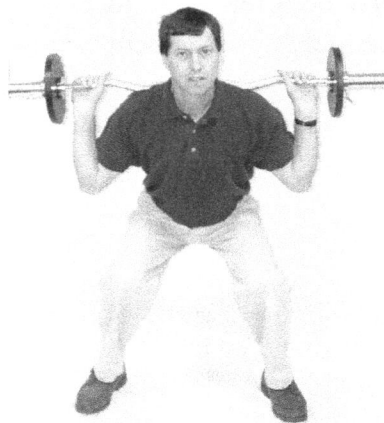

5. Keep knees neutral. Feet pointed straight forward.

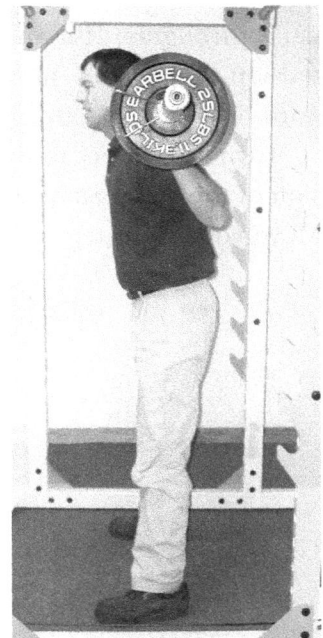

6. Back up to start position and repeat.

- Beginning weight 25–45 lbs.
- 3 sets of 12–15 repetitions.

AVOID PAIN!

Latex Band Exercises for the Hip

A good way to simultaneously work on coordination, balance, and hip strengthening is with this four way hip exercise.

If needed, hold on to something for balance. Use a three-to-four-foot piece of latex band or tubing. Attach it to a heavy piece of furniture and around your right ankle. Turn your back toward the piece of furniture. Stand up straight, feet are shoulder width apart. Position and keep your spine and pelvis in neutral. With your right knee straight, move the leg forward as if you are going to take a step forward and, without putting your foot down, let it return to the start position. Repeat the "step" forward. There should be a comfortable but challenging tension on the band throughout the movement. To adjust the tension of the band, move your whole body forward or backwards. Do 12 to 15 repetitions.

Turn 90 degrees to the right. Adjust the tension of the band. Stabilize your spine and pelvis. Move your right leg so that the foot crosses in front of the left foot and then back to the start position. Next, move the right foot so that it crosses behind the left foot and back to the start position. Repeat this pattern to do 12 to 15 repetitions.

Turn another 90 degrees to the right to face the piece of furniture. Stand up straight with the spine and pelvis in neutral. Move your right leg back with the knee straight. Return to the start position and continue to do 12 to 15 repetitions.

Finally, turn another 90 degrees to the right. Move your right leg as if you are going to step to the right and return it to the start position. Keep your pelvis level and neutral and do 12 to 15 repetitions. Turn to the right again and repeat the whole exercise again, and then switch legs.

Increase or decrease the amount of movement to suite your level of control. You may feel most of the work in the stance leg rather than the one doing the actual movement.

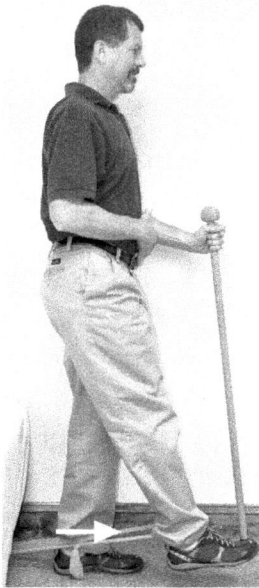

Forward

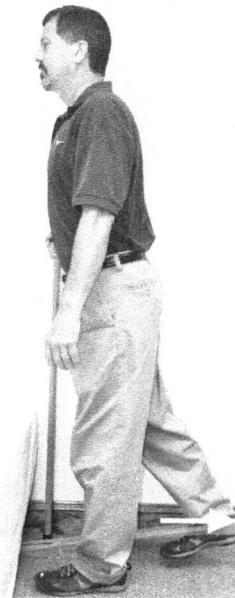

Backward

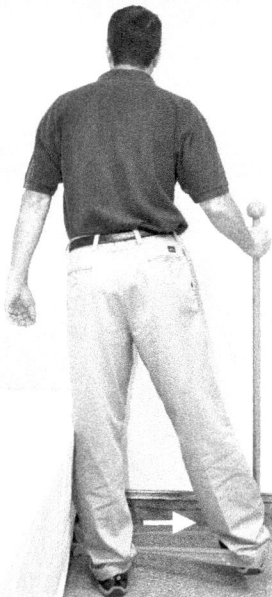

Abduction

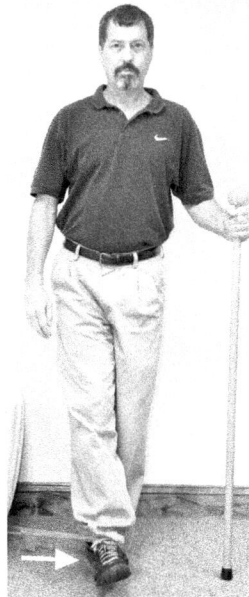

Adduction in front

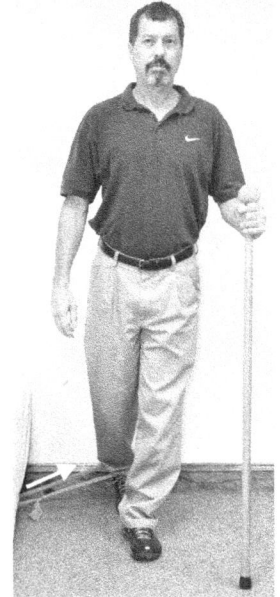

Adduction behind leg

- Use comfortable resistance.
- If needed, use chair for balance.
- 2 sets of 12–15 repetitions in each direction on each leg

AVOID PAIN!

Advanced Balance Training

Once you have things moving and the muscles appropriately recruited, you can work on balance training.

A simple balance exercise is to practice standing on one leg. If your balance is extremely poor, work on this exercise near your kitchen counter. Let your hands hover but not hold while you practice standing on one leg. Work up to 30 seconds on each leg with your eyes open, and then, if you are brave, with your eyes closed.

For more advanced training, stand on a two-to-six-inch step. Let your right foot hang off to the side of the step. Lower your right foot towards the floor. Keep your left shin almost vertical with most of your body weight on the heel. Keep your upper body vertical. Lightly touch your right heel to the floor and return to the start position. This is similar to the side step lunge (page 20).

Reach your right foot eight to ten inches forward and lightly touch your heel to the floor. Keep the shin and upper body as vertical as possible. Return to the start position.

Reach your right foot eight to ten inches back and touch the heel to the floor. This is like a reverse step lunge with the upper body and shin remaining as vertical as possible. Repeat the sequence eight to ten times. Do two to three sets on each leg. Most of the work should be felt in the buttock muscles—NOT in the knees. For a real challenge, do this exercise with your eyes closed.

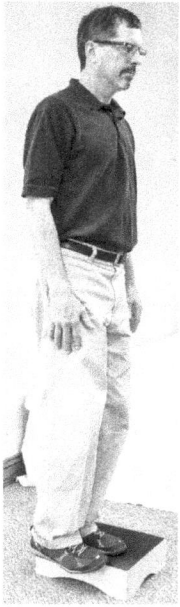

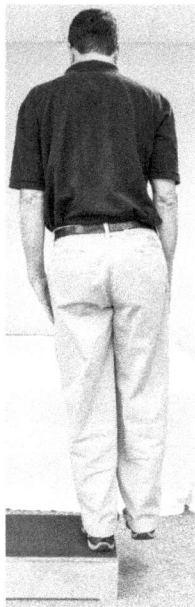

Start position
Begin on 2-inch block,
work up to 6-inch block.

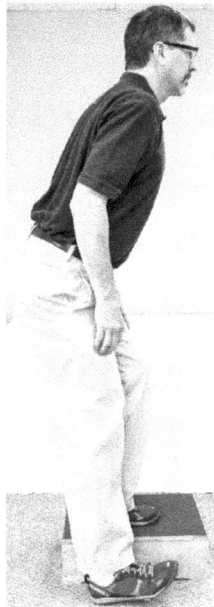

Lower your right foot
to the floor. Keep your
left shin and upper
body vertical.

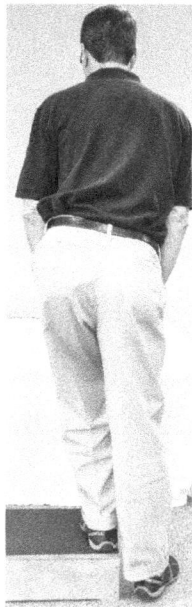

Let your pelvis push
back to the left.

Return to start position.

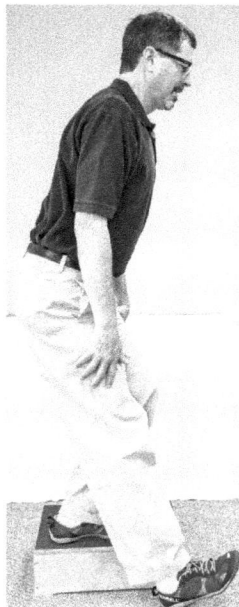

Reach your foot forward
10–12 inches and down
towards floor. Return to
start position.

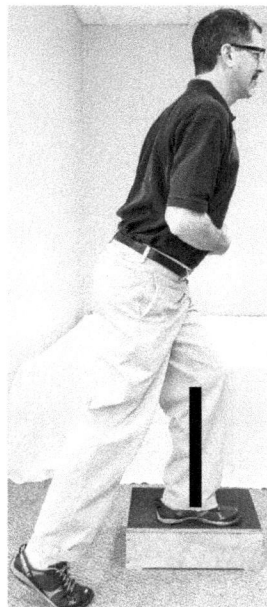

Reach your foot back
10–12 inches and
down to floor. Return
to start position.

AVOID PAIN!

III
Lower Extremity/Back Stretches
Stretching Guidelines

Stretching is an adjunct to a muscle re-education program. Stretching can decompress and restore full range of motion to joints. You can disinhibit muscles targeted for re-education.

Muscles that become tight and don't seem to loosen with regular stretching are overly recruited on a regular basis. Stretching is not going to make a long-term change in the length of the muscle unless the overload is removed.

A muscle may become inhibited from functioning if its opposing partner muscle is tight. Tight hip flexors along with other muscles on the front thigh may inhibit the gluteal muscles, causing problems in the back or legs. Tight pectorals (chest muscles) may inhibit scapular stabilizers, causing problems in the shoulder.

Stretching should feel good. Overly aggressive stretching may cause small injuries and soreness in the stretched muscle. This soreness results in more tightness, which is counterproductive to elongating the muscle. A gentle stretch should be held for a minimum of 15 seconds. A stretch can be held for 30 to 60 seconds or longer if it produces the desired result of lengthening the restricted musculature. Three to four repetitions of stretching with 15 to 20 seconds rest between stretches of the same muscle are generally sufficient for a session. If right and left sides are being stretched, one muscle gets a rest break while the opposite side stretches. Remember that overly aggressive stretching will actually slow the progress of elongation. Generally it is better to err on the side of a gentle stretch than stretching too hard.

Wall Squats

Wall squats can be thought of as a cousin to the wall-angel exercise. This exercise works by making backward bending uniform through the lumbar and thoracic spine. It is also a good way to learn correct form for Olympic squats that professionals use to lift heavy weights safely. The wall squat will help you master good lifting technique.

Begin by facing the wall with your toes touching the base molding. Point your feet straight forward slightly wider than shoulder width apart. Your hands can lightly touch the wall.

Start the exercise by slowly sitting down and pushing the pelvis back and away from the wall. Keep the knees neutral and the feet flat on the floor. At the bottom of the squat, most of your weight will be on the outside of your heels. Squat only as far as balance and control will allow. You can hold the down position for at least 15 seconds as you would for the wall angel, or do repetitions. When returning to the start position, keep your nose (or cheek bone) lightly pressed against the wall.

Placing a dowel or broom handle across the ridge of the shoulder blades will usually increase backward bending through the thoracic spine. Doing this exercise with the feet only two inches apart will help increase backward bending in the thoracic spine.

If pain or too much tightness is created in the low back, try adding a slight 12 o'clock or posterior tilt at the bottom of the squat to help neutralize the lumbar spine. Do not overcompensate and flatten the lumbar spine. Do the exercise within a comfortable range of motion.

Other exercises that will improve backward bending include the doorframe squat (page 18), doorframe backward bending (page 36), prone upper back extension (page 34), attention (pages 74 and 76), and wall angel (pages 80–85).

Stick

Target zone

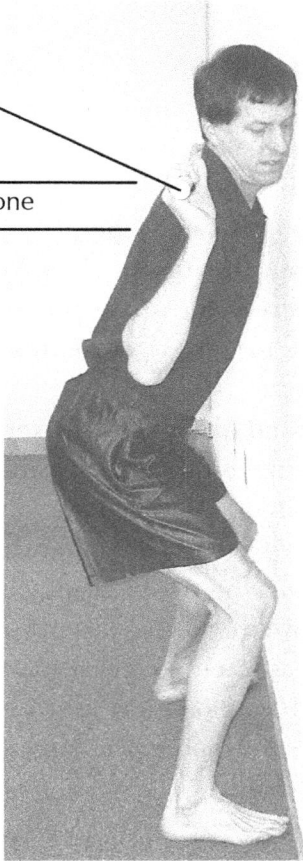

Wide base version

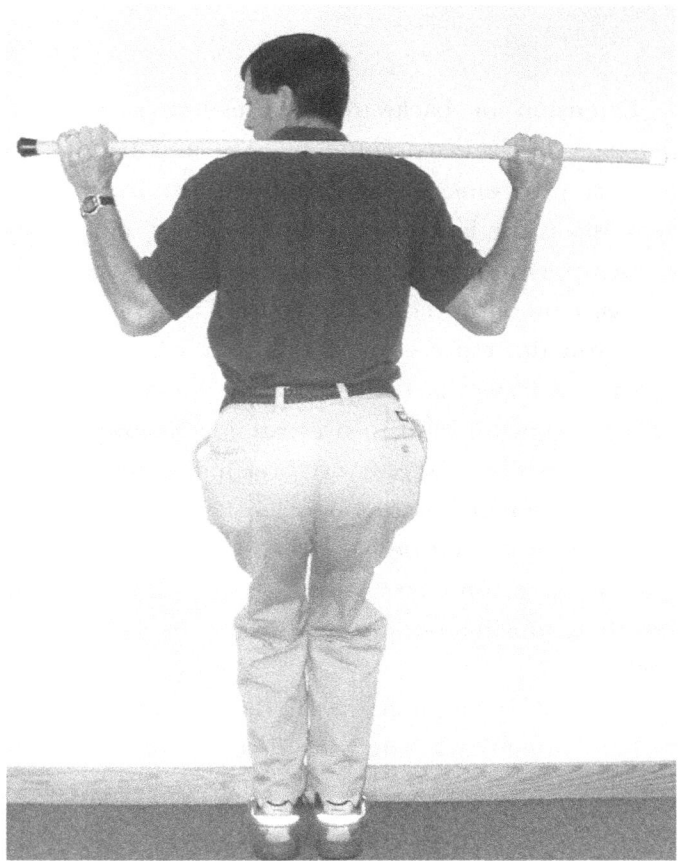

Narrow base version

- Cheek and toes touch the wall
- Keep knees neutral and feet straight forward
- Keep the chest up as you push your butt back
- If needed, do slight 12:00 tilt at the bottom of the squat
- Hold 15 seconds
- Can be used as an alternative to wall angel (page 80)

AVOID PAIN!

Prone Upper Back Extension

Extension or backward-bend exercises for the back are very common in yoga and back exercise programs. A major problem with these exercises is the lack of backward-bend mobility in the upper lumbar and thoracic spine, and the excessive mobility in the lowest part of the spine.

If you do a press up where your rib cage and pelvis leave the floor and your elbows are straight, you will tend to overextend the lower lumbar spine because the vertebrae higher up in the spine remain forward bent, or flexed, even though they should be backward bending. The goal of extension exercises is to have all of the vertebrae moving, not just the ones in the lower back.

There are a couple of ways to do this exercise to help upper-back vertebrae extend. In both versions, you lie on your stomach. If needed, use a pillow or two under your tummy.

To do the first version of the exercise, prop up on your elbows and push the front of your lower rib cage towards the floor. You should feel "work" or stretching above the low back. Move your elbows forward to move the "work" higher up your back.

The second way to do this exercise is to position your arms as though you were getting ready to do a push-up. As you push your upper body up, keep the front of your lower rib cage pressed firmly against the floor. Again, you should feel stretch above the lowest part of your back. Push up as high as you can comfortably.

Hold the position for at least 15 to 20 seconds. Relax 15 seconds and repeat two or three times.

Option A

1. Lie on tummy propped up on elbows.

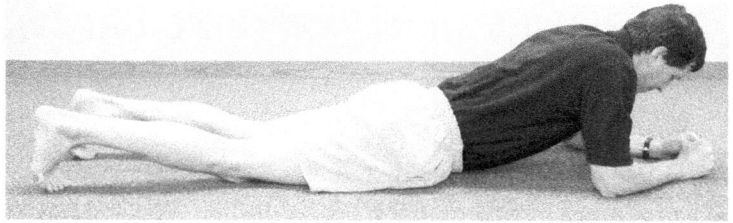

2. Press the lower part of the rib cage and/or breast bone down.

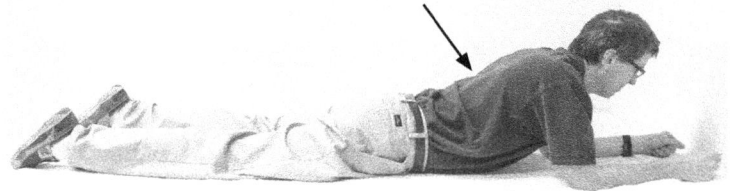

3. Try using a pillow under your stomach

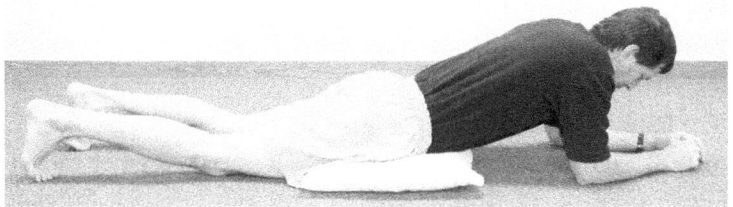

4. Keep the pelvis on the floor. Do not over extend your neck.

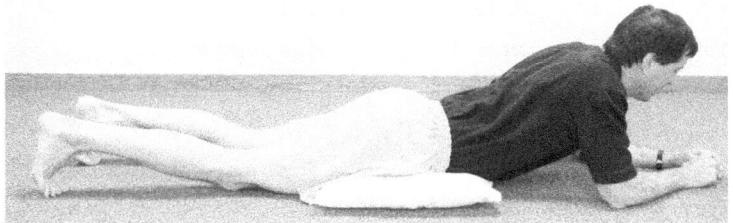

Option B

1. Start position for a prone pressup.

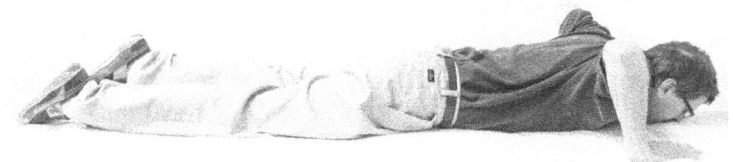

2. Press up, keeping the lower rib cage in contact with the floor.

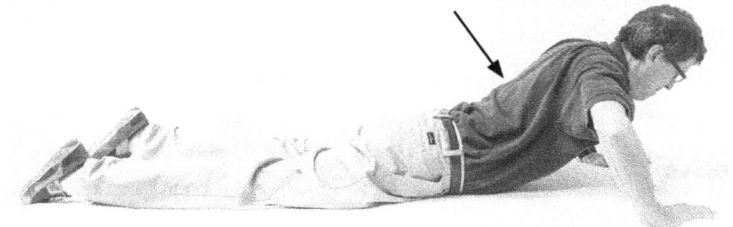

- Target: mid and upper back
- Hold 15–20 seconds
- Do 2–3 repetitions

AVOID PAIN!

Doorframe Backward Bend

This exercise can work for improving and maintaining sacral motion. It is an adjunct exercise for self-mobilization of the sacrum with a towel or tennis ball exercises, and it can be used as a generalized extension exercise. Since we tend to spend much of our time in a flexed position, sacral motion tends to become restricted. This restriction does not allow the top of the sacrum to move forward to a neutral position when we stand. This loss of motion of the sacrum then transfers more work to the lumbar spine.

Place your fingertips over the depressions just inside the pelvic bones at the bottom of your back. Each depression is a sacral sulcus. Test if your fingertip positioning is correct by bending forward slightly; you should feel the depressions become slightly shallower since forward bending of the trunk pushes the top of the sacrum backwards. Once your fingertip position is correct, back up to a doorframe so that your heels and upper back touch the doorframe.

Begin the exercise by letting your pelvis move away from the doorframe. As your pelvis moves forward, you should feel the depressions deepen as the top of the sacrum moves forward and the back muscles relax. Stay within a comfortable range of motion. Overall motion may be fairly small. Return to the start position and repeat this motion until you are comfortable with feeling the sacrum move. Moving too much may overextend the low back.

With your pelvis forward away from the doorframe, you can add a gentle sideways motion. When gently letting your pelvis move to the left, you should feel the right depression become slightly deeper. A slight left twist of the pelvis to aim the imaginary "headlights" on the front of the pelvis slightly left may also help. Gently moving the pelvis to the right and twisting slightly to the right should cause the left dimple to become slightly deeper.

If your sacral motion is very restricted, it may be difficult to feel movement. You are trying to feel for one eighth of an inch of movement through one inch of soft tissue. It can be frustrating because the landmarks that you are trying to feel are behind your back, and muscle guarding or spasms can obscure them as well.

Manual therapy or self-mobilization exercises can help restore sacral motion. The left sacroiliac joint is more often restricted in its forward motion than the right. The doorframe backward bend can be used to gently nudge the top of the sacrum forward from a restricted position.

This exercise can be done several times a day. Hold 15 to 20 seconds in the restricted direction or gently nudge the sacrum with small movements at the end range of its motion. Compare motion on the restricted side with the mobile side. If both sides are very restricted or if the side motions are painful, do just the first part of the exercise, and do not perform the left and right movements until more mobility is restored to the sacrum.

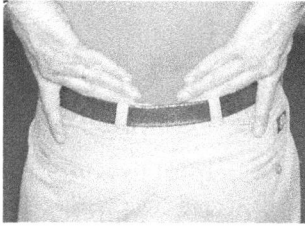

1. Finger tips in dimple area on back of pelvis

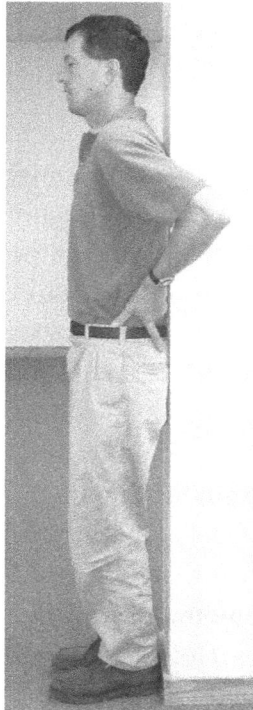

2. Back against doorframe. Heels against doorframe

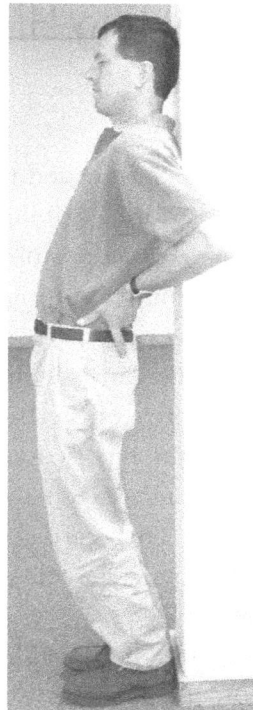

2. Let pelvis sway forward.

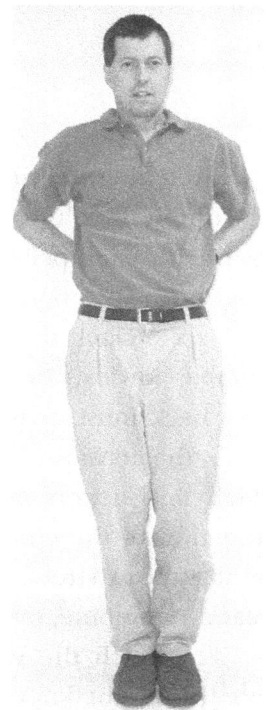

• Repeat steps 4 and 5, 2–3 times

AVOID PAIN!

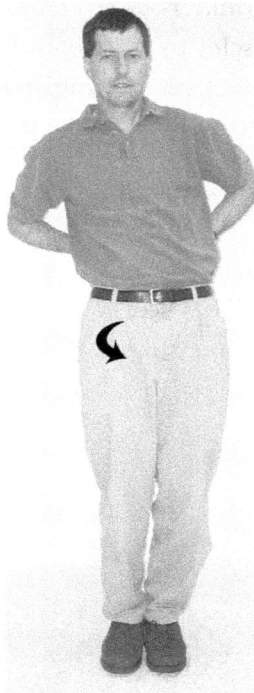

4. Then sway slightly to left, gently twist left, feel right dimple get deeper. Hold 10–15 seconds.

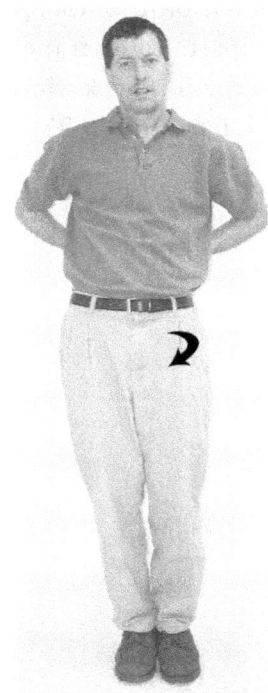

5. Then sway to right, twist right, feel left dimple get deeper. Hold 10–15 seconds.

Kneeling Hip Flexor Stretch

Stretching the hip flexors may be needed to disinhibit the gluteal muscles, restore flexibility to the hips and pelvis, and help correct posture. Tight hip flexors can cause too much anterior tilt (six o'clock tilt) of the pelvis and increase lumbar lordosis or swayback. The work of the low back muscles may increase to counterbalance the tension exerted by tight hip flexors. Tight hip flexors may inhibit and weaken the function of the gluteal muscles. There are several ways to stretch the hip flexors: kneeling, standing, supine, or sidelying.

To stretch the right side, start by kneeling on your right knee. Position the left leg with the hip and knee at 90 degrees each. The left foot is flat on the floor with the legs shoulder-width apart. Tighten the abdominal muscles to flatten the low back with a strong 12 o'clock or posterior pelvic tilt. Try not to lean the upper body back. You might find it helpful to bend the upper torso slightly forward. Use your hands to help with the pelvic tilt by putting your left hand on the front of the pelvis, and your right hand on the back of the pelvis. Pull the front of the pelvis up and push the back of the pelvis down. Tighten the right buttock muscle. You should feel some stretch in the front of the right hip and thigh. While holding the strong 12 o'clock tilt, the left leg can be used to pull your trunk slightly forward. This should increase the amount of stretch.

Hold a gentle stretch for at least 15 to 20 seconds. Repeat two to three times each side. Generally a 15 to 20 second rest is required between stretches. You can try the standing version of this stretch (page 40). The supine (page 42) or side lying (page 40) versions might work if you can't make these work.

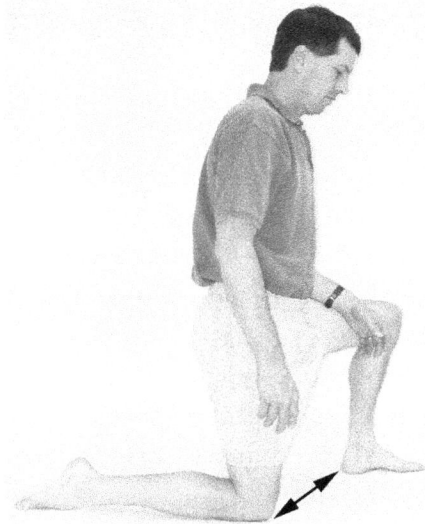

1. Have a wide base of support.

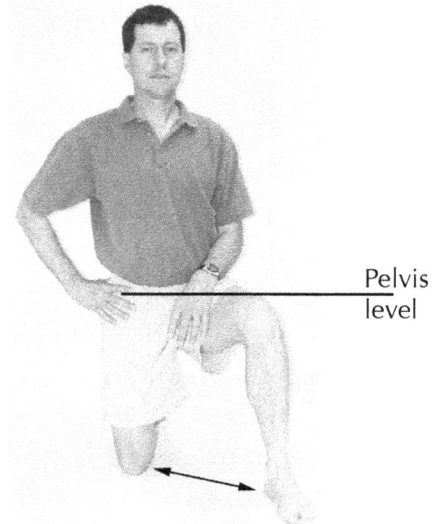

Pelvis
level

2. Begin with pelvis level.

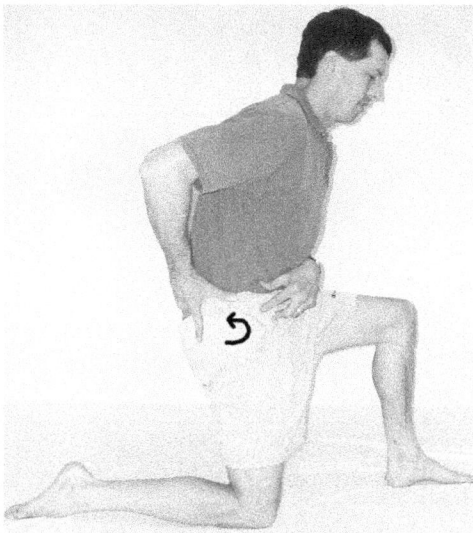

3. Strong 12:00. tilt. Use hands to help.
Strong gluteal contraction

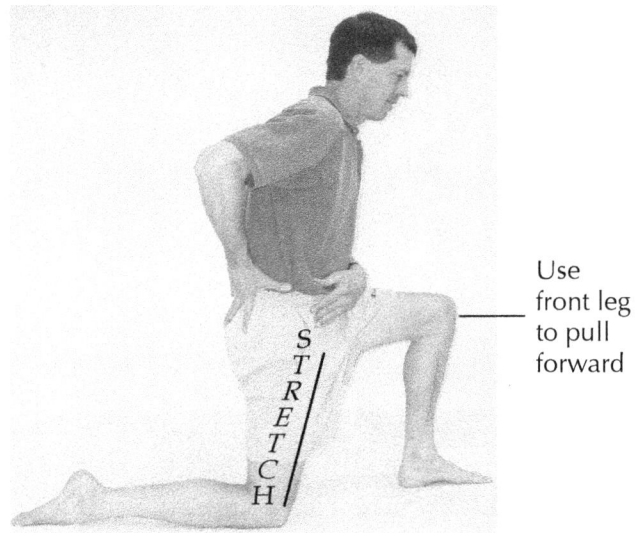

Use
front leg
to pull
forward

STRETCH

4. Feel stretch in front of thigh.

- Cushion under knee if needed
- Hold 20 seconds per side
- Do 2 per side

AVOID PAIN!

Standing Hip Flexor Stretch

The standing hip flexor stretch is similar to the kneeling stretch, but it is sometimes harder to isolate the stretch sensation to the top of the thigh.

Stand with your feet slightly wider than shoulder-width apart and with the stance length roughly equal to a normal step length. Toes pointed slightly inward or pigeon toed.

Tighten your stomach muscles by doing a strong 12 o'clock or posterior pelvic tilt to flatten the low back. Use your hands to help guide the movement. Hold the tilt, tighten the buttock muscle of the trailing leg, and straighten the knee. Slightly bend the front knee to help increase the stretch in the trailing leg. Make sure to maintain the strong 12 o'clock tilt.

If the exercise is done correctly, you should feel stretch in the top of the thigh of the trailing leg. Hold the stretch for at least 15 to 20 seconds. Try the side lying (page 44) or supine (page 42) versions if this one doesn't work for you.

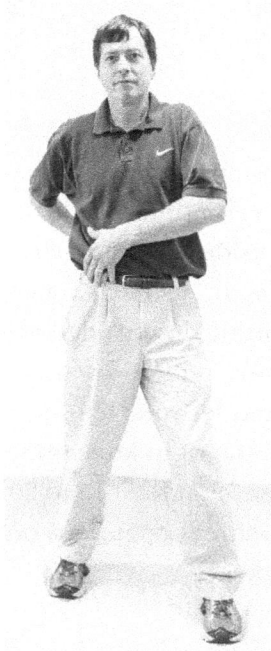

1. Stand with feet slightly wider than shoulder width. Back foot has toe turned slightly inward.

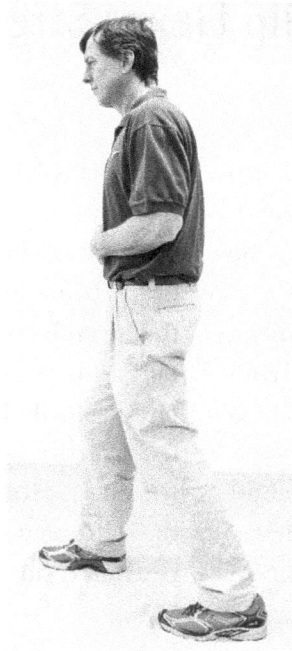

2. Make stance length same as width.

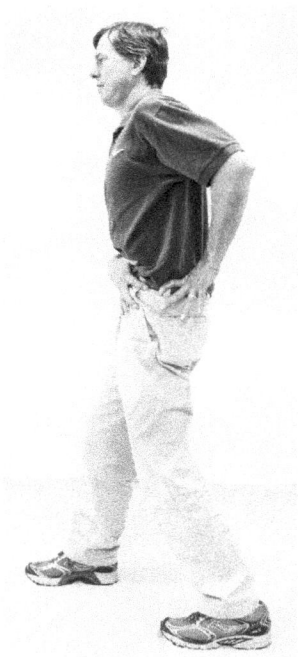

• Hold 15–20 seconds.
• Do 3 per side, 2 times per day.

Feel stretch

AVOID PAIN!

Keep knee straight

3. Perform a strong 12:00 tilt.

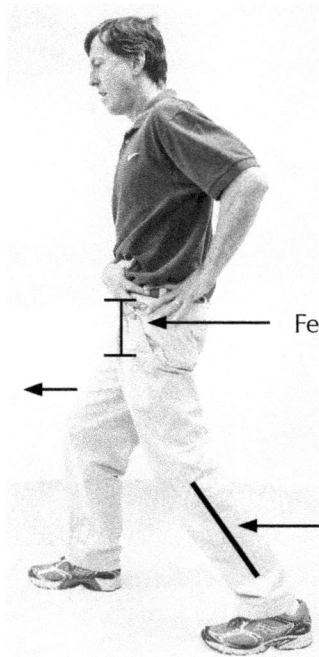

4. Strongly contract gluteal muscle of trailing leg and pull slightly forward with front leg.

Supine Hip Flexor Stretch

If a more gentle stretch is needed for the hip flexor, you begin the supine hip flexor stretch by lying on a bed or couch so the side to be stretched is at the edge of the bed.

Place your hips six to eight inches from the edge and your shoulders 12 to 18 inches from the edge. Bend your knees with your feet placed flat on the bed.

Bring your inside knee towards your chest and hold it with both hands. Let your outside leg ease off the edge of the bed towards the floor. Try to let this leg completely relax. Introducing some 12 o'clock or posterior tilt may increase the stretch. A partner can apply a light downward force above the outside knee if gravity does not provide enough stretch. A similar version of this stretch is done by sitting on the edge of your bed with your right knee pulled towards your chest. Slowly lie back and let your left leg relax towards the floor. Keep the right knee pulled to the chest. Hold stretches for at least 15 to 20 seconds. Repeat for two to three repetitions on the restricted side.

Option A

1. Lie on bed with hips 6–8 inches and shoulders 12–18 inches from the edge.

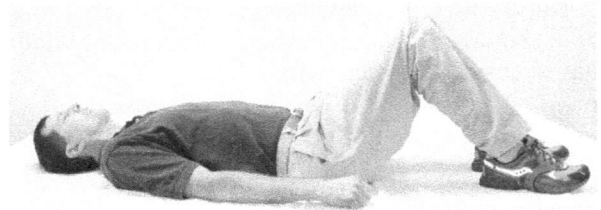

2. Bring inside knee toward chest.

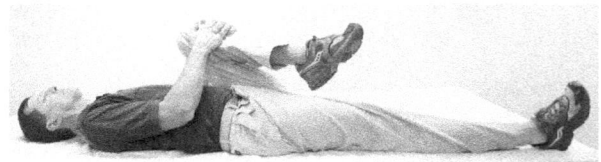

3. Ease outside leg off bed.

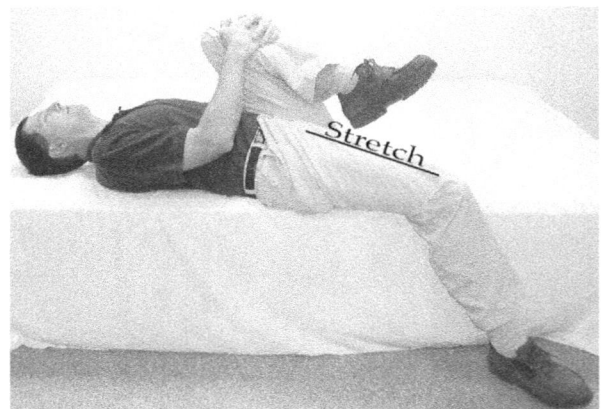

Option B

1. Sit on edge of bed with right knee pulled toward chest.

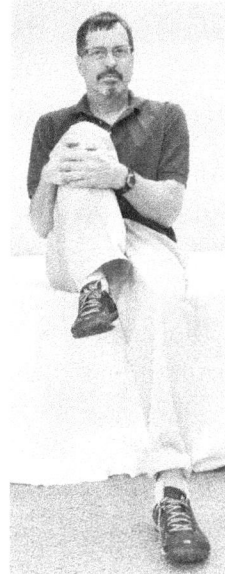

2. Slowly lie back. Pull right knee to chest.

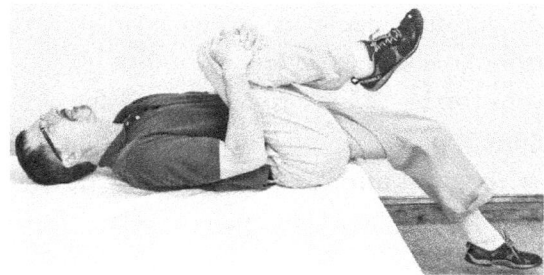

3. Let left leg relax to feel stretch in thigh.

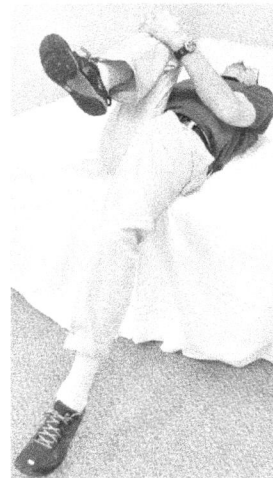

- Hold 15–20 seconds
- Do 2–3 times per side

A V O I D   P A I N !

Quadriceps and Hip Flexor Stretch in Side-lying

For athletes who need more aggressive work on their thigh and hip flexors, stretching can be done in side-lying. There are two versions of this stretch, both of which will also focus on the long muscles in the thigh: the sartorius, rectus femoris, and the iliotibial band (ITB). These are considered two joint muscles because they attach below the knee and to the front of the pelvis above the hip. Tightness in these muscles can affect the hip, knee, low back, and pelvis. To stretch these muscles, you must simultaneously flex the knee and extend the hip.

In the first side-lying stretch, you pull your bottom knee towards your chest, bring the foot of your top leg behind you, and grab above your top ankle with your top hand. Bring your foot as close to your buttock as you can. Let your thigh go back as far as it will go and try to get your knee to the floor. Stay on your side. Avoid the tendency to roll back.

With the second version of the stretch, you pull the top knee towards the chest, and bend

bottom leg back so that you can grab above the ankle with your top hand. Pull the bottom foot toward the buttock to flex the knee, and let your thigh go back to extend the hip. Keep your pelvis rolled forward.

With each stretch, you should feel a comfortable stretch somewhere between the knee and pelvis. If your hip and/or knee range of motion is so restricted that you can't reach your ankle, use a belt or strap to help you reach and pull it. You can change how much knee flexion versus how much hip extension you do by changing the pull at the ankle, or how far back you let the thigh go. This may allow you to stretch the upper thigh without causing knee pain. Hold each stretch for at least 15 to 20 seconds and do two to three stretches on each leg. There is a subtle difference in how each of these stretches affects the target muscles. You can do one or both versions in a given stretching session.

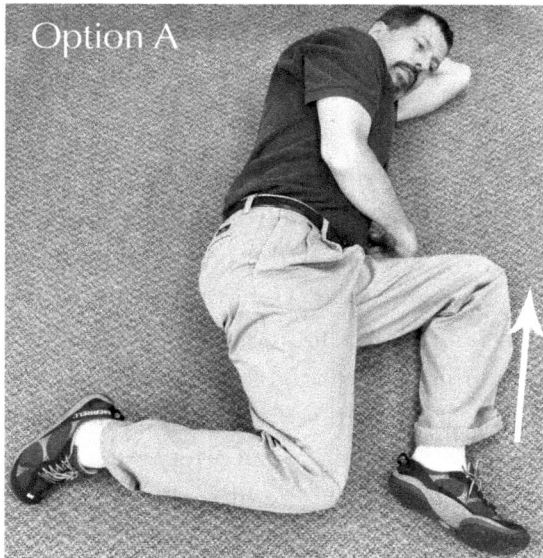

Option A

1. Lie on side. Pull bottom leg toward chest.

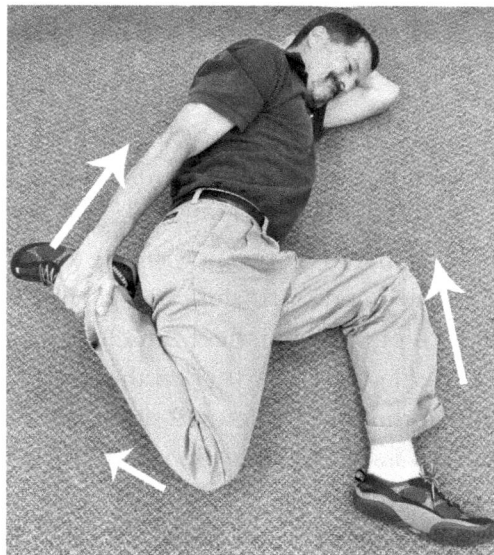

2. Pull top thigh back and heel toward buttock. Try to get knee to floor.

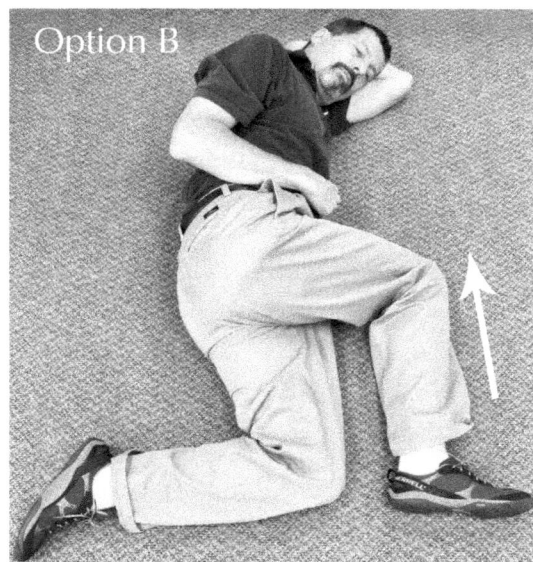

Option B

1. Lie on side. Pull top leg toward chest.

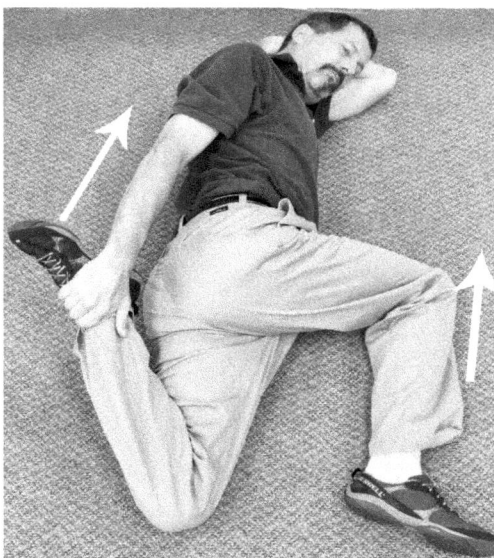

2. Pull bottom thigh back and heel toward buttocks. Roll slightly forward.

- Do not over-arch the low back
- Hold stretches for 15–20 seconds
- Do stretch 2 times on each side

AVOID PAIN!

© Brian Lambert

Lower Extremity/Back Stretches | 45

Massage the Front of One Hip with a Ball on a Stick

The front of the hip is a very busy place. Long muscles from the thigh cross this area to attach to the front of the pelvis. These include the iliotibial band, sartorius, and rectus femoris. An inch or so inside these muscles, you have part of the iliopsoas. Farther to the inside, you have hip adductors. Prolonged sitting positions, mechanical issues in the spine and pelvis, and poor posture can cause the muscles in the front of the hip to get tight. Massage can help loosen these tight muscles.

Use a one-inch diameter by 48-inch dowel. Make a one-inch slice in two tennis balls and put them on each end of the dowel.

Put one end of the stick on the floor against a wall. Position yourself in a front stance, and place the other end of the stick so that it pushes against the muscles in front of the hip of the trailing leg just below the pelvic bone. Tender areas are tight areas. Use your hands to move the end of the stick to massage these areas while maintaining a comfortable pressure by pushing your pelvis forward. Work each tight area for 30 to 60 seconds. The femoral artery and nerve are in a space in front of the hip called the femoral triangle. If you press on an area and feel pulsations or feel tingling in the front of the thigh, avoid massaging directly on that area. You may also try using the foam roller to loosen the front of the hip (page 194).

1. Make a ball on a stick with a 1-inch by 48-inch dowel. Cut 1-inch holes in each tennis ball and place them on the end of the stick.

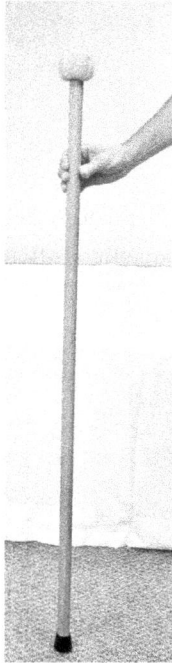

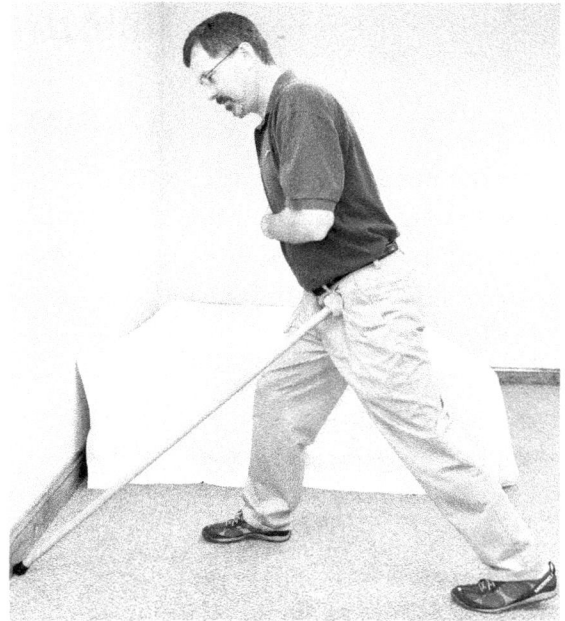

2. One end of stick against wall

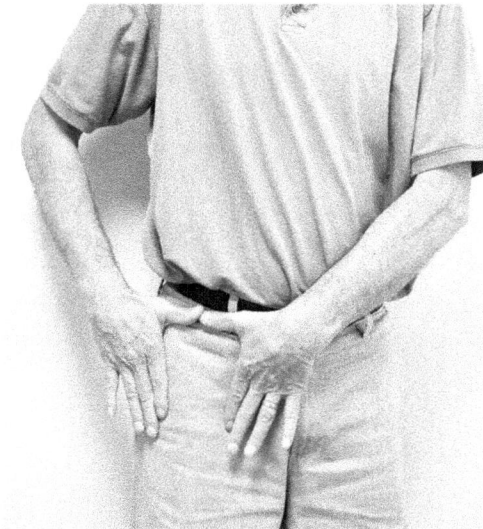

3. The other end of stick will be on muscles on front of hip of trailing leg.

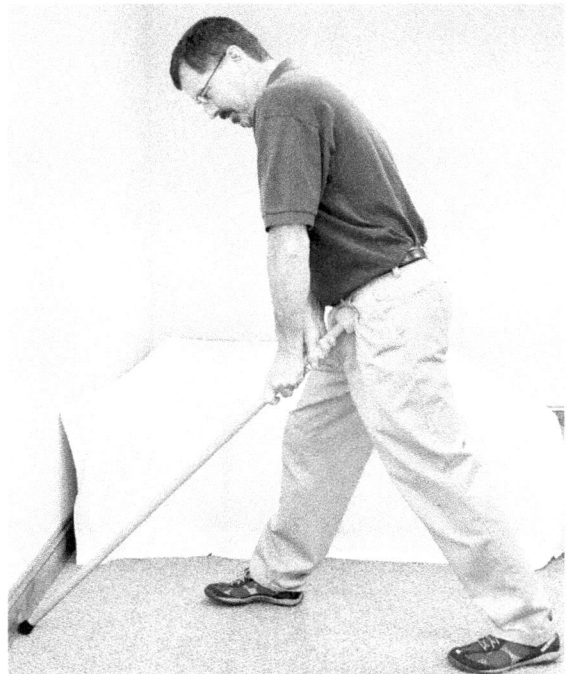

4. Lean into stick with enough pressure to get a deep massage by moving stick against tight muscles for 30–60 seconds.

AVOID PAIN!

Hamstring Stretches

The hamstring muscles run down the back of the thigh. The upper ends attach to the lower part of the pelvis and back of the thighbone. The lower ends attach below and to either side of the knee. There are many ways to stretch hamstrings. Generally, to lessen the stress placed across the low back, you want to maintain neutral or a slightly increased sway to the low back when doing either the seated or standing stretches.

The door-frame (or column) stretch may be used if you want your back completely unloaded, or if you want a stretch that involves movement and stretch of the sciatic nerve. A belt placed over the ball of the foot can be used to apply extra force to the stretch. See page 50 for more specific instructions on stretches for the sciatic nerve. A gentle static stretch is held for at least 15 to 20 seconds. Stretches can be repeated two to three times on each side.

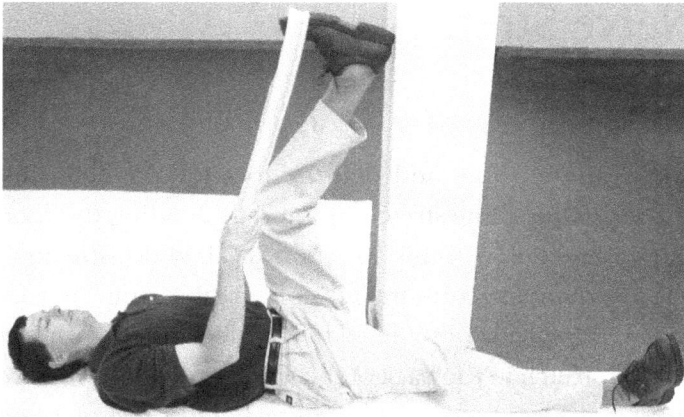
1. Doorframe or column stretch

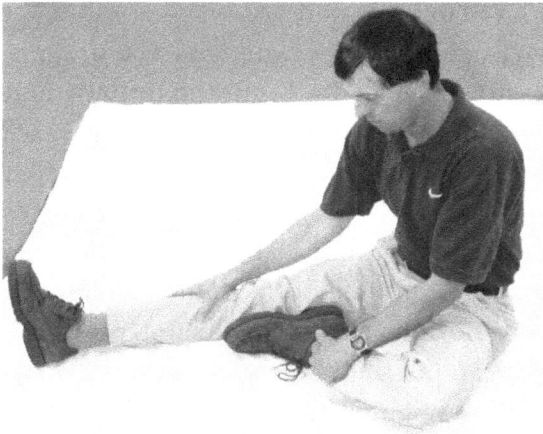
3. Lean forward from hips.

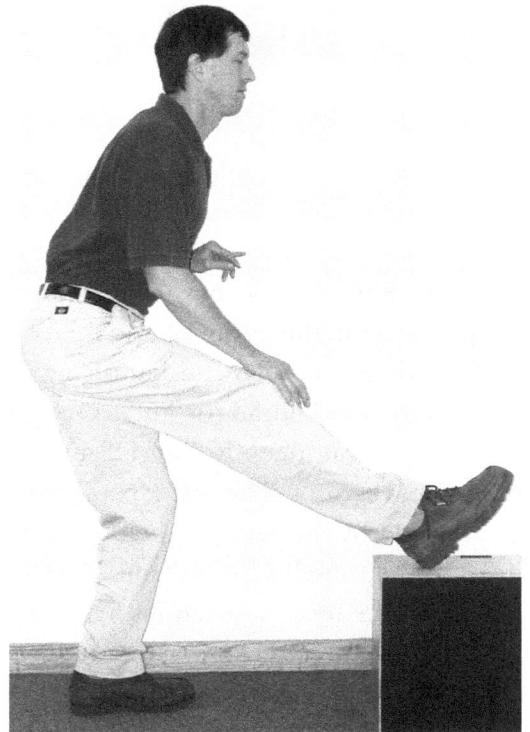
2. Push tush back.

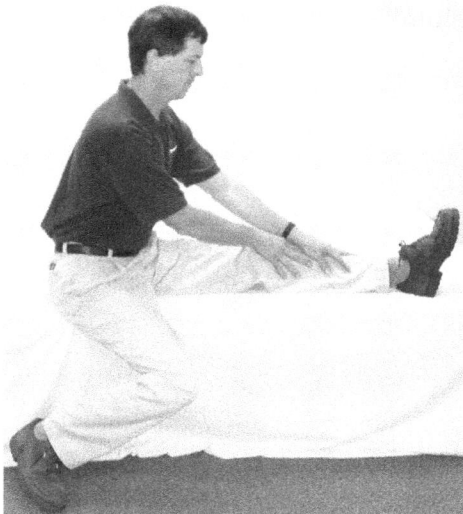
4. Lean forward from hips.

- 2–3 stretches per muscle
- Hold for 15–20 seconds
- Some experimentation may be needed to find the stretch that best suits your abilities

AVOID PAIN!

Sciatic Nerve Stretch

Sometimes it is helpful to pull the sciatic nerve through its channels on the back of the leg. Each sciatic nerve (one each leg) starts as nerve roots in the low back, comes through the deep muscles in the buttocks, and then down the back of thigh between the hamstring muscles. The nerve splits behind the knee. One part goes behind the shin, deep in the calf muscle to the bottom of the foot. The other part goes around the outside of the leg, just below the knee, to deep in the muscles in the front of the shin to the top of the foot. Restrictions in movement of the sciatic nerve can cause pain, numbness, and "pins and needles" sensation in the legs and feet. If you have these symptoms, try these stretches.

To stretch the left sciatic nerve, lie in a doorway with your right leg through the door with the knee straight. Move in or out of the doorway and then to the left so that you can prop your left leg up on the outside of the doorframe, and the inside of your right thigh touches the inside of the doorframe. Put a strap over the ball of the left foot and pull the toes towards the shin to feel some stretch in the calf. Bending the foot and ankle in this direction is called dorsiflexion. Maintain constant tension on the strap as you straighten your left knee to feel a comfortable stretch in the back of the left leg. Hold the stretch (15 to 20 seconds) or gently bend and straighten the knee in small movements at the end range of motion (10 to 15 repetitions).

You can alter this technique by first straightening the knee to its comfortable limit and then pulling on the strap to gently increase ankle dorsiflexion. You can hold the stretch or gently "pump" the ankle with small changes in the strap tension. If you are very inflexible, move away from the doorface. Individuals who are very flexible (and who do not need this stretch) can put their buttock against the doorface, fully straighten their knee, and dorsiflex their ankle. Repeat stretches two to three times on each leg. Use whichever technique seems the most helpful.

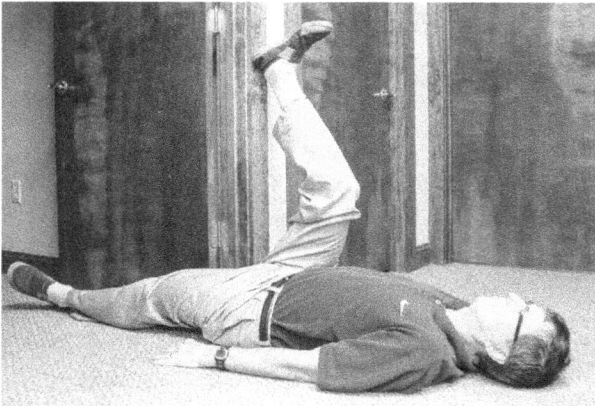

1. Lie on floor with leg through doorframe and other propped on wall.

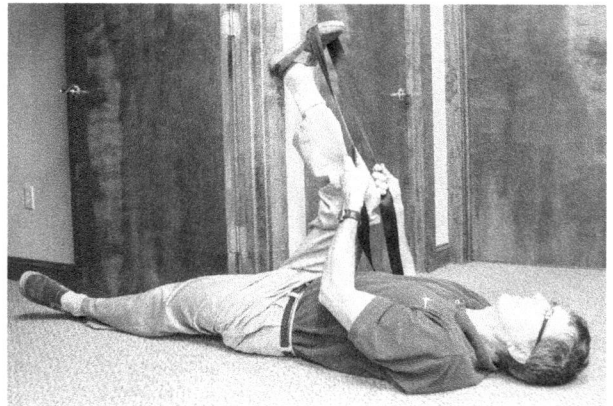

2. A belt is looped over foot on wall.

Option A

1. Pull toe toward knee

2. Then gently straighten knee.

Hold stretch for 15-20 seconds or gently straighten and release knee 10-15 repetitions.

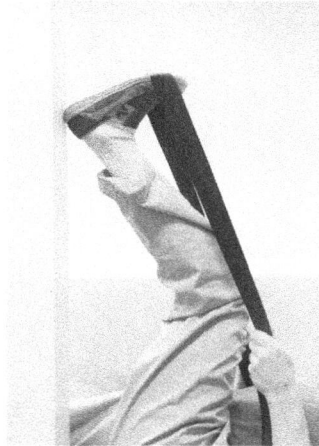

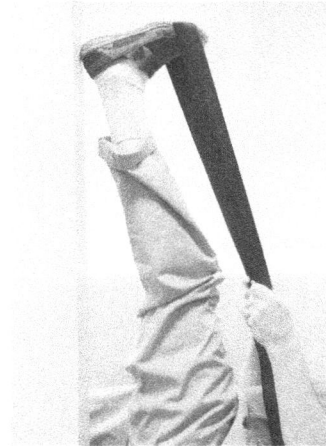

Option B

1. Straighten knee to feel stretch

2. Then gently pull toes toward knee.

Hold for 15 seconds or "pump" ankle with belt.

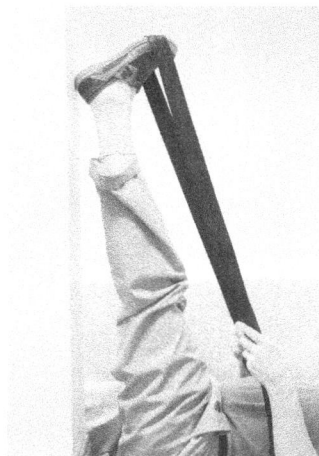

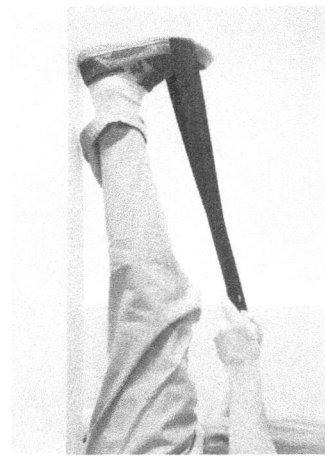

- 3 repetitions per leg
- 1-2 times per day.

AVOID PAIN!

© Brian Lambert

Quadriped Stretch For The Piriformis

A more aggressive stretch for the piriformis and other small rotators of the hip may be accomplished in a quadriped position. It is essentially the upside down version of the piriformis stretch used as one of the basic exercises for the low back (page 2).

Begin the exercise on all fours. Position left leg so that your knee is under the center of your body, with the shin at a 45 degree angle to the long axis of the body. Slide the pelvis and right leg back so that your body flattens down. Try to keep your pelvis level and square. It may be helpful to rotate the right side of the pelvis downward towards the left ankle as you slide your right leg back. To make the stretch more comfortable, you can rest on your elbows and forearms.

Gently roll to the left to get out of the stretch. As with other stretches, hold the position for a minimum of 15 seconds. Generally three repetitions are sufficient.

1. Start on hands and knees.

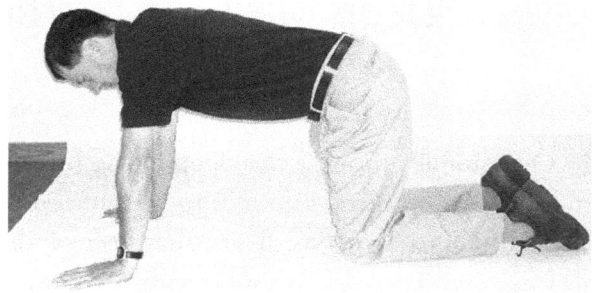

2. Straighten one leg and move other under center of body. Shin should be at 45° angle to floor.

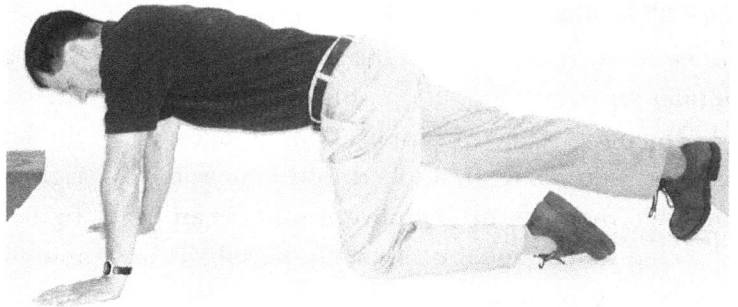

3. The foot of leg under should be under opposite side of pelvis.

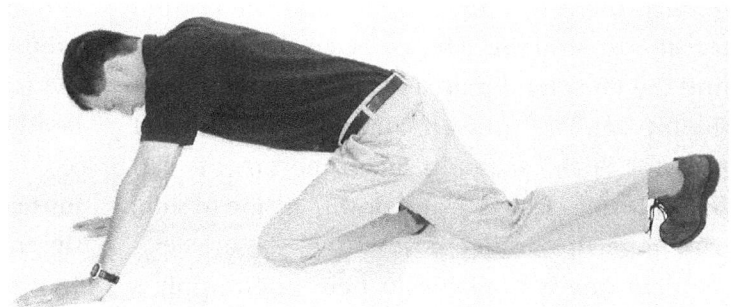

4. Now slide pelvis and leg back so that chest is over underside knee.

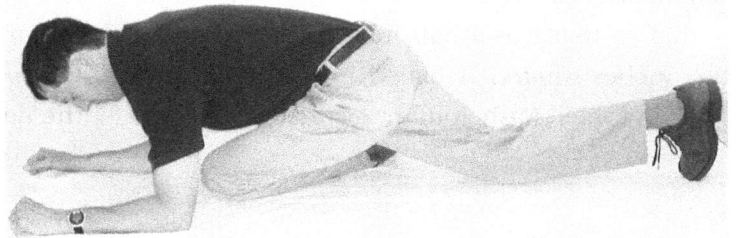

- Hold for 15 seconds
- Do 3 per side
- Keep pelvis level. Keep knee in center of chest

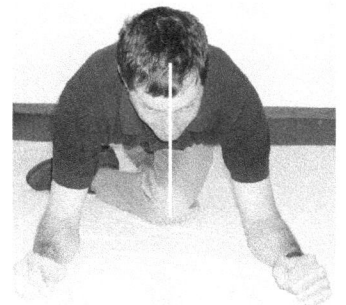

AVOID PAIN!

Deep Massage Of The Piriformis Musculature

Occasionally the muscles deep in the hip are too tight, or even too knotted, to be affected by stretching. Piriformis syndrome may occur if the sciatic nerve becomes trapped within the muscles. This situation can feel like a pinched nerve. Deep massage is helpful if the piriformis is very tender and won't loosen up with stretching.

The most effective application of massage is done with a stretch applied to the muscle. A massage therapist or "significant other" can be directed to massage the area with the subject in a side-lying position and the top leg pulled up towards the center of the chest and the bottom leg almost straight. The massage therapist will find the most tender area deep in the buttock of the top leg. Use pressure almost to the point of pain for 30–60 seconds. Small movements can be made in a circle, up and down, or side to side, with fingertips or an elbow.

If no one is available to help, then apply a self-massage using a tennis ball or a washcloth folded so that it is a half inch thick and about two inches square. A balled up sock may also work. A folded washcloth may work best because a wiggling movement will create a shearing force that will break up tight tissue. To work on the right side, the ball or cloth is positioned just behind the right hipbone. Rest on your right forearm and elbow. The right leg is pulled up a 45 degree angle so that the knee comes towards the center of the chest and is then crossed over the left leg at the knee. Roll your pelvis to the right so that the cloth is under the back of your right hip. The cloth is now under the piriformis muscle. Adjust the location of the cloth so that you find the area that is most tender. Small oscillations or wiggling will provide a deep massage. Adjust the thickness of the cloth depending on the tenderness in the hip. Sit up straighter and bend both knees more to increase the pressure.

Massage can be applied to the piriformis muscles one to two times per day. Sometimes the initial massage session will make the muscle very tender. Some people will start out doing this exercise every other, or even every third day, until the muscle will tolerate daily massage. Once the muscle has loosened, you can massage the muscle only on an "as needed" basis.

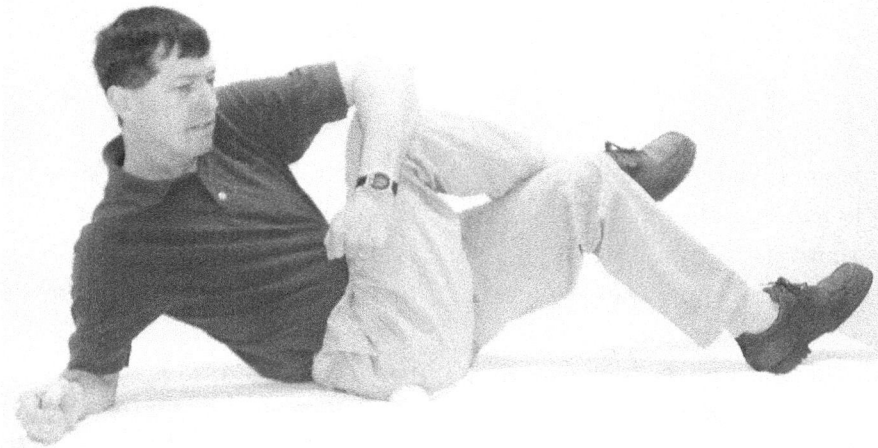

Position balled washcloth or sock under hip in tender area. Roll or move in small motions to deeply massage piriformis muscle for 30–60 seconds.

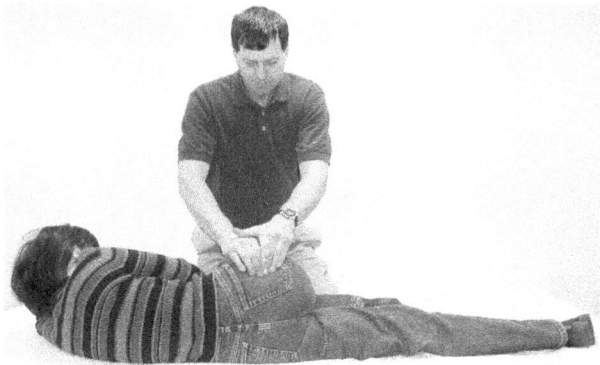

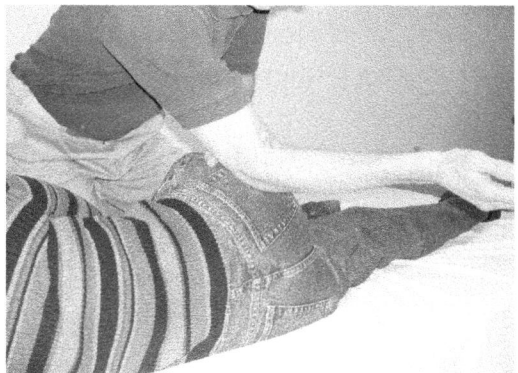

Have a signficant other massage the area. Push almost to the point of pain.

• Do 1–2 times a day

AVOID PAIN!

Standing Calf Stretch

Occasionally it's necessary to stretch the muscles on the back of the leg between the knee and the ankle with a standing calf stretch.

Stand 12 to 18 inches from a wall. Your feet will be slightly wider than shoulder-width apart. Place your hands on the wall at approximately chest height. Position the foot of the leg to be stretched 18 to 24 inches back from its original starting position. Turn the toe of this foot slightly inward and gently lock the knee straight. Keep the heel in contact with the floor. Bend the knee of the front leg slightly. Lean in towards the wall to increase the stretch in the calf. Keep your body straight. If more stretch is desired, move the trailing leg farther back. To stretch the lower calf muscles, let the back knee bend slightly, but keep your heel on the floor.

As an alternative, you can stretch your calf on a step by having one foot fully on the step while the other foot is back so that the ball of the foot is on the edge of the step with the toe turn slightly inward. Gently let your heel down. Keep your body straight. Resist the tendency to lean backwards. Keep one half to three quarters of your body weight on your front foot. To focus more stretch on the lower calf, slightly bend your knee. Bent and/or straight knee stretches should be held for at least 15 or 20 seconds each. Again, two to three repetitions per side are optimal.

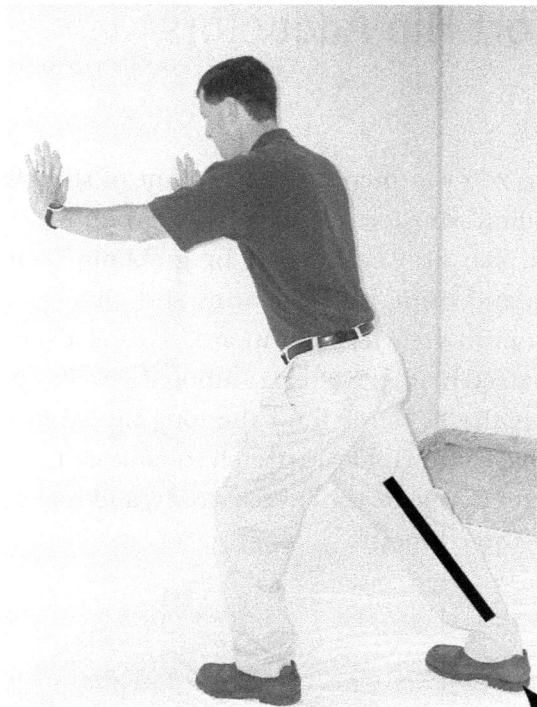

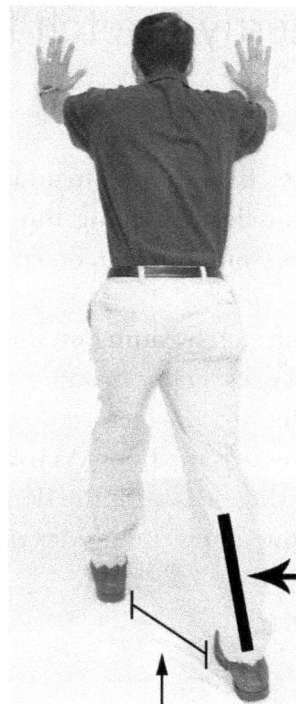

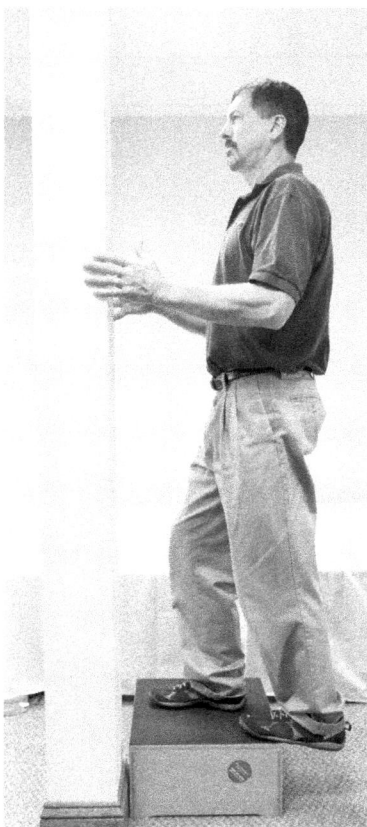

Stretch ←

Heel down

Rear foot toe turned in ←

Shoulder width

Alternative:

Stand with ball of one foot on the edge of step. Let heel down. Keep body vertical and knee straight.

To stretch lower calf muscle (soleus), let knee bend but keep heel down.

- 2–3 stretches per muscle
- Hold 15–20 seconds

AVOID PAIN!

Butterfly Stretch for the Short Hip Adductors

Occasionally, stretching of the hip adductors is helpful. These muscles run along the inside portion of the thighs from the groin down to the knee.

Start a butterfly stretch by sitting on the floor with your pelvis and back against a wall. Position your legs so the soles of your feet are together. Lower your knees towards the floor. As you push the outsides of your thighs towards the floor, you should feel stretching along the insides of your thighs. You can increase the amount of stretch by pulling your feet closer to your groin. More stretch can also be applied by grabbing your ankles and using your forearms and elbows to gently push your legs downward. This is a very good stretch to do after running or walking. Also try the "V" stretch for the long hip adductors (page 60). Hold the stretch for at least 15 to 20 seconds, release the stretch slowly, and repeat two to three times.

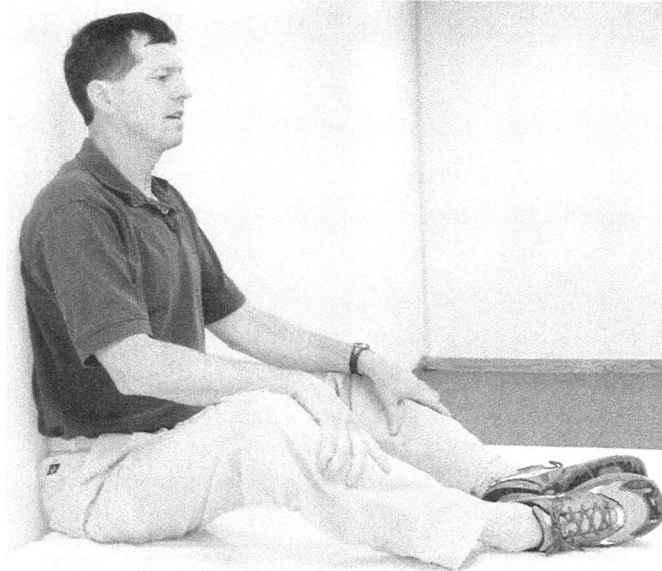

1. Sit with back and pelvis against wall.

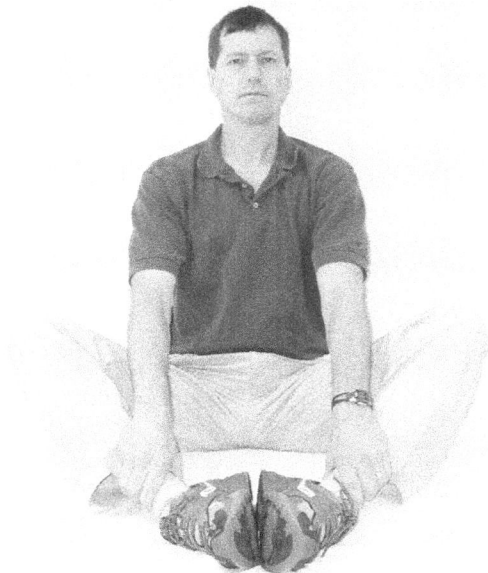

2. Draw feet towards groin.

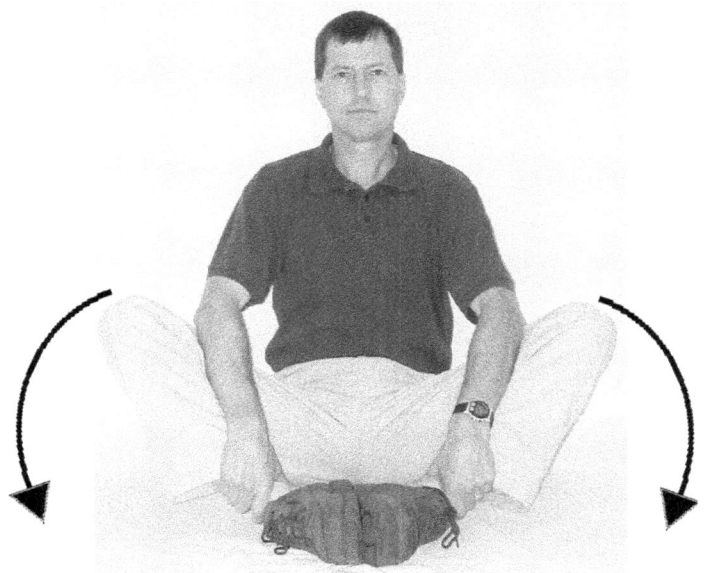

3. Use forearms to push legs down, to feel stretch on the insides of the thighs.

- Hold 15–20 seconds
- Repeat 2–3 times

AVOID PAIN!

"V" Stretch for the Long Hip Adductors

The long hip adductors run from the groin to below the knee. The "V" stretch will also stretch the hamstrings.

Start by sitting on the floor with your back and pelvis flat against a wall. With your knees straight, use your hands to push your feet as far apart as you can get them. Some people will feel enough stretch just by assuming this position. You can increase the amount of stretch by reaching towards one leg, left hand to right foot and vice-versa. This will also stretch the muscles in the sides of the torso. Hold the stretches for at least 20 seconds, and do two or three times on each side.

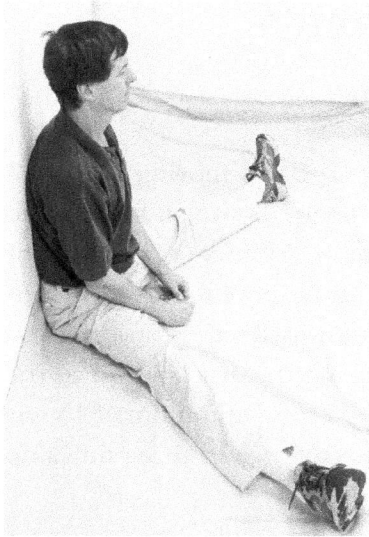

1. Sit with back and pelvis flat against wall.

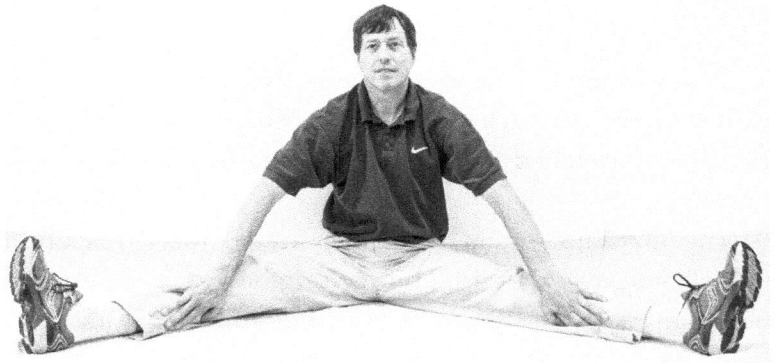

2. Push legs apart as far as comfortable.

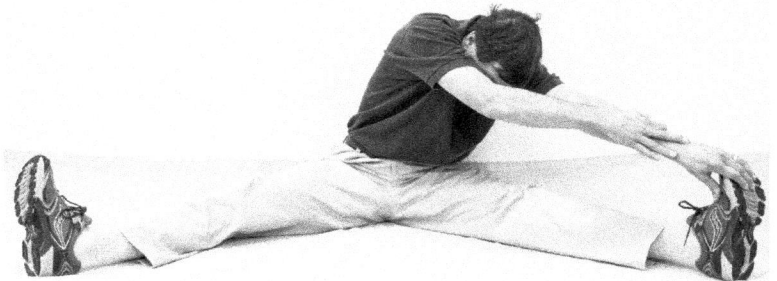

3. Reach over towards one leg and then the other. Hold 15–20 seconds.

- Repeat last 2 steps 2–3 times
- 1–2 times per day

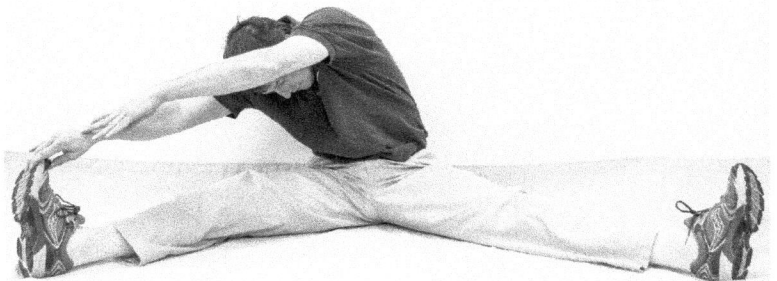

4. Push legs farther apart and repeat previous step.

AVOID PAIN!

Quadruped Latissimus Dorsi Stretch

The latissimus dorsi is a large muscle that runs from the low back to the armpit. This muscle can be stretched from a sitting or standing position.

The quadruped version of this stretch for the left side is accomplished by getting on your hands and knees an arm's length from a heavy object or doorframe. Align your right shoulder with the doorframe. Grab the doorframe with the left hand. Grab low to the floor with the thumb down. Now sit back, moving your buttocks towards your heels. As you sit back, try to increase the amount of "C" curve of the back by moving your left buttock more towards your left heel. If the latissimus muscles are restricted, you will feel a stretch along the arm and down the side of the body. Hold for a minimum of 15 seconds. Repeat this stretch two to three times on each side of the body.

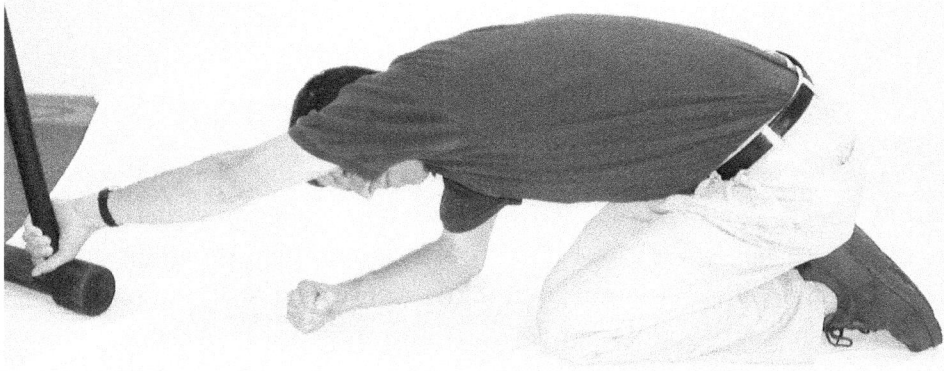

1. Grab heavy object with thumb pointed down.

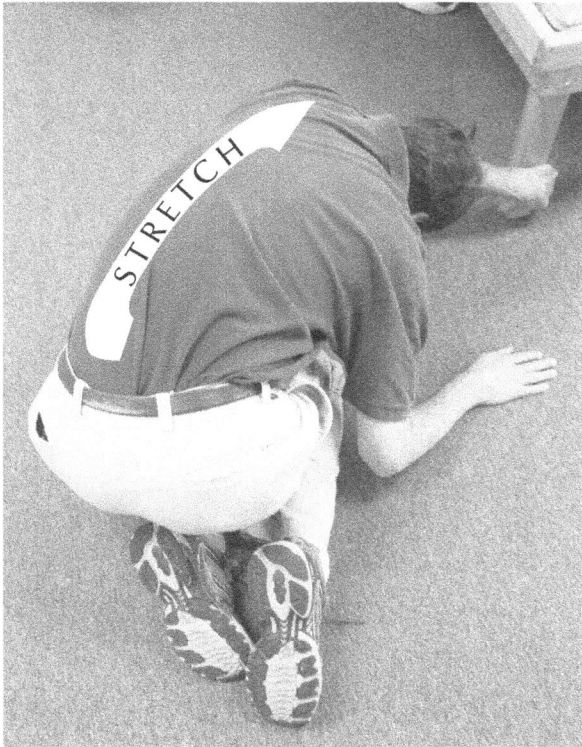
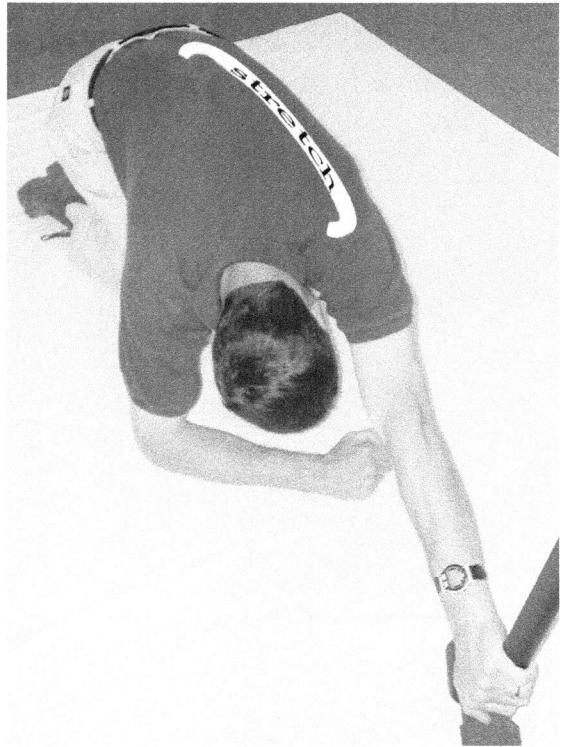

2. Sit buttock back toward heels to make a "C" curve in back. Feel stretch along "C".

- Hold 15 seconds.
- Do 3 per side.

AVOID PAIN!

Latissimus Dorsi Stretch With A Chair

This stretch may also help increase thoracic extension. Start by kneeling in front of a bench or chair. You should be far enough from the bench so that when you lean forward with your elbows bent, five to six inches of your upper arm will rest on the bench. Rest your arms on the bench so that your elbows are touching each other and are bent to 90 degrees. Rest your forehead on your arms. Contract your abdominal muscles and move the pelvis into a 12 o'clock or posterior tilt. Then lower your chest towards the floor. This movement will be fairly small. You should feel stretching through the sides of the rib cage and central portion of the thoracic spine. You can increase the amount of stretch with a slight lowering movement of the hip towards the heels. Be careful not to cause pain in the shoulders. Hold this stretch for at least 15 seconds and it repeat two to three times.

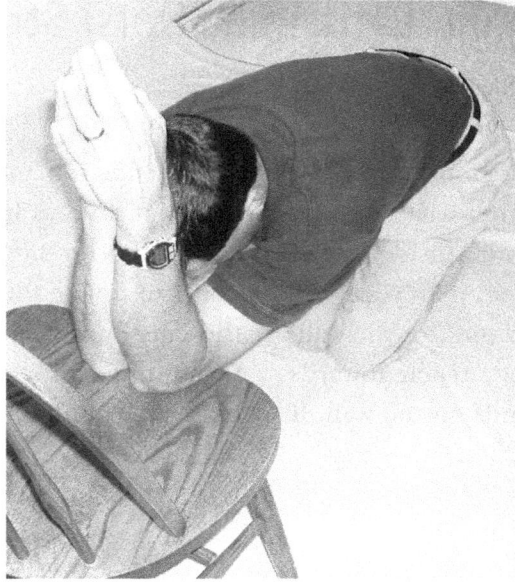

1. Kneel with elbows together on chair. Place elbows and 5–6 inches of upper arm on chair.

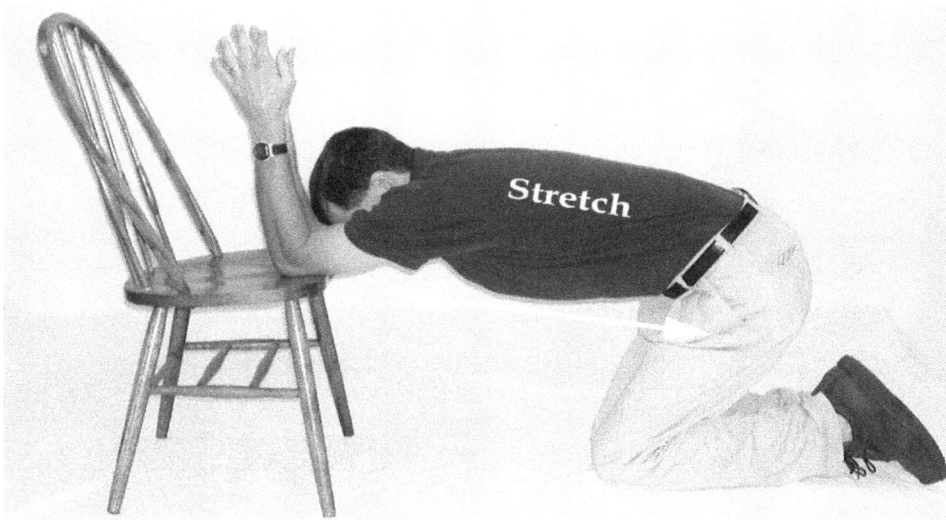

2. Keep tummy tight (12:00 tilt) and slightly lower chest. Move buttocks toward heels to increase stretch.

- Hold for 15 seconds
- Repeat 3–4 times

AVOID PAIN!

Standing Latissimus Dorsi Stretch

You can also stretch the latissimus dorsi from a standing position. Stand with a wall 24 to 36 inches from your side. Cross your outside foot in front of or behind the inside leg. With your outside arm, reach over your head towards the wall. With the side-bending motion, reach towards the wall and position both hands on the wall. If no stretch is felt, move your feet farther from the wall or push your hips farther from the wall. You can also move the hips slightly forward or backwards to isolate the stretch to different fibers of the latissimus dorsi. Repeat this stretch two to three times on each side. Each stretch can be held for a minimum of 15 seconds.

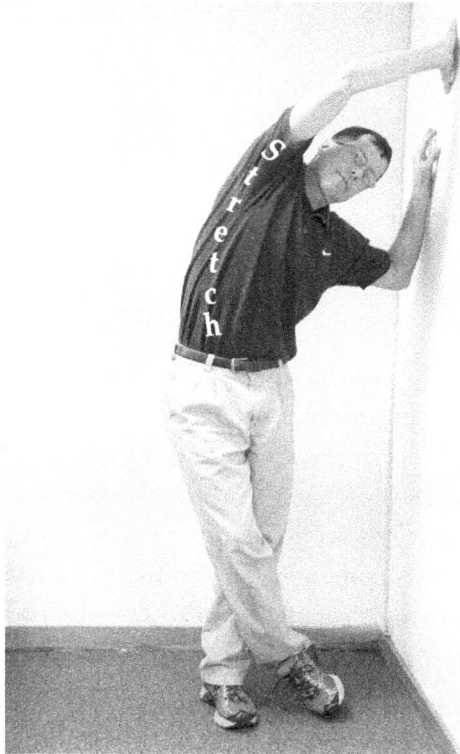

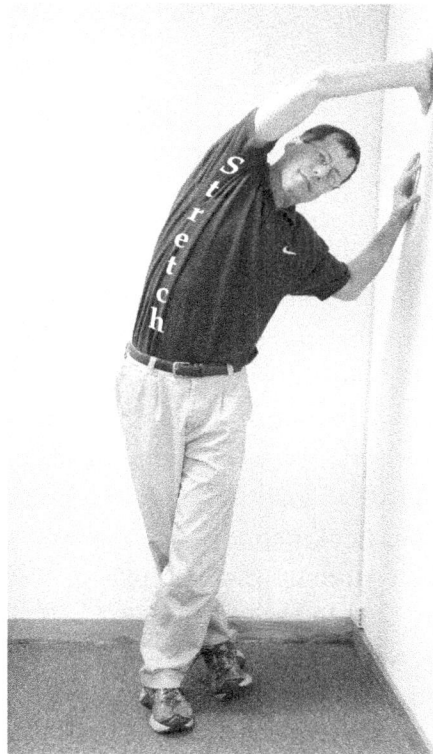

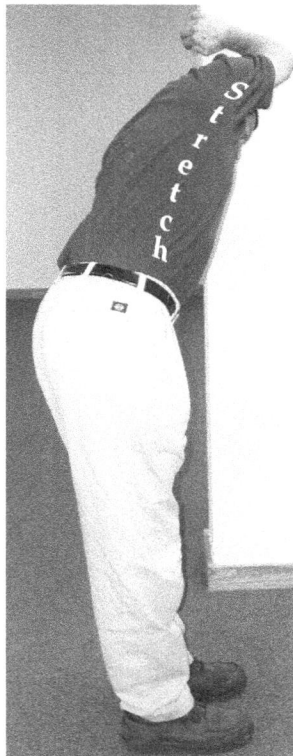

- Position yourself to feel stretch along rib cage
- Cross outside leg in front of or behind inside leg
- Hold 15 seconds
- Do 3 per side

AVOID PAIN!

Low Back Stretches

The sway in the low back is called lordosis. When you bend forward, this lordosis should completely reverse so that the curve of your low back goes from concave to convex. Tight back muscles (erector spinae) may limit movement and contribute to pain.

Lying on your back and using your hands to pull one or both knees toward your chest can help stretch very tight back muscles. Pull from behind your knees if knee pain is a problem.

A "prayer stretch" can be used if you can kneel with your buttocks on your heels. From there, lean forward to rest on your outstretched arms. Tighten your stomach muscles to help push your back up to increase the amount of pull in the back muscles.

"Plow pose" is a more advanced stretching technique and is not recommended for everyone. Begin by lying on your back. You must then roll up and back on to your shoulder blades so that your feet and legs end up over your head. Grab your feet or ankles. You should feel stretch in your back muscles as you relax into the position. Sometimes an assistant can help pull and then hold your legs over your head. Hold the stretch for at least 15 seconds and do two to three repetitions.

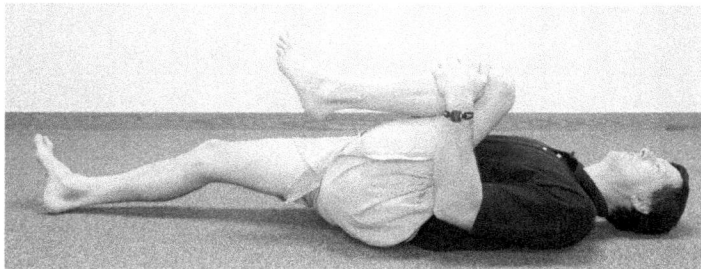

Single knee to chest for hip and low back

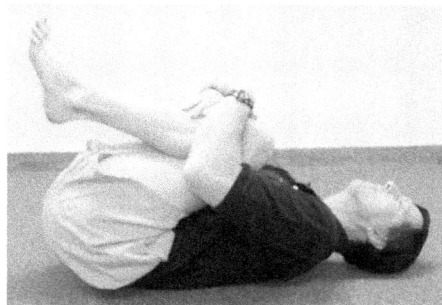

Double knee to chest for hips and low back

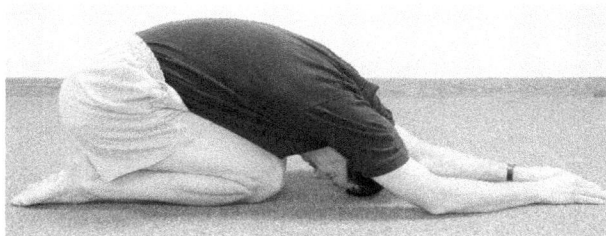

Prayer stretch for low back
Push low back upward.

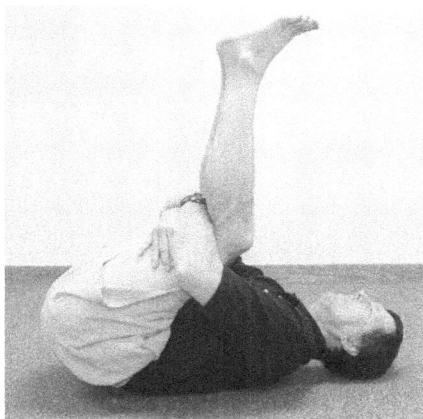

Partial plow pose

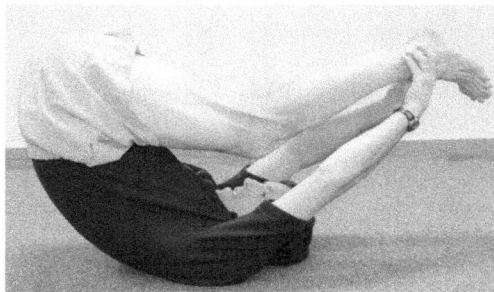

Advanced unassisted plow pose

- Hold stretches for 15–20 seconds
- Do 2–3 repetitions

AVOID PAIN!

IV
Neck and Posture Exercises

The following exercises balance muscular control and restore mobility in both the neck and upper back. These are key elements for postural control. Imbalance in the cervical region involves overuse of the scalene, levator scapulae, upper cervical extensors, and trapezius muscles, which then become tight, as well as underuse of the deep neck flexors and thoracic extensors, which then become weak. Poor backward bending mobility in the thoracic spine perpetuates forward head posture. To level the head, the scalenes and muscles in the back of your neck are overused.

The scalenes, in addition to providing dynamic support for the head and neck, can assist in breathing. They help lift the chest when extra lung volume is needed. Many people tend to breathe by lifting the upper chest rather than efficiently using their diaphragm. The upper-chest breathing pattern can be reinforced with sedentary and/or stressful lifestyles. An upper-chest breathing pattern adds work to the scalene muscles, which may increase the tendency toward poor posture. It may also cause the upper rib cage to remain in an elevated position.

The scalenes and upper rib cage are intimately associated with the nerve and blood supply to the arms. The nerves that go to the arm or, brachial plexus, start out as nerve roots exiting the spinal column. These nerves pass through the scalene musculature, over the first and second ribs, under the collarbone, and under the pectoral muscles to get to the arm. With dysfunction in any of these areas, you can get symptoms in the arm that could include weakness, pain, tingling, burning, or numbness.

The muscles in the back of the neck include, among others, the levator scapula, upper trapezius, and the deeper muscles that make up the cervical extensors. With forward head posture, these muscles may become overused, which causes them to get tight and sore.

The levator scapulae and trapezius muscles attach to the head and neck and to the scapulae or shoulder blades. They help control shoulder blade movement as well as head and neck movement. If too much of their work is devoted to the head and neck control, they are less effective at controlling the shoulder blade.

If posture is poor, mechanical dysfunction may occur at the base of the skull in the suboccipital joints and in the vertebrae in the upper part of the neck. This can aggravate and/or cause problems with headache and the temporal mandibular joints. The temporal mandibular joints are located where the jawbone attaches to the sides of your head. They are in front of the ear canals on either side of your face.

Retraining the function of the deep neck flexors must be done in conjunction with improving function in the thoracic spine. Since most of our daily activities involve some degree of flexion or bending forward of the thoracic spine, we tend to lose the ability to return this part of the spine back to a neutral position. Using a towel roll or foam roller will help passively restore motion. The attention and wall angel exercises will help restore muscular control. Occasionally, the pelvic clock is needed if control of the abdominal muscles is poor.

Stretching of the scalenes and/or levators may be helpful. The following exercises can be done in any order, and are generally done twice a day. The wall angel can be done several times during the day as a "microbreak". The other exercises in this section are adjunct exercises for neck, shoulder, and upper back problems, and each one can be used on an as-needed basis.

Play Dead

Retraining the deep neck flexors is paramount for correcting poor posture. Play dead is one of the better exercises for isolated retraining of these muscles.

Why is it called "play dead?" Imagine playing a game with a six-year-old. You are playing dead. You think that the child is near your feet. If the child sees you lift your head and look towards him, then you are out of the game. So, a very subtle tuck, very small lift, and slow setting down of your head are required to keep playing.

Start by lying on your back on the floor looking at the ceiling. Your knees can be bent or straight. Without lifting your head, tuck the chin by nodding the head downward to look toward the toes. Pause for a second or two. Continue the tucking movement to slowly lift the back of your head no more than one-eighth of an inch from the floor. Hold this position for only two to three seconds, and then slowly relax. Imagine an axle or rod placed through the ears; this nodding motion causes rotation around the axle. The slight lift is a continuation of the rolling motion. You should feel "work" on either side of your throat, and possibly some stretching in the back of your neck.

Once you do the tuck, pause, lift, and relax sequence to the center, turn your head slightly to one side and repeat the tuck, pause, lift, and relax sequence. Turn the head only far enough so that one eye is looking straight up. Do not turn too far, or you will be out of the game! Repeat the same sequence with the head turned slightly in the other direction. Lifts to center, left, then right equals one repetition. Do five repetitions.

If needed, place a folded towel under the head. This may be required with severe forward head posture and/or very weak deep neck flexors. The exercise can be further modified by eliminating the lift portion. Gently tuck the chin and hold this position for four to five seconds. Turn slightly, re-tuck and hold, and then repeat in the opposite direction. When the tuck portion of the exercise becomes easy and comfortable, gradually add the lift. To make play dead more challenging, fold a bath towel so it is five to six inches wide, and place it under the upper back so the top edge of the towel runs across the top of the shoulders.

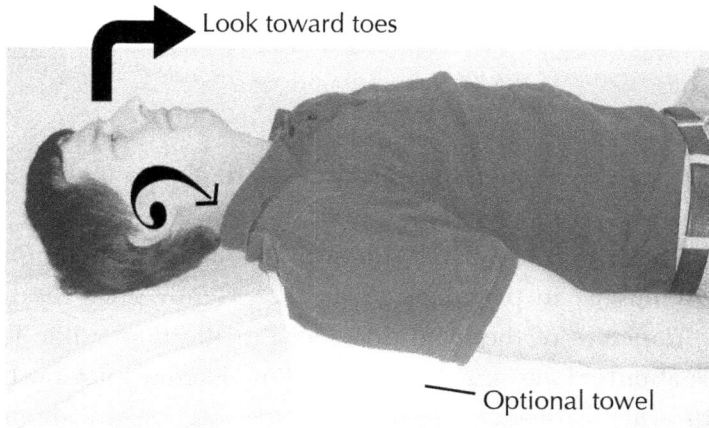

Look toward toes

Optional towel

1. Tuck chin in a rolling movement. Imagine an axle running from ear to ear. Pause 2 seconds. Continue the rolling movement to lift head less than ⅛ inch. Hold lift 2–3 seconds. Relax slowly.

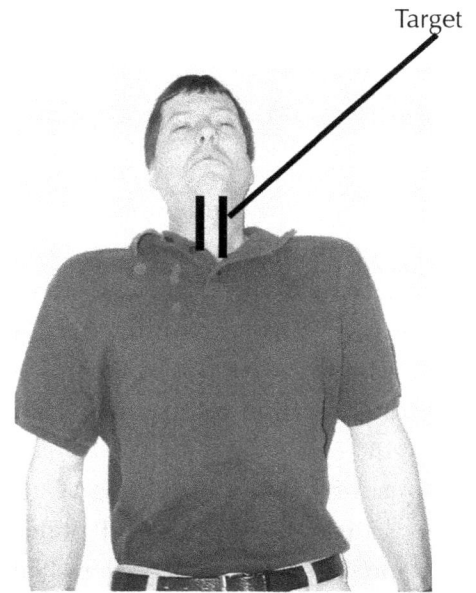

Target

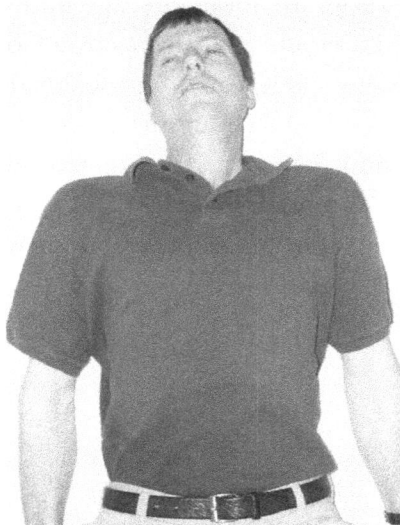

2. Turn very slightly to right, tuck, pause, lift, relax.

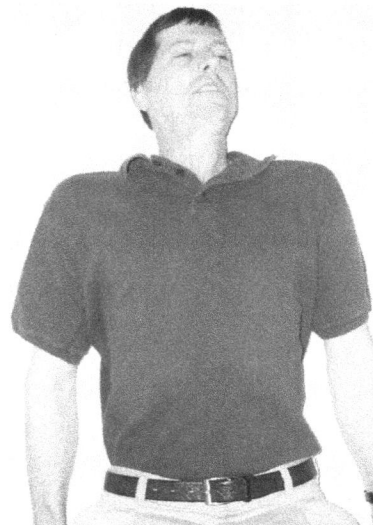

3. Turn very slightly to left, tuck, pause, lift, relax.

- Repeat sequence 5 times, 2 times per day
- Target: deep neck flexors

AVOID PAIN!

Attention: Supine Version

Since the upper back tends to be stuck in a forward bent or flexed position you may no longer properly use the muscles in this area. This is essentially a communication exercise. You must use finesse to isolate the muscles in the upper back. The focus on this exercise is more about restoring function to a specific area, not brute strength.

Imagine a soldier standing at attention. His chin is tucked with his head pulled back over his shoulders. His stomach is pulled in and his upper chest is lifted with the shoulders pulled back. In this exercise, you lie on your back like a soldier "at attention." The supine attention exercise is used to retrain the muscles in the upper thoracic spine just below the neck.

Lie flat on your back. Your knees can be bent or straight. Fold a small washcloth so that it is about four inches long and one to two inches wide. Place it vertically under the center of your upper back between the upper portions of your shoulder blades. If needed, place a folded towel or small pillow under your head.

Tuck the chin with the same nodding motion in play dead. (page 72). Gently press the back of the head down against the floor while looking straight at the ceiling. Flatten your low back against the floor. Gently squeeze the shoulder blades together towards the center of the spine towards the cloth. This squeeze should cause the upper part of the breast bone to gently rise toward the ceiling. Try to focus the work or tension on the upper back muscles adjacent to the cloth. Keep the lower back flat. Do not arch the low back or let the lower rib cage push upward. If you feel a gentle isometric contraction in the vicinity of the cloth, you are probably doing the exercise correctly. Hold this position for five seconds, and then relax for five seconds before repeating. Generally, five to six repetitions are sufficient. As it becomes easier, you may want to try the prone version.

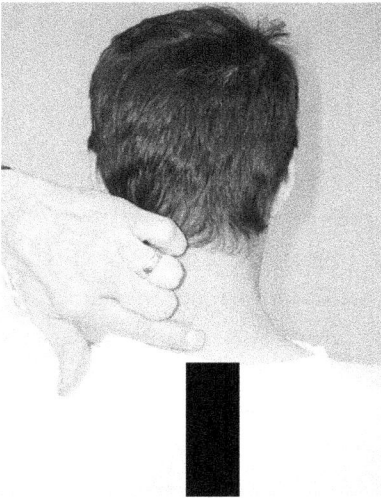

1. Place 1-inch by 4-inch folded cloth between shoulder blades.

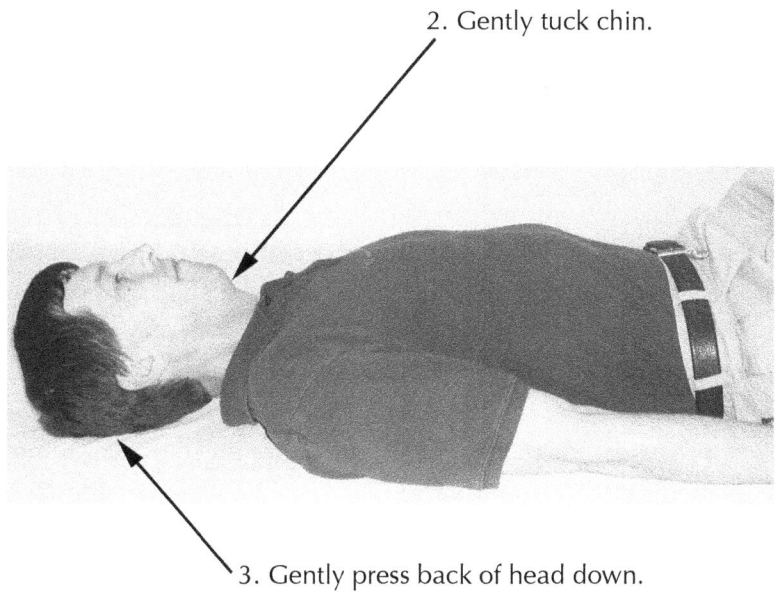

2. Gently tuck chin.

3. Gently press back of head down.

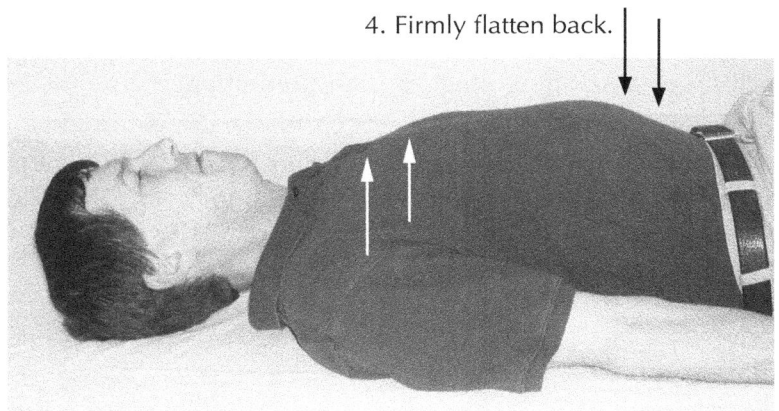

4. Firmly flatten back.

5. Gently pinch shoulder blades toward cloth to push the breastbone upward to feel an isometric contraction on either side of cloth.

- Hold 5 seconds
- Rest 5 seconds
- Do 5–6 repetitions twice per day

AVOID PAIN!

Attention: Prone Version

The prone attention exercise is usually harder that the supine version, and is designed to isolate the function of the upper thoracic spine extensors and, to some degree, the scapular stabilizers. The scapular stabilizers on the back of the body help pull the shoulder blades towards the center of the back. If the prone version proves either painful or just too difficult to coordinate, try the supine version.

For the prone attention exercise, you need one or two pillows, a rolled-up hand towel, and a "lump." This lump can be an ace wrap, folded washcloth, or a balled up sock.

Lie face down with the pillow under the stomach area, generally no higher than the bottom of the rib cage. The lump is placed under the upper part of the breastbone below your throat. Your forehead rests on the rolled towel. Your arms will be at your sides.

Once positioned, begin by pressing your breastbone down against the lump. Without lifting from the lump, retract your shoulder blades by pulling them to the center of the back and slightly downward toward the low back. Do not lift your hands. Now lift your head very slightly while keeping the chin tucked, and then press down into the lump again. At this point, you are lying face down at "attention." You should feel work or tension between the shoulder blades. Hold this position for five seconds and repeat five to six times, with at least five-second rests between repetitions.

The exercise may be modified by eliminating the head lift portion. Adding an extra pillow under the abdominal area and/or repositioning the pillow may also help. If this version still proves too difficult, the supine version may be better for you.

1. Press chest down to "lump."

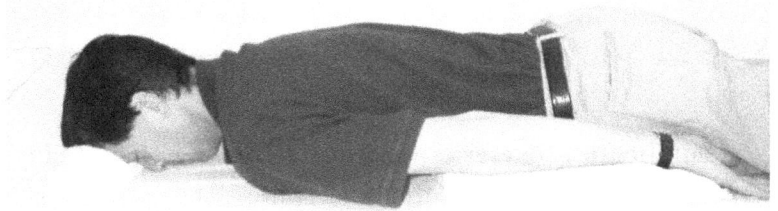

2. Retract shoulder blades.

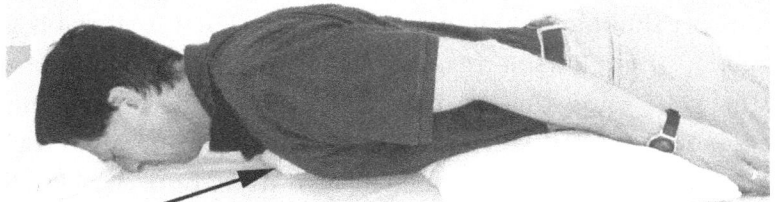

Do not lift hands

Lump

3. Lift head slightly with chin tucked.

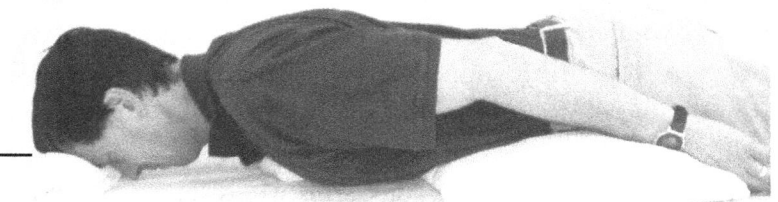

Slightly ————

4. Press chest down again.

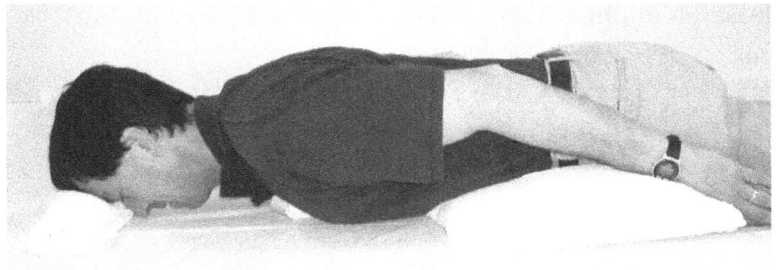

- Hold 3–5 seconds
- Don't look up
- Focus tension between the shoulder blades
- Do 5–6 repetitions twice per day

AVOID PAIN!

Towel Roll

The attention exercises work on increasing muscular control in the thoracic spine. The towel roll works on increasing mobility. Raising the arms over head while on the towel can also improve shoulder mobility, and stretch the chest and latissimus dorsi muscles.

Do the towel roll exercise on the floor. An exercise mat may be used. You will need one or two hand towels and a folded bath towel or small pillow for supporting your head. Roll two hand towels together, widthwise, so that the roll is about 15 inches long. Place them on the floor and position yourself on the towel roll so that it is centered in your back, and running from the base of your neck down to the bottom of your rib cage. Your head should be supported in a comfortable position with your pillow or folded bath towel. Your legs can be bent, straight, or propped on a chair. Place your arms wherever they are comfortable. Lie on the towel roll for at least ten minutes. Every one or two minutes, you can stretch your arms over your head.

Before raising the arms, tighten the tummy slightly to perform a 12 o'clock or posterior pelvic tilt. Slightly tuck the chin, and then raise the arms over your head as far as they will comfortably go while keeping the elbows straight. If discomfort occurs in the top of the shoulders, move the arms either closer together or farther apart, or do not raise them quite so far. If you have a shoulder injury, this prevents you from raising one of your arms. Use a stick or wand to let your good arm help you raise the bad one. Hold this stretch position for at least 15 seconds and repeat every one to two minutes while on the towel roll.

When your thoracic spine begins to loosen up, you may increase the size of the towel roll up to three towels. When towels no longer provide a good push, you might consider the foam roller exercises described later in this book (page 173).

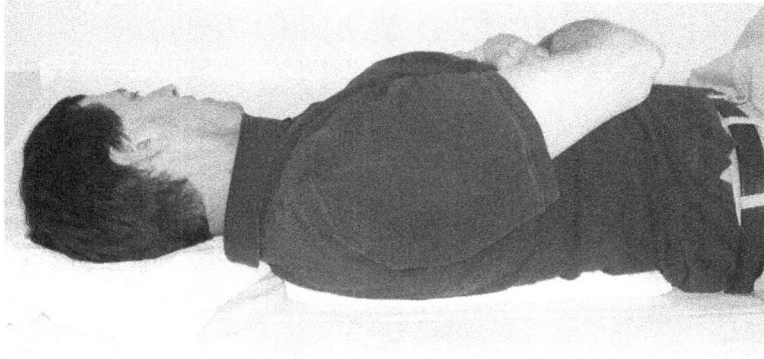

1. Lie on 1–2 hand towels rolled up width-wise and placed lengthwise under spine. Start towel at base of neck. Support head.

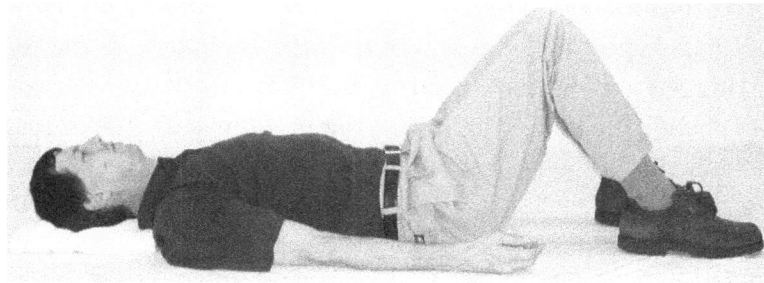

2. Lie on towel for total of 10 minutes.

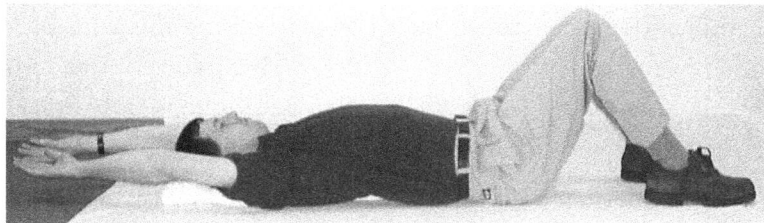

3. Every 2 minutes, raise arms over head and hold for 15 seconds. (Hint: tighten tummy, and tuck chin when raising arms.)

• Lie on towel 2 or more times per day

AVOID PAIN!

Standard Wall Angel

Sometimes poor posture is a key part of neck and back pain. Try the "wall angel." If it is challenging to do and/or makes you feel better, then include it in your exercise program. Keep in mind that posture happens all the way down to the ground. Ideal posture is a stacking process where key points are aligned one over the other. The wall angel works by moving from a slouched posture to the opposite extreme by flattening out the curves in the spine. When one relaxes from the wall angel, posture is usually slightly improved. Doing the wall angel several times a day will start to change the body's default settings, so that eventually posture gets closer to the ideal.

The wall angel combines all of the neck exercises into one stand-up version. When we are vertical, we need our parts to be able to stack themselves up; and then the muscles control things when we move. Lie-down exercises can improve muscle function and mobility, but the change in postural reprogramming must be done in the vertical mode.

Start by standing with your back against the wall with the feet six inches or more from the wall. Try to flatten your low back against the wall so that there is no space between the wall and your lower back muscles. If needed, move your feet farther from the wall; bending your knees will help you flatten your low back. While keeping your low back as flat as you can get it, look straight ahead and push your head back towards the wall as far as it will comfortably go. If you

can, touch the back of your head against the wall. Keep the low back flat and your head back with the chin down. Ideally, at this point you should be looking straight ahead. You can hold at this point or add in your arms.

Next, raise your arms to the side, along the wall, to 90 degrees at the shoulders with the palms facing the floor, and then bend the elbows to 90 degrees. The back of your upper arms should remain in contact with the wall. Keep your head pushed back towards the wall and the low back flat; and now rotate the back of both arms up towards the wall. There may be a tendency for the low back to be pulled away from the wall. Rotate the arms up to get the hands as close to the wall as you can with good control and comfort. Hold this position for 15 to 20 seconds. You may do one or two wall angels five to six times throughout the day.

If coordinating the angel is too difficult, there are several variations. Make the wall angel easier by only raising the arms part way or not at all. If the low back and/or head will not touch the wall, then get them as close as you can without undue discomfort. Try the straight arm version (page 85) if this positioning hurts your shoulders.

This exercise does not have to be executed perfectly to be beneficial. If you feel work or stretch with this exercise, it is probably taking you in the right direction. If the standard wall angel proves too difficult, try the seated wall angel.

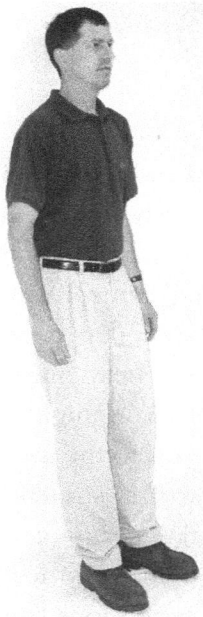

1. Stand with back to wall, feet 6 inches or more from wall.

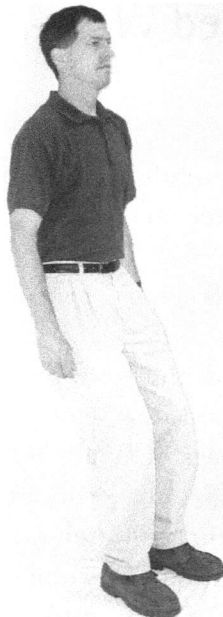

2. Tighten your tummy muscles to flatten your low back to the wall. Bend knees if needed to get back flat. Keeping the back of your head on the wall, bring your chin down.

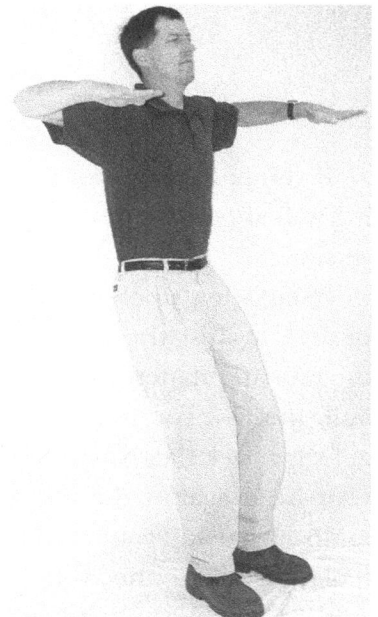

3. Start with palms facing floor.

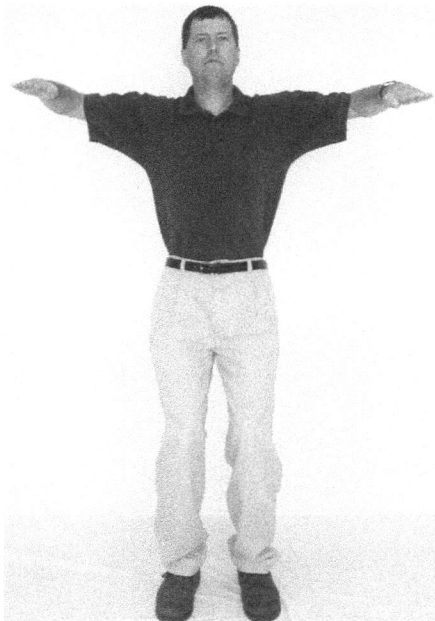

4. Keep back flat and head on wall with chin down.

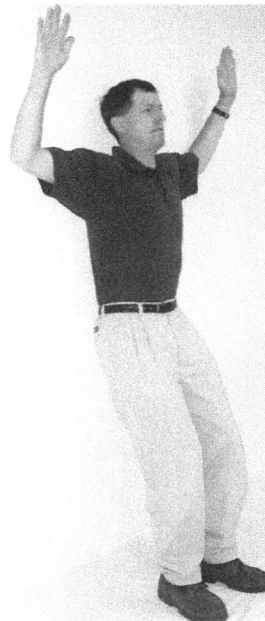

5. Move backs of forearms to wall.

- Hold 15–20 seconds
- Do 5–6 times per day

AVOID PAIN!

Seated Wall Angel

If you have very poor posture and the standing wall angels are too hard, then try the seated version.

Using a low stool or sturdy chair with its side pushed against the wall, sit with your back to the wall and flatten your lower back against the wall. Initially, you may need to lean forward to get your back flat. Now, try to touch the back of your head against the wall while keeping your low back flat and your chin down so that you are looking straight ahead. If you find it too difficult to touch the wall with either the low back or the head, then come as close as you can without undue stress and strain. Hold this position for 15 to 20 seconds, and do one or two repetitions five to six times during the day.

If you can touch your head to the wall and keep your low back flat, slowly raise your arms to the front with your elbows straight. Raise the arms as far as comfort and control will allow. If you are very tight, the arms may only get to horizontal. The low back and head must stay as close to the wall as possible. You might eventually be able to touch the arms to the wall above your head. A sensation of work or stretch may be felt through the upper back, neck, or across the shoulders. Hold this position for 15 to 20 seconds, and do one or two repetitions five to six times during the day. Try the standing versions when this one becomes easy.

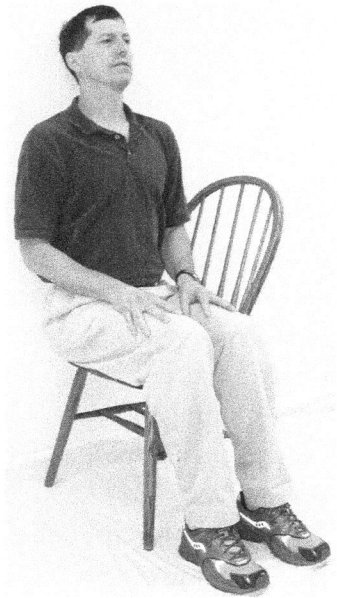

1. Sit with back to wall. Tighten tummy muscles to flatten low back to wall.

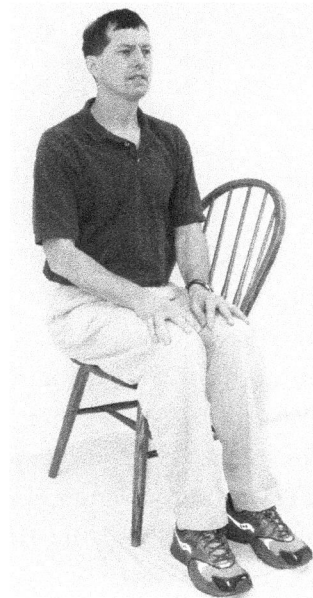

2. Keeping back of head on wall, bring chin down.

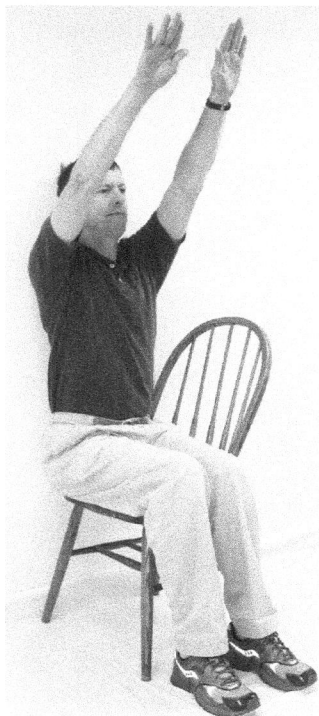

3. Start with palms facing floor, elbows straight. Raise arms as high as they will comfortably go.

- Do 1–2 repetitions
- Hold 15–20 seconds
- Do 5–6 times per day

AVOID PAIN!

More Wall Angel Variations

The straight elbow version of the wall angel may be used if shoulder problems prohibit movement or positioning used in the standard wall angel. If raising the arms with the elbows straight still causes shoulder pain, the exercise can be further modified by using a cane or stick so that one arm can help the other. Only raise the arms as far as they will go comfortably. As with the other versions, you want to keep the low back flat against the wall and the head against the wall with the chin down so that you look straight ahead.

Another wall angel technique might be called the "Martian variation." Start with the low back flat and the chin tucked as before. Raise your arms in front of you with the elbows fully bent and the elbows as close together as possible. Your palms can be turned towards the ceiling and the backs of your fingers will touch the wall beside your head.

Keeping the fingers on the wall and your elbows close together, push your hands toward the ceiling, causing the elbows to straighten. Stretch may be felt between the shoulder blades or along the sides of the chest. Take the arms as high as they will comfortably go. Hold a comfortable stretch for 15 to 20 seconds.

Avoid the tendency for the elbows to push out to the sides. A single arm version can be employed if the double arm version is too difficult. Use your free hand to help push the arm upward. If the arms are very weak, a helper may assist by pushing the arms upward. Again, hold the positions for 15 to 20 seconds and repeat two to three times. This exercise can be done several times during the day.

Variation 1: Martian

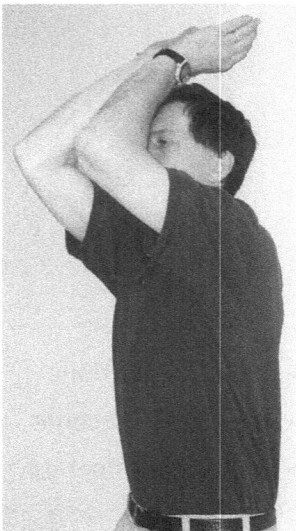

1. Elbows bent, touch fingers to wall just overhead.

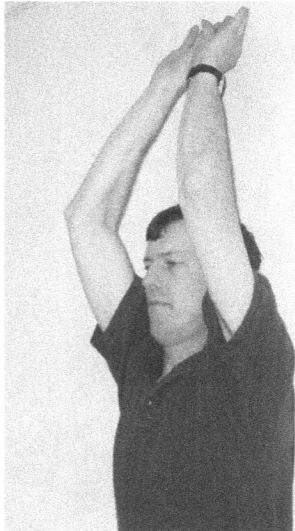

2a. Elbows in, push hands up the wall.

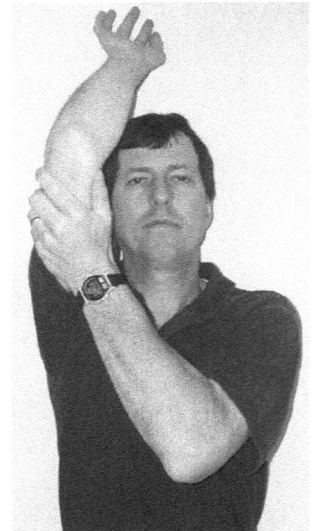

2b. If both arms are difficult, do single arm.

Variation 2: Straight Elbow

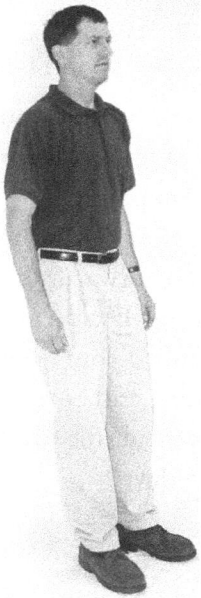

1. Stand with back to wall, feet 6 inches or more from wall.

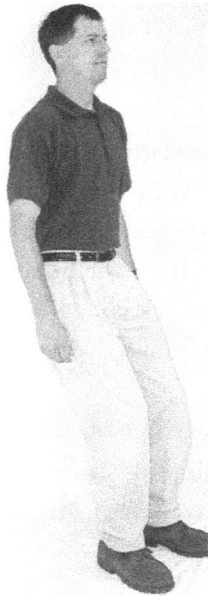

2. Tighten tummy to flatten low back to wall. Bend knees if needed to get back flat. Keeping back of head on wall, bring chin down.

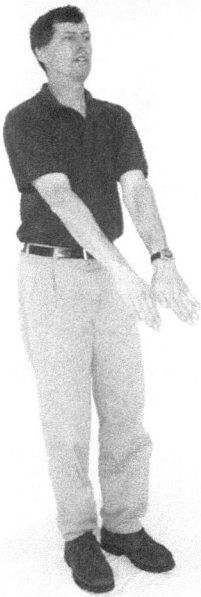

3. Start with palms facing floor.

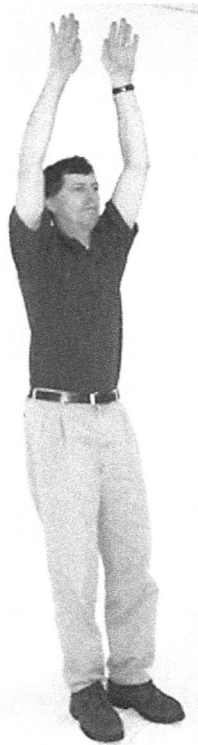

4. Raise arms overhead towards wall.

- Hold 15–20 seconds
- Do 5–6 times per day

AVOID PAIN!

Cueing for Posture

For retraining posture, you can use the foot tap, look-ahead exercise. To determine if this exercise will help you, try to tap your feet alternately. Can you lift the ball of your foot? Do you have to shift your weight back onto your heels, or throw your shoulders back, or rock your body side to side? If so, this exercise may help with posture correction.

Start by looking at your shoestrings or at the top of your socks. For most people, this shifts the pelvis back so you can now tap your feet. Keeping the pelvis back, lift the chest and head so you are looking straight ahead. Do not let the pelvis come forward. This may entail keeping a little tension in the stomach muscles. Now shrug the shoulders up and down and then forward and back two to three times. Can you still tap your feet? Initially this may feel awkward, but with practice, default setting will change, and correct posture will feel more natural. Repeat this exercise several times throughout the day.

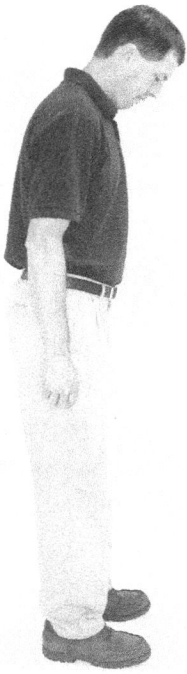

1. To correct poor posture, look down at shoe strings or top of socks.

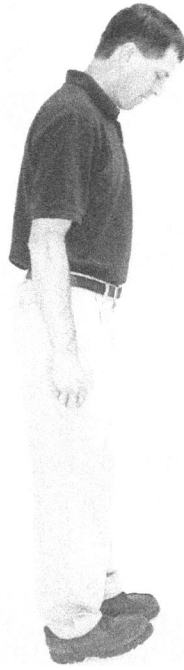

2. Tap feet. Note that pelvis is back.

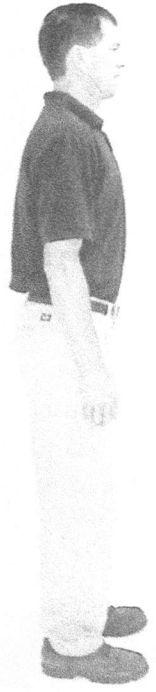

3. Look ahead, but don't let pelvis come forward.

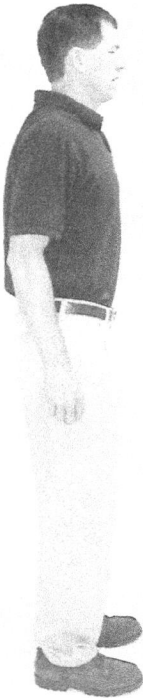

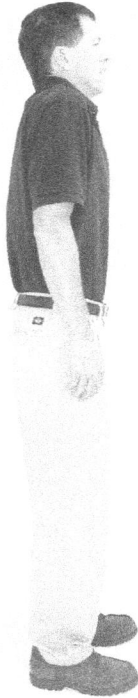

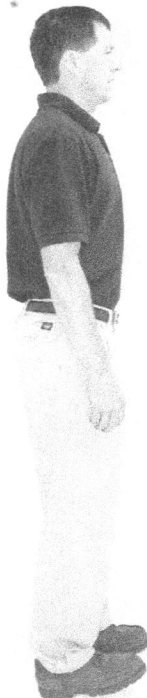

• Repeat every 30 minutes when standing

AVOID PAIN!

4. Roll shoulders in a circle, 2–3 times.

Relax slightly. Make sure you can tap your feet with shifting body position.

Arm Stretch

Tightness in the chest and upper arm is probably the result of compromised posture and not participating in activities that use the full motion of these muscles. Once tight, these restrictions may pull the shoulders forward and hold them in this protracted position. Tightness in the pectoral muscles may inhibit the use of shoulder blade stabilizers. These include the rhomboids and lower and middle trapezius muscles. This results in overuse of the upper trapezius and rotator cuff muscles. This exercise will stretch your chest and upper arm muscles.

Begin the stretch standing beside a wall. The little toe of your right leg should touch the base molding with the foot at a 45 degree angle to the wall. Your left foot should be parallel to the right and shoulder width apart. Your chest should be at a 45 degree angle to the wall. Position your right arm with the palm on the wall, elbow straight, so that it is at a 45 degree angle. If you start with the arm at your side and raise it up along the wall, stop when it's approximately halfway up. Your right shoulder should remain in contact with the wall. Now place your left hand on the wall in front of your chest.

Stand up straight. Do not rest your head on the wall. At this point, you may feel some stretch in the front of the right arm. To increase the stretch, gently push against the wall with your left hand to rotate the upper body to increase the angle of your chest in relation to the wall. Try not to twist the hips without the upper body. If you can rotate your upper body so that it is 90 degrees to the wall and without feeling a stretch, then reposition the chest back to 45 degrees and move the right arm three to four inches up the wall. Push again to rotate the upper body away from the wall. If you can get your arm to horizontal and your body to 90 degrees to the wall, you probably do not need to do this stretch.

If pain is felt in the shoulder, you can lower the arm below 45 degrees. The right arm can be rotated so that the thumb and forefinger are against the wall. If this does not make the exercise comfortable, try doing the stretch by grabbing a doorframe and turning your body so that stretch is applied. When this can be done comfortably, try the wall again.

Hold each stretch for a minimum of 15 seconds. Repeat two to three times per side. This exercise can be done several times during the day.

Push to rotate body

45°

A

1 month

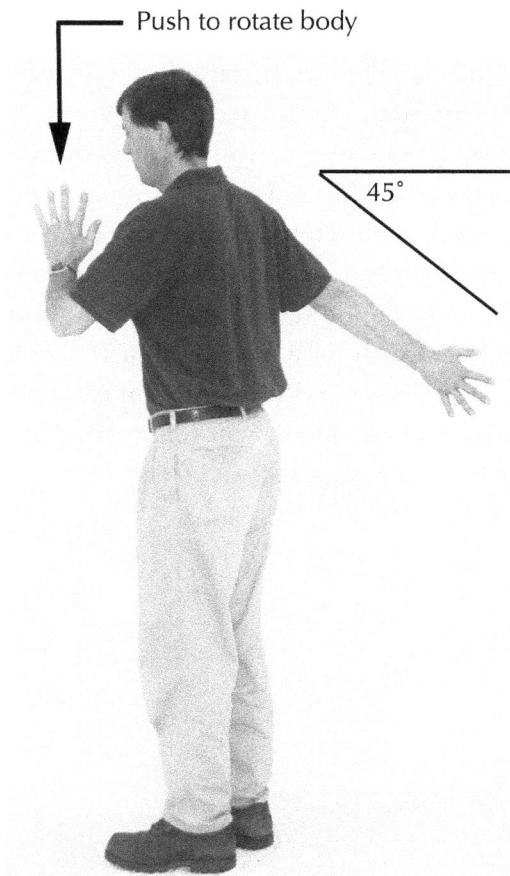

1. Starting position:

- Little toe against baseboard
- Feet 45° to wall
- Arm 45° from horizontal

2. Push with front hand to rotate body to increase stretch in front of arm that is on wall.

- Hint: keep shoulder "A" in contact with wall
- Hold 15–20 seconds
- Do 2–3 per side 2 or more times per day

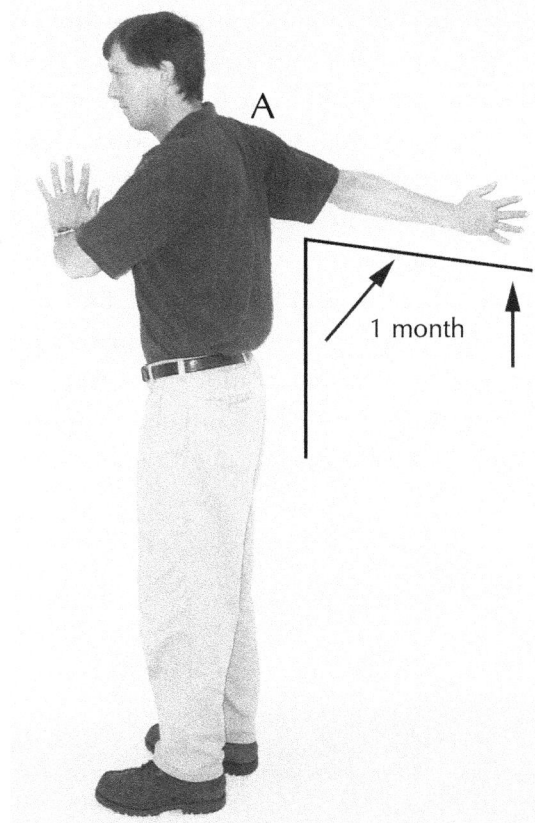

AVOID PAIN!

Pect Minor/Shoulder Stretch

A variation on the arm stretch for the chest and upper arm focuses more on the deeper muscles in the chest. The pectoralis minor is under the pectoralis major, and when tight, it pulls the front of the shoulder blade downward.

Start by standing in a doorway in a lunge position so you are close enough to one side to position your forearm and hand on the face of the doorframe. Adjust your position in or out of the doorway so that your shoulder is comfortable. Reach up the door facing so that you feel some stretch in the front of your chest and shoulder.

While keeping your raised arm stationary, slightly increase the lunge movement by bending your knees so that your body moves down and forward. This movement should increase the amount of stretch in the front of the shoulder. If you have shoulder pain, you can vary the down movement versus forward movement. Hold the stretch for a minimum of 15 to 20 seconds, and do two to three times on each side. If this stretch feels good, you might try the side-lying stretches (pages 92 and 94).

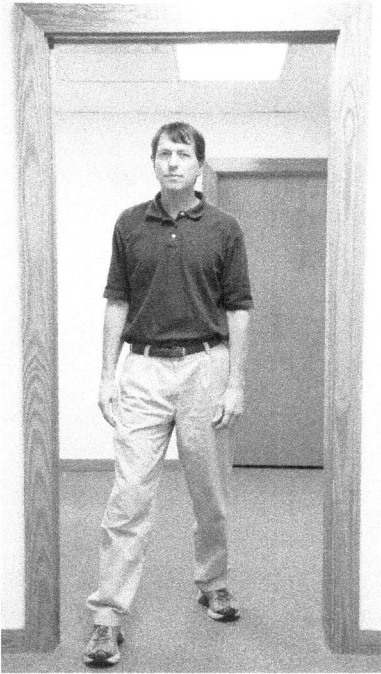

1. Stand in doorway in a "lunge" position.

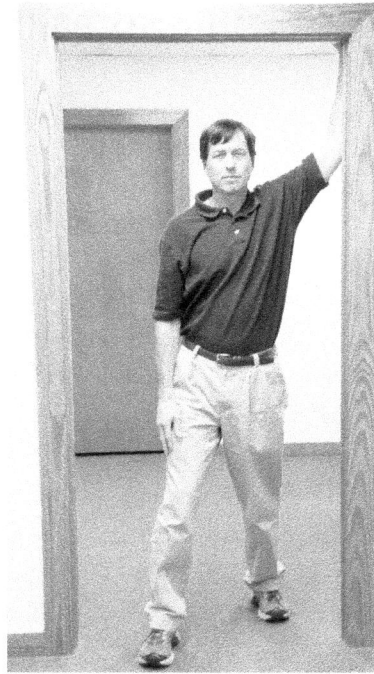

2. Put forearm on inside of doorframe.

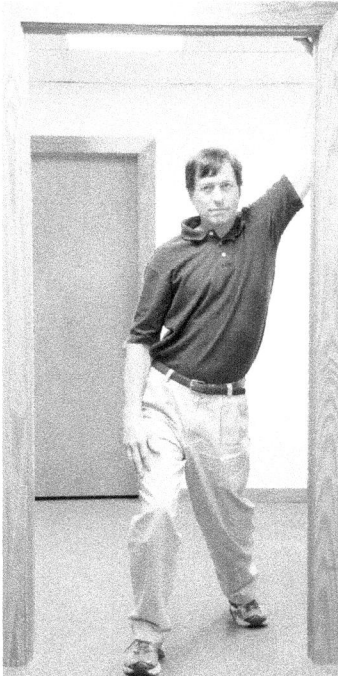

3. Slowly bend knees and move down and slightly forward.

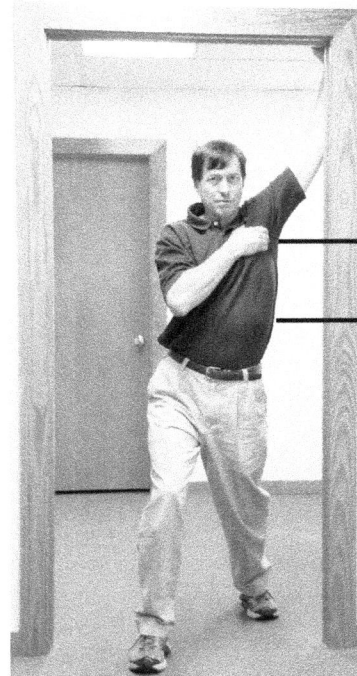

Stretch

4. Apply pressure over ribs while exhaling to enhance stretch.

- Hold 15–20 seconds
- Do 2–3 per side

AVOID PAIN!

Side-Lying Rotation Stretch I

To stretch the chest and upper torso muscles, you will lie on your side with your hips bent to 90 degrees. Your top knee is straight and your bottom knee is bent. Arch your back by pushing your lower rib cage forward. Point your top elbow towards the ceiling and let your upper torso roll back towards the floor. You are trying to move the back of the top shoulder blade towards the floor, not just your arm. Maintain the arch in the back. You should feel stretch in the chest and upper torso, not in the low back. You can hold at this point or increase the stretch by straightening your elbow. For even more stretch, move your upper arm towards your ear.

Be careful to avoid any pinching in the shoulder. Try pointing your thumb towards the floor. When we were little kids, we were able to get the back of the top shoulder blade flat on the floor. Since we do not use this motion, we lose it along with our good posture.

If your back or hip is uncomfortable, keep the top knee bend and do not roll back quite so far. Hold the stretch for at least 15 to 20 seconds. Do two or three stretches on each side. Slow deep breaths may help relax tight chest wall muscles. For a more aggressive stretch, try version II (page 94).

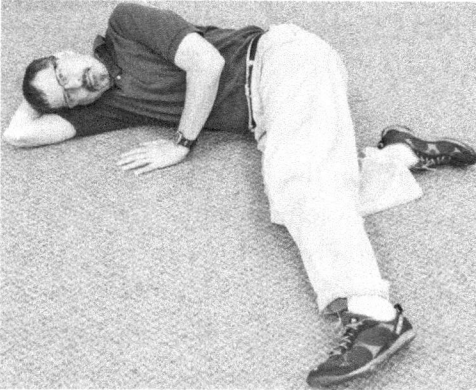

1. Lie on side with your thighs at 90°. Top knee straight. Bottom leg bent.

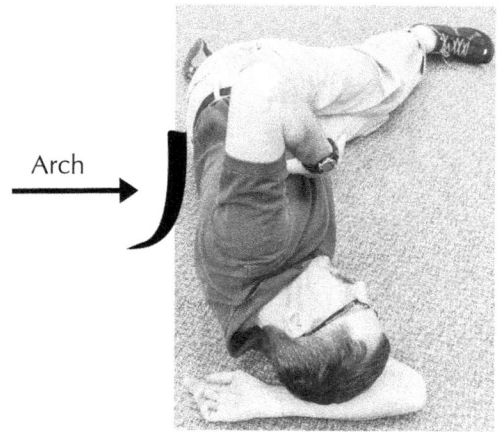

Arch →

2. Arch upper body by pushing breast bone forward. Point elbow toward ceiling.

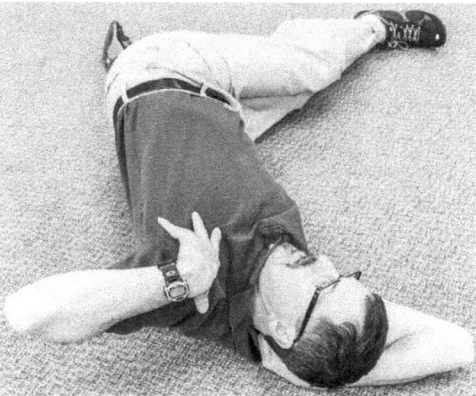

3. Let upper torso roll back toward floor. Maintain arch and hold posiiton.

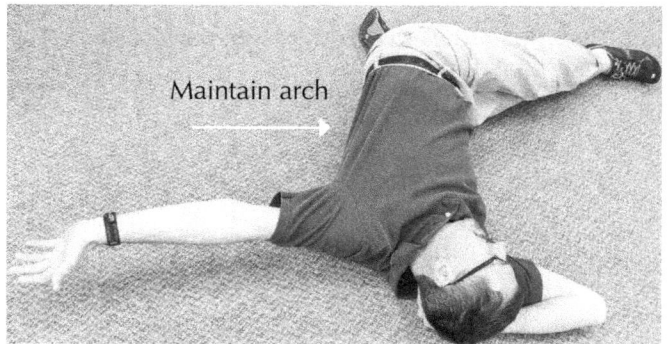

Maintain arch →

4. Or straighten elbow to increase stretching.

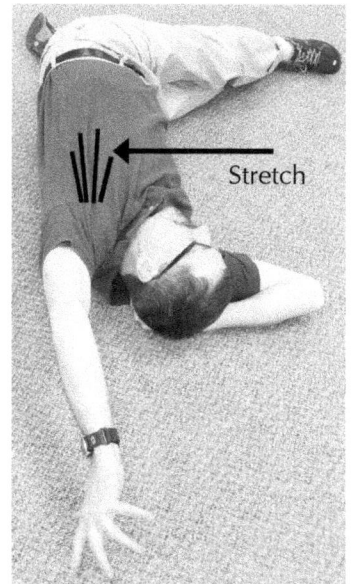

Stretch

5. Bring arm toward ear and reach to further increase stretching.

- Hold 15–20 seconds
- Breathe
- Do 2–3 times each side

AVOID PAIN!

Side-Lying Rotation Stretch II

This is a more aggressive stretch for the upper body.

Lie on your back with your knees bent and your feet flat on the floor. Position your left arm straight out from the side of your body so that you can get your hand under a heavy piece of furniture, or you can use a 20 to 30 pound dumbbell. Your left arm should be at a 90 degree angle to your body. Arch your back by pushing the lower part of your rib cage towards the ceiling. Let your knees fall to the right towards the floor. Maintain the arched back. Use your right hand to pull the left lower ribs forward. You should feel stretch in the left side of your chest and through the whole upper torso. Slow deep breaths may help you relax. Increase the stretch by straightening the top knee. Hold for at least 20 seconds, and do two to three times each side.

You can modify this stretch by starting on your back. Angle your body so that your arm is about a 160 degree angle to your body. Arching your back and rolling your knees towards the floor from this position should stretch additional muscles down the side of your body. You can straighten your top leg for more pull.

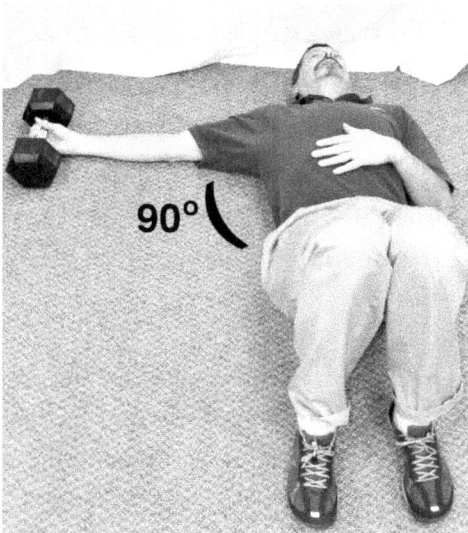

1. Lie so that fingers reach under door or something heavy.

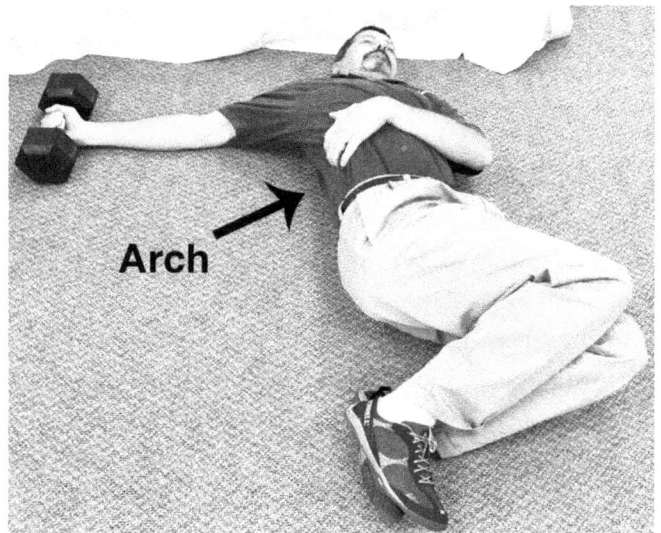

2. Arch low back and let bent knees lean to opposite side. Pull your ribcage forward.

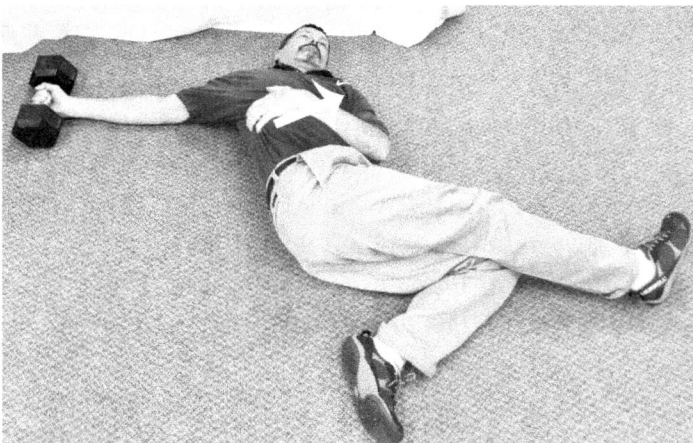

3. Straighten top leg. If needed to increase stretch, pull ribcage forward and try to touch your foot to the floor.

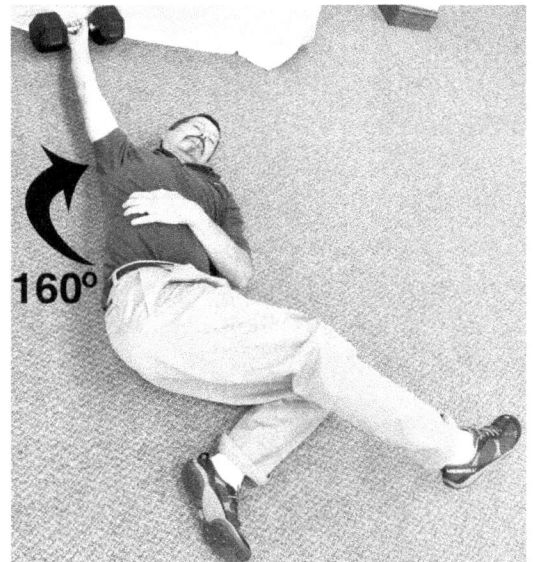

4. Experiment with different angles. Relax with deep breathing.

- Hold 15–20 seconds
- Do 2–3 repetitions on each side

AVOID PAIN!

Massage Your Pit with a Ball on a Stick

The soft tissue in your arm pit should be loose. Look at how your shirt is made. There is extra material under your arm to allow you to reach upward. Tight armpit tissue can restrict movement and cause alterations in movement patterns that will lead to shoulder problems.

To loosen this tight tissue, put tennis balls on either end of a one-inch diameter, 48 inches-long dowel. A broom stick or mop handle will do as well. To fit the ball on the stick, make a one-inch slice in each ball. Put one end of the dowel on the floor against a wall. People over six feet tall may put the end of the stick on a step or use a longer stick. The other end goes in your arm pit. There are three areas to massage. Work on these areas for 30 to 60 seconds each.

First, the subscapularis muscle is on the front of the shoulder blade. It can be very tender. Raise your arm, and rest your hand on the wall. Angle the ball on the stick so that you push on the front of the shoulder blade between the shoulder blade and the rib cage. Search for tight and tender areas along the border of the shoulder blade. Push almost to the point of pain. Use your other hand to grab the stick near your arm pit, and move that end of the stick to knead the arm pit tissue.

Next, the pectoral muscles make up the front border of the arm pit. Angle the ball on the stick and your body to massage tender areas on the edge of the chest muscles. The nerves that go to the rest of your arm run under this muscle near where it attaches to the upper arm. You may feel some transient tingling or "numbness" in your hand if you overwork this area.

The top of your upper arm bone is called the "head of the humerus." There should be a soft gap between it and the rib cage. Angle the ball on the stick into the space between the head of the humerus and the rib cage. Avoid pushing directly on the bone. Spend 30 to 60 seconds loosening tight tissue in this area. You can do this technique up to three times a day.

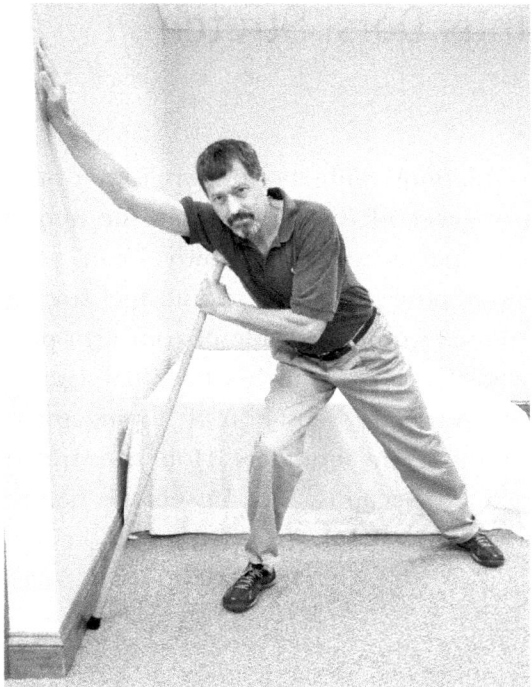

Make a stick with a 1-inch x 48-inch dowel. Cut a 1-inch hole in each tennis ball and place on end of stick.

Areas to Massage

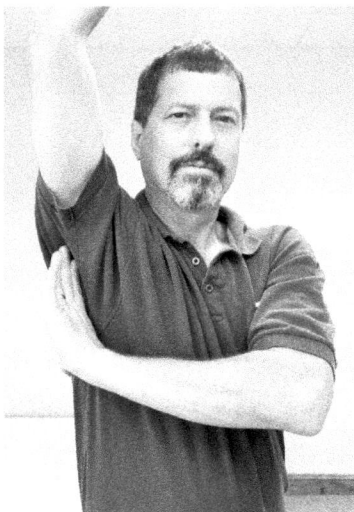

1. Front of shoulder blade subscapularis muscle

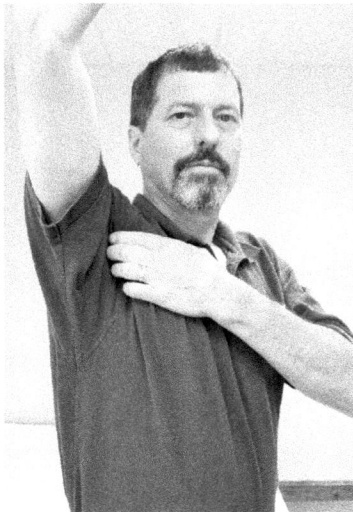

2. Pectoral muscles

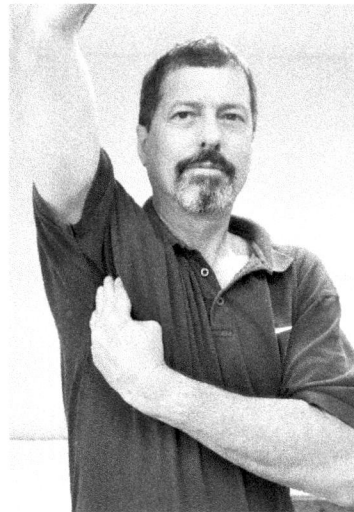

3. Between head of humerus and rib cage. Note: not directly on head of humerus.

- Use opposite hand to move stick to massage tight areas
- 30–60 seconds per area
- 1–2 times per day

AVOID PAIN!

Supine Shoulder and Latissimus Dorsi Stretch

If your upper back is bent and your shoulders are tight, try lying on your back with your elbows straight and your arms raised over your head. If your hands are more than 12 inches from the floor, you need to do this stretch.

Lie on your back with your knees bent with a heavy piece of furniture or a 30-pound dumb bell about six inches beyond the reach of your hands that are stretched over your head with the elbows straight. Lift your hips up to get your arms to the floor. Slide, bottom up, towards the weight or piece of furniture. Grab the weight with your palms up, then slowly lower your hips towards the floor. You should feel stretch in the muscles on either side of your arm pits. If you can, try to get your low back flat against the floor. Avoid the sensation of impingement or pinching in the shoulders. Hold the stretch for at least 15 seconds. Rest 15 seconds before repeating. Do two to three repetitions.

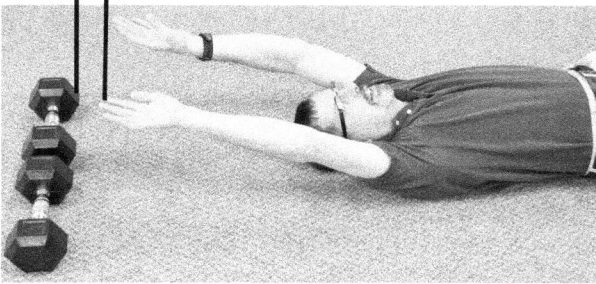

6 inches

1. Lie on back so that finger tips are 6 inches away from weights.

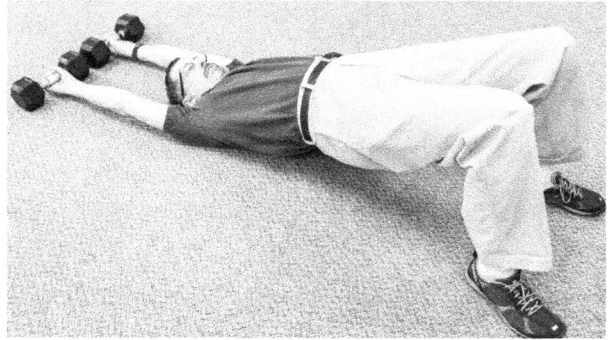

2. Lift pelvis and stretch arms to reach weights.

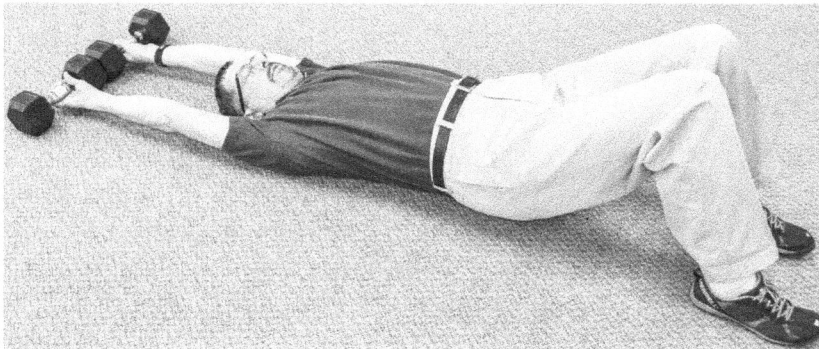

3. Slowly lower hips to feel stretch in upper arms and latissimus dorsi.

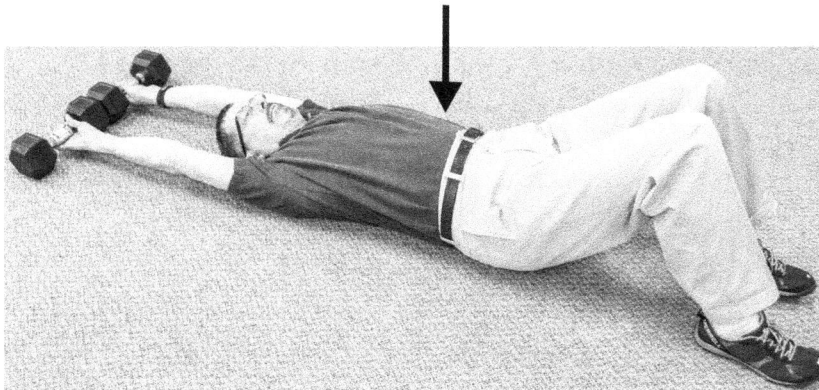

4. Work to get low back flat on floor.

- Avoid pinching in shoulders
- Hold at least 15 seconds
- Repeat 2–3 times

AVOID PAIN!

Self Stretch for Median Nerve Distribution

(After David Butler)

The nerves that service our arms start as nerve roots exiting the spinal column at the mid and lower portion of the neck. The nerve roots join together to form the brachial plexus that passes through the scalene muscles, then over the first and second ribs. From there, the plexus passes under the collarbone and chest muscles. The median nerve begins at the border of the chest muscle at the upper arm. From there, it travels along inside the upper arm to the front of the elbow. It then dives into the muscles of the front of the forearm and travels through the carpal tunnel to anchor into and innervate the thumb, index, and middle finger. Restrictions in movement of the median nerve through this course can cause numbness and tingling, and can be a contributor to carpal tunnel syndrome. The median nerve stretch will help move the nerve through its tortuous course, and restore the movement needed for optimal function.

Begin by positioning your arm like a waiter carrying a tray on one hand. Keep your palm facing the ceiling and your fingers pointing to the side away from your body. Keep your shoulder down by placing the opposite hand on top of the shoulder and exerting a downward pressure. Extend your arm by straightening your elbow directly to the side. Keep your hand at the same height as your shoulder with the wrist fully extended. Straighten your arm to the point of feeling a stretch in the forearm or front of the elbow.

Looking in a mirror may help maintain ideal positioning. Keep the shoulder down and the wrist fully extended. The arm should be moved directly out to the side of your body. A stretch can be held for at least 15 seconds. You can also use a pumping motion in which you straighten the arm to the limit of stretch, then relax it slightly and repeat the straightening. Do this for eight to ten repetitions. Leaning the head away from the arm being stretched will increase the amount of pull. This exercise can be repeated several times during the day. If this area seems especially tight, you may try the forearm massage (page 102).

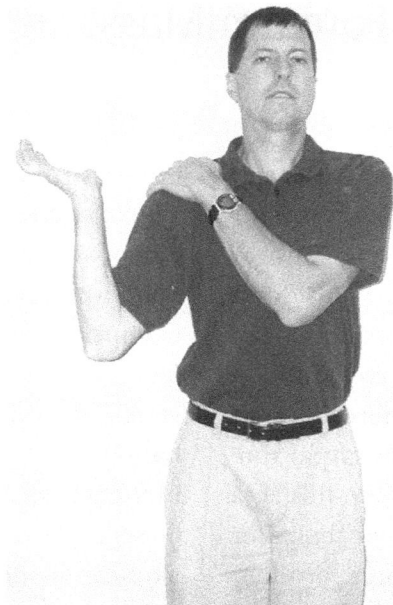

1. Hold shoulder down, wrist fully extended.

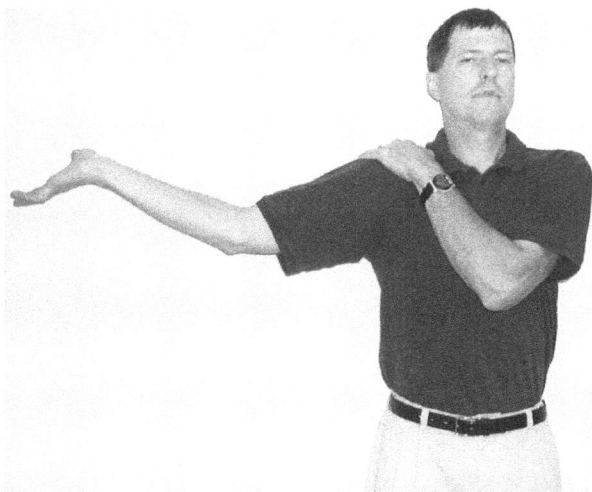

2. Straighten elbow. Keep shoulder down and wrist extended. Feel stretch in forearm.

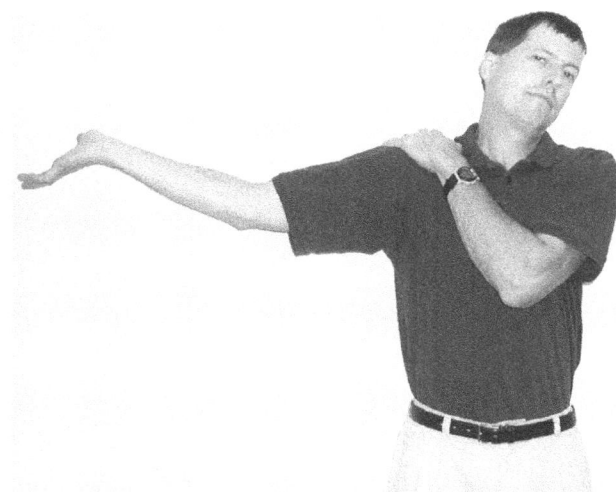

3. Increase stretch by leaning head to opposite side.

- Hold 15 seconds
- Or bend and straighten elbow or wrist several times

AVOID PAIN!

Forearm Massage

The upper part of the front of your forearm is a busy place. The muscles that give power to your grip attach to the inside of your elbow. Muscles that bend your wrist and turn your palm down are also there. The biceps tendon attaches deep in front of the elbow. The ulnar nerve (think of your funny bone) goes through there, as does the median nerve on its way to the carpal tunnel and thumb side of the hand. When this area gets tight, you can have symptoms of tennis or golfer's elbow, carpal tunnel syndrome, or ulnar nerve entrapment.

To loosen this tight tissue in your left upper forearm, you sit with your knees apart and rest the left arm against the inside of your left thigh. The arm should contact the leg just below the elbow and six to eight inches from the knee. Start with the palm facing the right leg, then extend or bend the wrist back so that the palm faces the floor. Rest your right elbow on top of your right thigh. Use the knuckles of the right hand to find and massage tight and tender areas in the left forearm. Massage these areas for 30 to 60 seconds, pushing almost to the point of pain. This can be done three to four times in a day. If the muscles on the back of your arm are tight, you can turn your arm around, flex the wrist, and work on this area too.

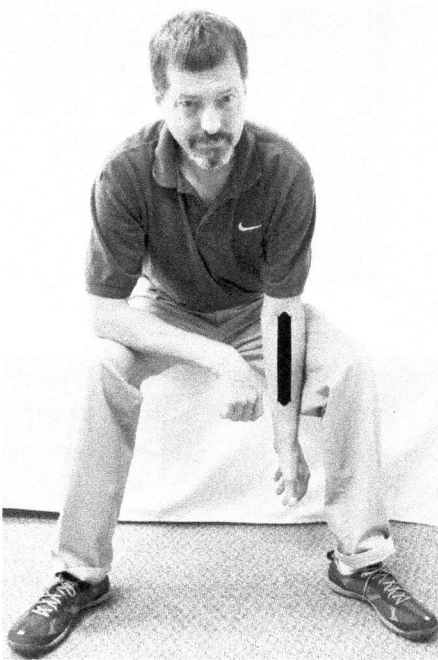

1. To massage left forearm, put right elbow on right thigh

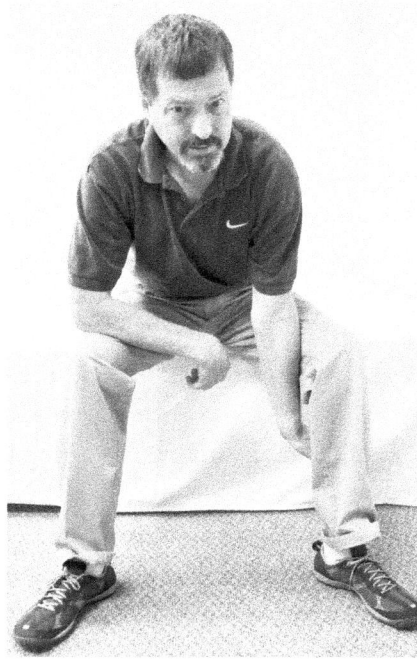

2. Rest back of left arm against inside of left thigh

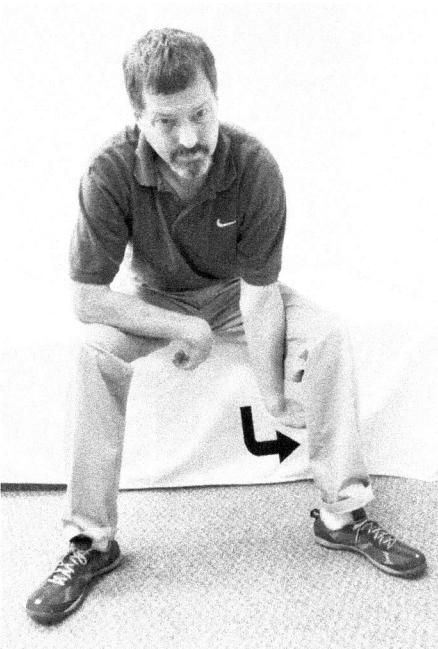

3. Pull wrist back.

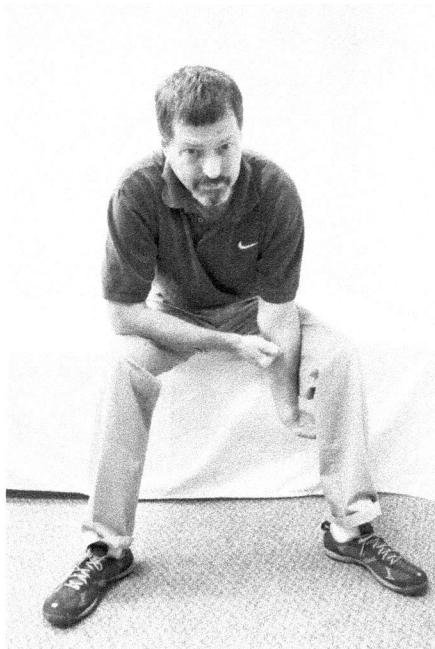

4. Massage muscles just below elbow. Push almost to the point of pain.

- Massage for 30–60 seconds
- 1–2 times per day

AVOID PAIN!

Upper Cervical Soft Tissue Release

Occasionally deep soft tissue work will be beneficial in loosening the suboccipital muscles located along the back of the neck just under the base of the skull. Impingement on the suboccipital nerves by tight muscles may contribute to headaches, neck and jaw pain, and restrictions in motion in the neck. This exercise can be done either from an upright or a side-lying position.

The side-lying technique is probably the most effective because you can more easily relax the muscles, but good results can be obtained either standing or sitting. If one side is more restricted, then lie on the opposite side so that the sore side is up. Do not use a pillow unless absolutely necessary. Position your head so that the area above your lower eye is resting on the surface of whatever you are lying on. Your top arm will rest along your side, and the hand of the bottom arm will be used to massage the suboccipital muscles. The spots that will benefit most from the massage are usually very tender. Massaging for the purpose of loosening is most effective when a slight stretch is applied.

Knead the restricted area for 30 to 60 seconds per square inch. Apply pressure that is sufficiently firm to work on the underlying tissue. This pressure may be almost to the point of pain.

To work on the left side of the neck when standing or sitting, turn your head to the right, and tip your head down like you are looking at the ground near your right foot. Reach with your right hand to the back of the left side of your neck. Search for and massage the tender and tight areas.

This technique can be repeated several times a day on any area that you find that needs work.

Sit/Stand Version

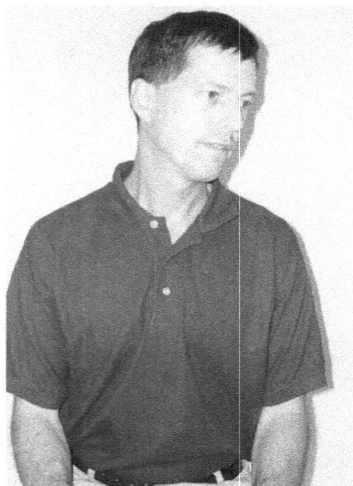

1. Rotate head slightly to one side.

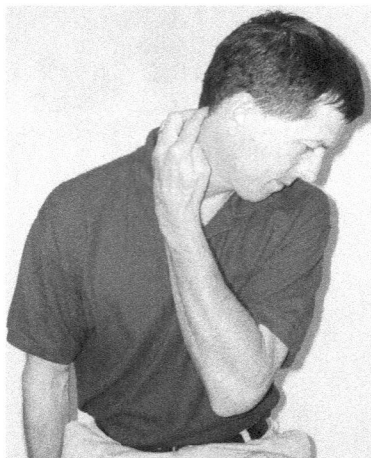

2. Look down. Reach around with opposite hand to provide deep massage to upper neck.

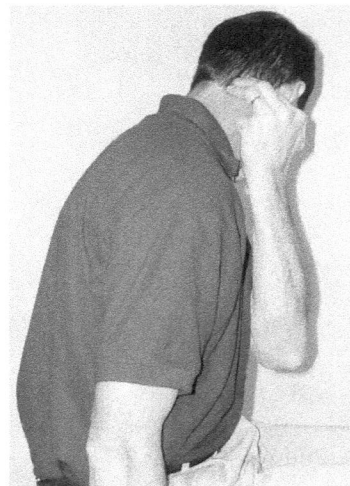

3. Adjust rotation to get best stretch

Side-lying Version

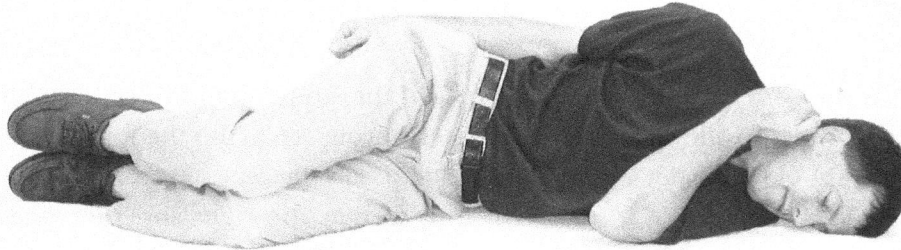

1. Lie on side with top arm resting along top side of body.

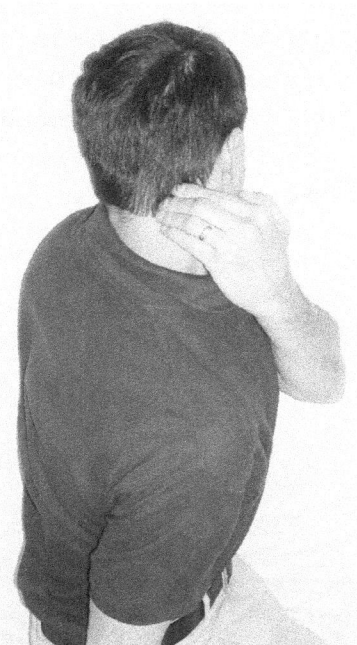

2. Rotate slightly downward to obtain best stretch. Work on any areas that feel tight or tender.

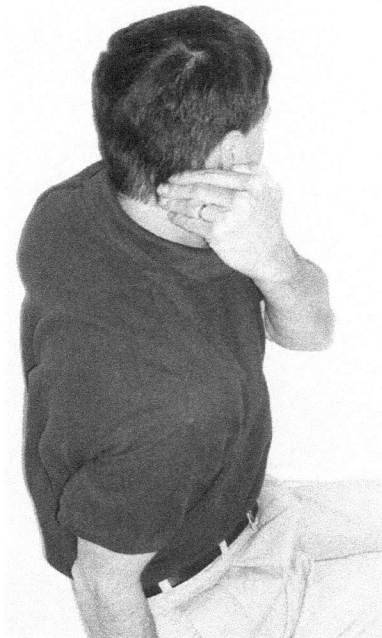

3. Use opposite hand to reach behind neck to provide deep soft tissue massage.

> • Press hard enough to provide a deep massage but not so hard as to elicit pain
>
> • Work on restricted areas for 30–60 seconds
>
> • 2–3 times per day

AVOID PAIN!

Upper Trapezius/Levator Scapulae Stretching

The upper trapezius attaches to the back of the neck and base of the skull, and runs down to attach along the top of the shoulder blade. The levator scapulae attaches along the back of the vertebrae of the neck and to the top, inside corner of the shoulder blade.

Stretching these muscles can be done from either a standing or sitting position.

Start by sitting in a chair. If you are stretching the right side, your right arm will be at your side. Turn your head 45 degrees to the left, tip your head slightly to the left, and now look down towards your left leg. Adjust the rotation and side bending to find the stretch that will be best felt along the back of your neck into the top of your shoulder blade. Grab the seat of the chair with the right arm so that the right shoulder does not come up. You can also rest the left hand on top of your head and let just the weight of your arm increase the amount of stretch. Reverse the directions to stretch the other side.

Each stretch should be held for at least 15 to 20 seconds, and can be repeated two to three times per side. Stretching can be done several times a day.

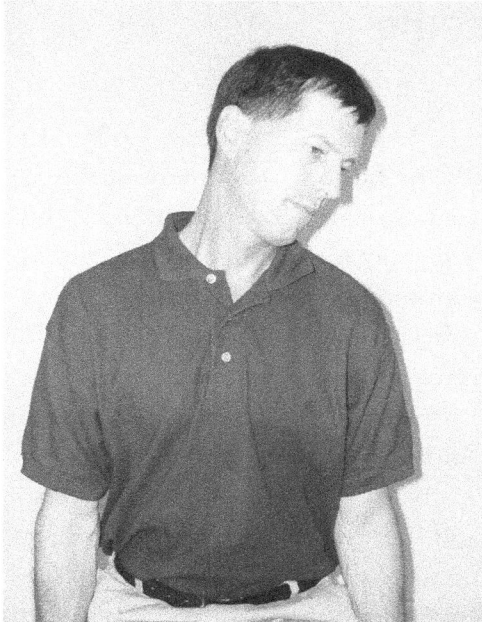

1. Tip your head to side. Rotate slightly to the same side.

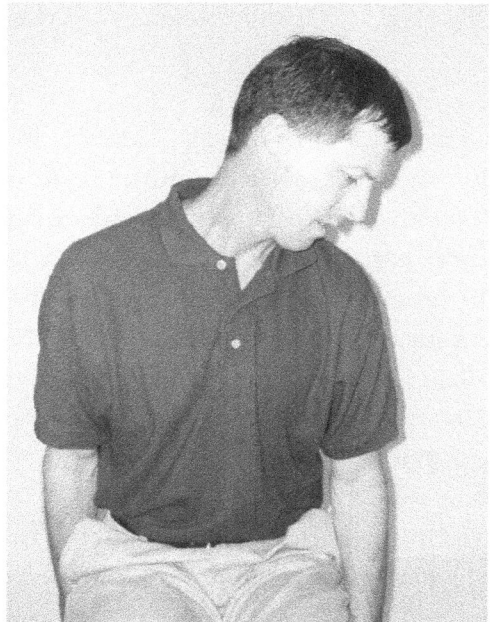

2. Look downward. Reach downward with opposite arm.

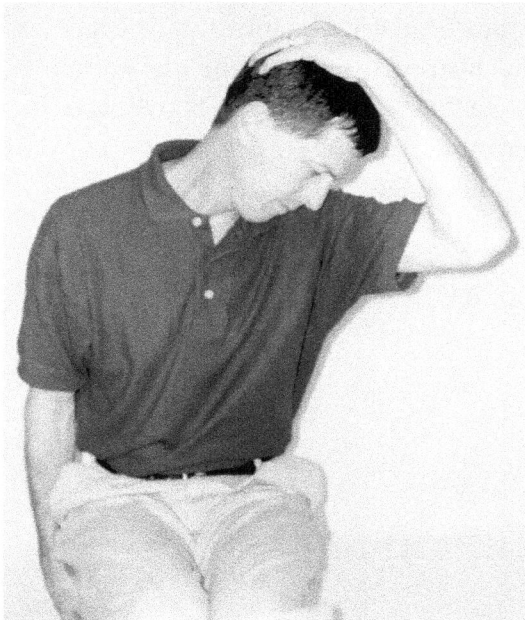

2. Place hand on head to provide extra stretch.

- Hold 15–20 seconds
- Do 2–3 per side

AVOID PAIN!

Scalene Stretching

The scalene muscles are in the front of the neck on either side of the throat and are divided into three parts. The posterior scalene is on the side of your neck and runs from the vertebrae below your ear almost straight down to the second rib. The anterior and middle scalenes run from the sides of the vertebrae down and forward to attach to the first rib just behind the collar bone.

Stretching of the scalene muscles can be done from either a standing or sitting position.

The right posterior scalene is stretched by placing the base of the left thumb in the soft area above the right collarbone at the base of the neck. The rest of the palm cups over the collarbone so that the inside border of the little finger is on the underside of the collarbone. Apply a downward pressure, not on the collarbone itself, but over the portion of the rib cage above and below it. This downward pressure stabilizes the bottom attachment of the scalenes.

With the bottom attachment of the scalenes stabilized, tip your head to the left and "lift" your right ear away from your right shoulder. Keep the downward pressure on your upper rib cage, and resist the tendency to turn your head to the right. Hold for at least 15 seconds.

To stretch the right middle and anterior scalenes, hold the upper rib cage down, tip your head slightly to the left, and rotate it slightly to the right. Let your head tip back as if you were looking up with only your right eye. "Lift" your jaw away from your collar bone. The back of the head will be aiming downward towards the back of the left shoulder. This should provide a stretch from the jawbone down to the collarbone on the right side. Adjusting rotation, tipping, and lifting your head will fine-tune the stretch.

Each stretch should be held for a minimum of 15 to 20 seconds and can be repeated two to three times per side. Stretching can be done several times a day.

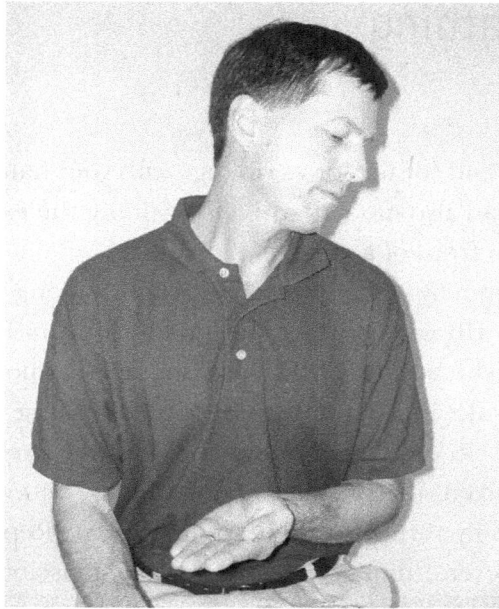

1. Align thumb with index finger.

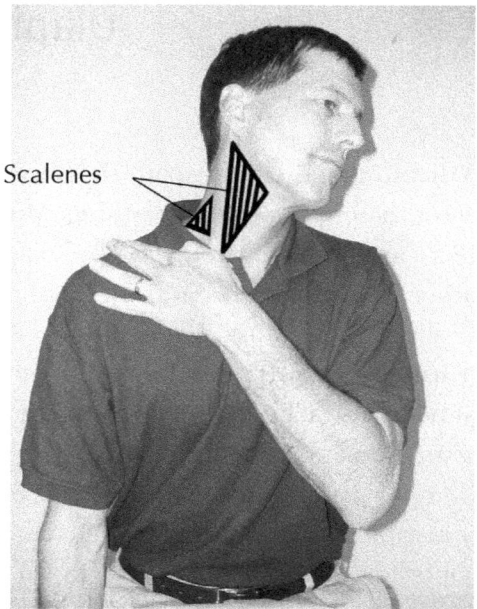

2. Place palm of hand over collarbone so that thumb is above the bone.

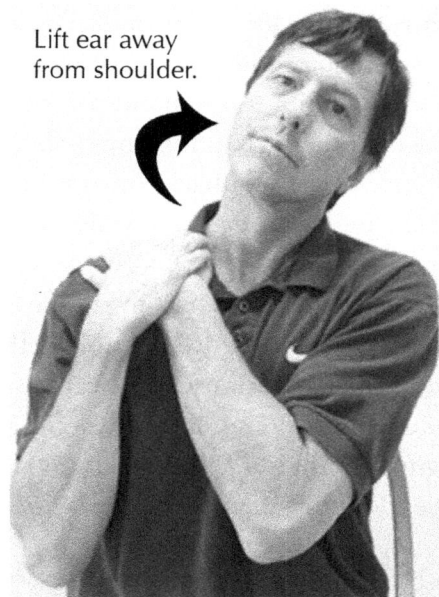

Scalenes

Lift ear away from shoulder.

3. Press downward with hand. Tip your head to the opposite side, without rotation for posterior scalene stretch.

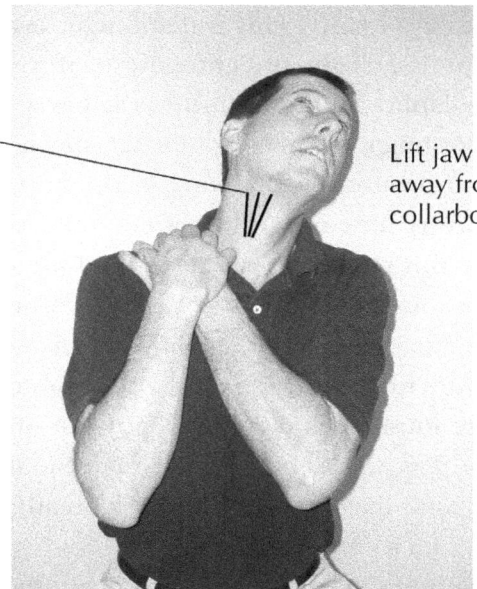

- Hold 15–20 seconds
- Do 2–3 per side

Stretch

Lift jaw away from collarbone.

4. For anterior and middle scalenes, tip head back. Adjust rotation of head and neck to get best stretch. Use other hand to add support.

AVOID PAIN!

© Brian Lambert

Diaphragm Breathing

A diaphragm-breathing pattern is much more efficient than upper-chest-breathing. Musicians, singers, and athletes tend to be diaphragm breathers. Using the respiratory diaphragm to draw air into the lungs is much more effective than using accessory muscles to lift the upper chest because the lungs are bigger at the bottom than they are at the top.

Compromised postural habits, stress, and poor aerobic capacity may lead to a change from a diaphragm breathing pattern to an upper-chest-breathing pattern.

Ideally, when one takes in a deep breath, the lower rib cage and upper abdominal area expand outward. This is diaphragm breathing. There is a slight straightening of the spine as the diaphragm draws air into the lower portion of the lungs. In an upper-chest pattern, a deep breath causes mostly lifting of the upper chest with very little expansion of the lower rib cage. With this pattern, the scalenes and some of the deep muscles in the upper back and neck provide much of the rib cage lift. This pattern contributes to overuse and subsequent tightening of these muscles, and subsequently the upper rib cage gets stuck "up." People who breathe like this look like they took a deep breath in, but never let it completely out.

Retraining of the breathing pattern can be done by monitoring movement of the upper chest and/or the lower rib cage with your hands. You can also monitor visually by doing the exercise in front of a mirror.

Begin by placing your hands lightly along the lower rib cage so that the middle fingers line up at the bottom of the sternum or breastbone. Now take in a slow, deep breath by making the lower rib cage push outward. When the breath is relaxed, the ribs and abdominal area should naturally return to their starting point. Repeat this several times. You may have to consciously inhibit the tendency to move the upper chest.

Another technique would involve inhibiting the upper chest movement by placing your hands on the upper chest and consciously restricting the movement in this area during inhalation. Sometimes one hand on the upper chest and the other across the upper abdominal area will give better feedback. Any of the above hand placements can be used while looking in a mirror.

With a little practice, retraining of the breathing pattern will help reduce overuse of the scalenes and upper back muscles. It can also be a good relaxation exercise. If this exercise proves challenging and helpful, do four to five repetitions several times a day.

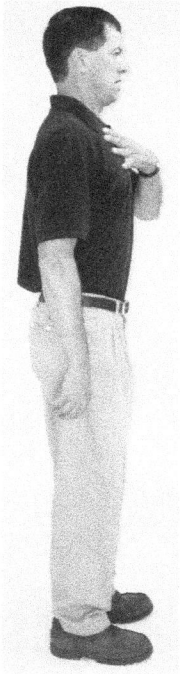

1. In a stress pattern of breathing, upper chest lifts with inhalation.

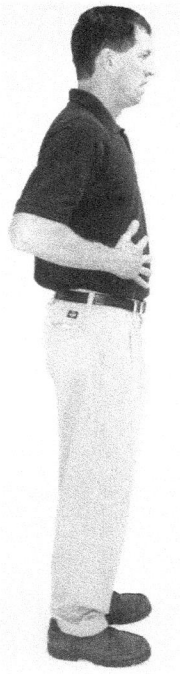

2. With an optimal breathing pattern, lower ribs move out with inhalation.

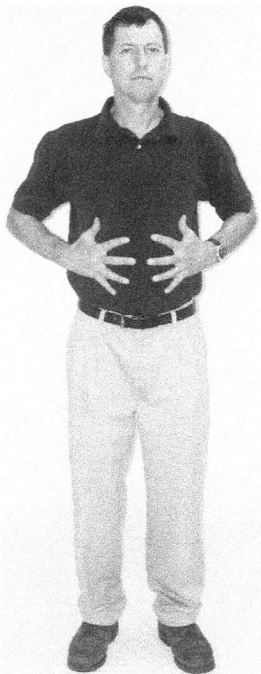

3. Correct breathing by monitoring movement of chest and ribs with hands.

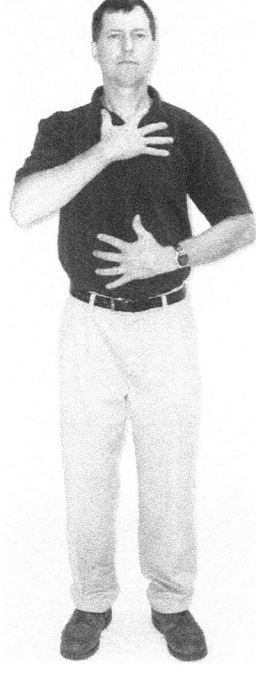

4. Emphasize movement of lower ribs while lessening the movement of the upper chest.

> • Monitor several times during the day.

AVOID PAIN!

Doorframe Pull Down

This exercise is designed to activate the back extensors and scapular stabilizers. You will need a four-foot piece of latex band or bicycle inner tube.

Tie a knot in the center of the latex band, and place it over the top of a door. Close the door to hold the knot. Face the door, and grab the band at eye level with your palms facing forward, little fingers on top, and thumbs pointing downward. Bend your elbows so the arms form a circle. You can be sitting or standing.

Your elbows remain bent at a constant angle as you squeeze the shoulder blades back and down toward the center of the back. Let the movement of the arms open the circle as your hands move apart. You should feel work between your shoulder blades. Slowly relax to the starting position. Repeat for two sets of eight to ten repetitions. Adjust your arms up or down to get the best work out of the exercise.

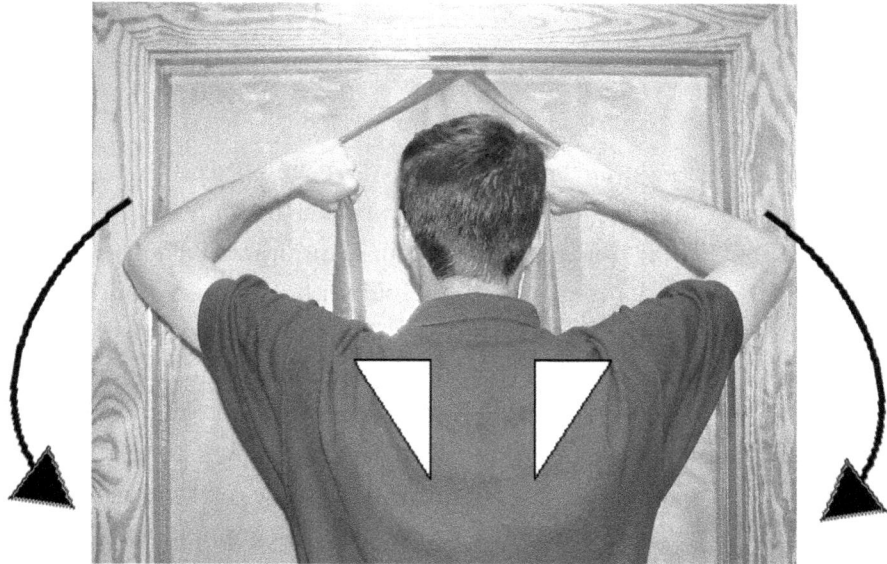

1. Grab band with thumbs down. Start motion by squeezing shoulder blades.

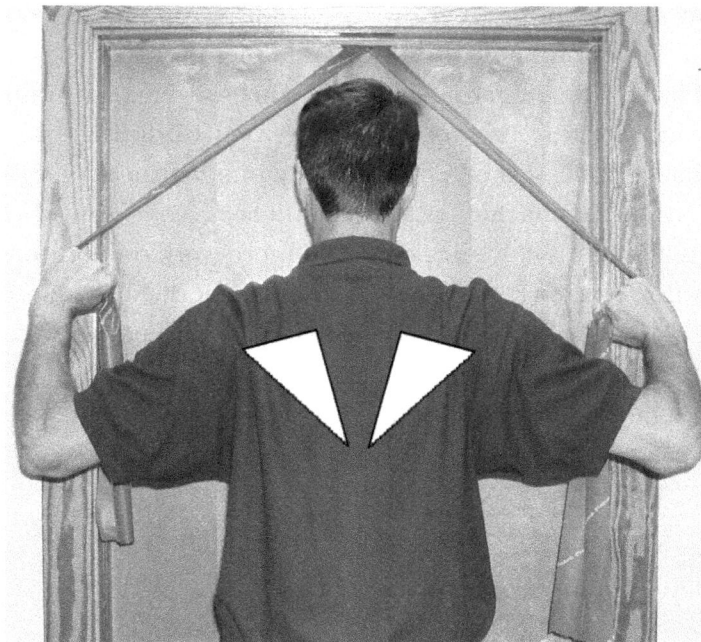

2. Let arms move in a circular motion. Keep elbow angle constant. Return to start position.

- Do 2 sets of 8–10 repetitions.
- Rest 30 seconds between sets.

AVOID PAIN!

Upper Thoracic Segmental Retraining

Restrictions in backward bending motion of the upper thoracic spine tend to pitch the head forward and contribute to a "hump back" appearance. The foam roller and rolled towel techniques will help loosen the area (pages 78 and 193). The following technique will help you regain active control. This exercise might be thought of as a vertical version of the attention exercises.

Sit in a straight-back chair. Place your index fingertip in the space between two of the largest big bumps at the base of your neck. Nodding your head in a slight up and down motion will help in identifying the correct position. Now place the fingers of the opposite hand on top of the first fingers, and bring your forearms forward to hold under your jawbone or around the sides of your face. Your elbows should point straight forward. Tighten your stomach muscles and hold your lower trunk in a 12 o'clock or posterior pelvic tilt. From this position, the arms, head, and neck should move as a solid unit with most of the motion localized to the segment under your fingers. The motion is small. Individual vertebrae only move four or five degrees.

Move your arms (head and neck) slightly downward to feel the space open. Now move your arms upward. Feel for the small movement. Hold for one to two seconds, and then relax back to neutral. Now lift your elbows slightly up and to the right, hold, and relax. Lift slightly to the left, hold, and relax. Position the head and neck back at the center, and then reposition your fingers down into the next interspace. Repeat the above exercise. If a segment is extremely restricted, you may repeat the lift/relax sequence several times at that segment. You can use this technique as far down as your fingers can reach. If significant relief is provided, this exercise may be done several times per day.

This can be a frustrating exercise. It can be very hard to distinguish any movement of the vertebrae with a very tight upper back. If you don't seem to get anywhere doing this exercise do more work on the towel or foam roller exercises. See if the attention exercises will help you regain control of this area.

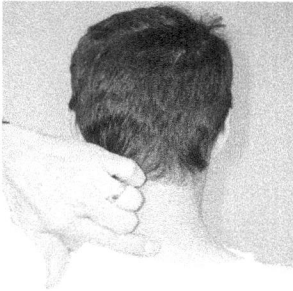

1. Start at interspace where good movement is identified.

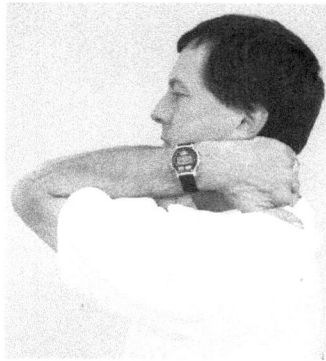

2. Hold jaw and neck with forearms. Hold spine and pelvis in a 12:00 or posterior tilt.

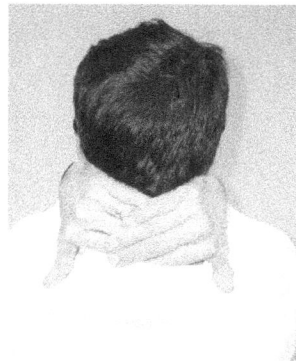

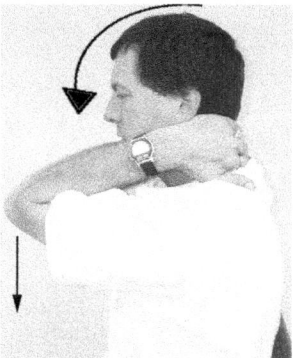

3. Arms, head, and neck should move as unit. Move down slightly. Feel the interspace open.

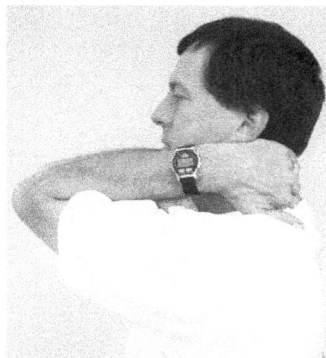

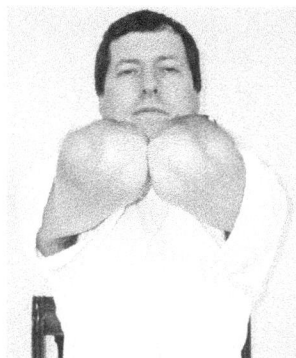

4. Then move up slightly. Feel the interspace close. Go back to neutral.

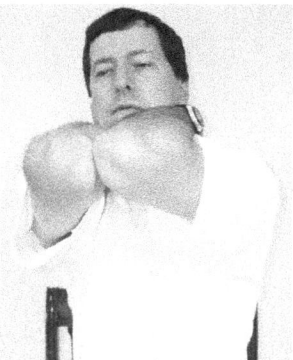

5. Then lift at a slightly left angle.

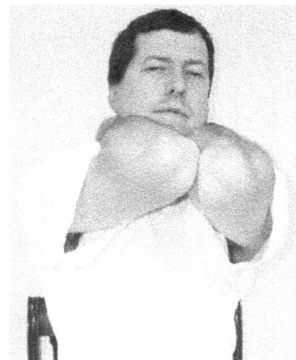

6. Then lift at a slightly right angle.

- Repeat lifts to center, right, and left 4 times at each level that you can reach.

- Do this exercise 4–5 times per day.

AVOID PAIN!

V

Advanced Abdominal Exercises

The following exercises strengthen and train the abdominal muscles in ways that are similar to how we use them when we are vertical. During upright activities, the muscles that surround the trunk from the rib cage to the pelvis function as a guy-wire/cylinder system. The only time the abdominal muscles function as a sit-up or crunch muscle is when you get out of bed in the morning. Once you are up, you need these muscles to balance the tension of the back muscles, not to bend you forward.

Sit-ups, crunches, and many "ab" machines have a tendency to increase flexion or forward bending of the upper back. Any time you lift your head and shoulders off of the floor, you tend to use all of the muscles in the front of the neck and chest. Tight scalene, pectoral, and intercos-tals (the muscles between the ribs) contribute to poor posture. Sit-ups and crunches also can tighten the hip flexors, which can pull on the low back, pelvis, and knees. Most activities in our modern society will cause these problems for us anyway. Therefore, exercises that promote trunk flexion should be minimized.

The following exercises are designed to strengthen the abdominal muscles using methods that will not increase flexion of the thoracic spine. With the heel touch-down exercises, you learn to control the abdominal muscles when your legs are moving, which happens when you are walking or running. You might want to master the Pelvic Clock (page 8) before starting any of these exercises.

Supine Heel Touchdown

A basic stomach exercise is the "Supine Heel Touchdown." Start by lying on your back on the floor with your knees bent and your feet flat. You can use your hands to help with feedback by placing your finger tips under the back between the rib cage and the pelvis. Slightly tuck your chin, but do not lift your head off the floor. Perform a strong 12 o'clock or posterior tilt. The tummy muscles should be pulled flat and tight so your finger tips are smashed against the floor under your back. With the posterior tilt established, bring one thigh and then the other towards your chest with the knees relaxed. Retighten the 12 o'clock tilt, and re-tuck your chin. Now slowly lower one leg to lightly touch the heel to the floor, and slowly return it to the start position. Do not straighten your knee. Repeat the process on the other side. Concentrate on keeping your tummy tight, so that you keep firm pressure on your fingers under your back. Continue alternating heel touchdowns to complete at least eight to ten repetitions. You can do up to 25 or 30 repetitions. After resting for a minute, try to do another set. If you are enjoying the exercise, do a third set.

If abdominal control is poor, take the heel only halfway towards the floor before returning it to the start position, and do fewer repetitions. The primary work of the exercise should be felt in your stomach muscles, not in your legs or back. Go back to the pelvic clock exercise if you do not feel significant work in the stomach muscles. As the exercise gets easier, straighten your knee to touch your heel down a little farther away. Always make sure your back is flat against your fingers, and the abdominal muscles are the primary muscles working.

If this exercise is too easy, try doing the version of this exercise on the foam log (page 120).

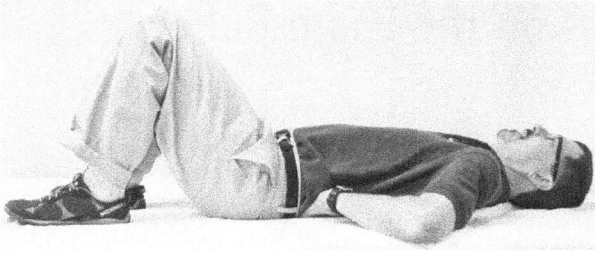

1. Lie on back with knees bent. Place fingers under small of back.

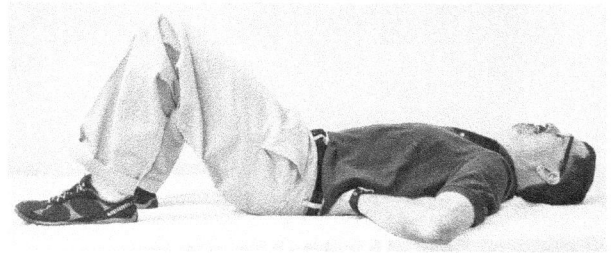

2. Do a strong 12:00 tilt to flatten low back and mash fingers.

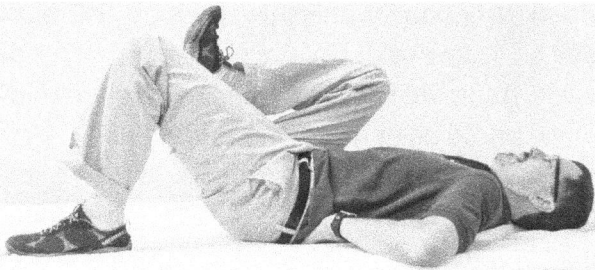

3. Bring one leg toward chest with knee relaxed.

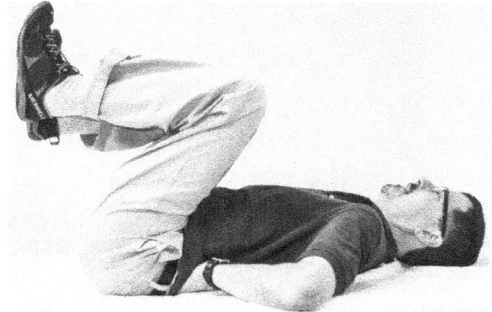

4. Bring other knee up. Retighten the 12:00 tilt and tuck chin.

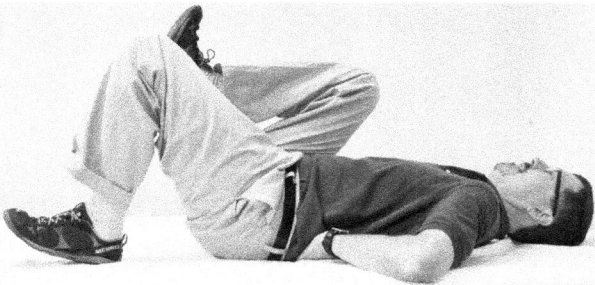

5. Slowly lower one heel toward floor. Lightly touch the heel down. Keep your back mashed against your fingers.

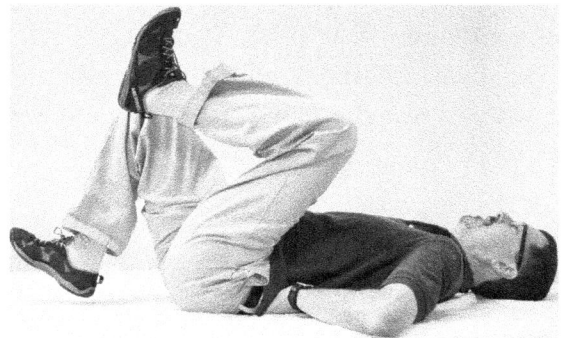

6. Bring leg back toward chest and repeat on other side.

• Do 2–3 sets of 8–10 repetitions.

AVOID PAIN!

Supine Heel Touch Downs on the Foam Roller

This is a more advanced exercise for the stomach muscles than the previous one. With this exercise, you stabilize the spine and pelvis, and engage the upper back while the legs are moving. This needs to happen when you are walking and running.

Begin by lying lengthwise on a 36- by 6-inch foam roller. Both arms are placed straight out from your body to form 90 degree angles. Your palms are up. The elbows are straight, and the backs of your hands are pressed against the floor. Flatten your low back against the roller. Tuck your chin without lifting your head. Look straight at the ceiling. Slowly bring one leg towards your chest and then the other one. Keep knees relaxed. Flatten your back again, and re-tuck your chin.

Once you feel stable, slowly lower your right leg, without straightening your knee, to let your right heel lightly touch the floor. Keep your left leg pulled towards your chest to help keep the low back pressed against the roller, and better engage the abdominal muscles. After lightly touching the floor, slowly return the right leg to the start position. Repeat the sequence by slowly dropping the left leg keeping the right one pulled towards the chest. If you have trouble keeping the back flat against the roller, then move your foot only half way to the floor.

Beginners might start with two to three sets of eight to ten repetitions per leg. Straightening your knee as you lower your leg will increase the difficulty. Make sure that your low back stays pressed against the roller and your chin tucked. If this exercise is easy, try the advanced exercises.

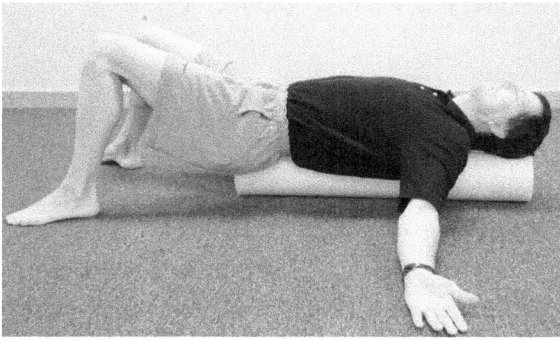

1. Lie on foam roller with arms perpendicular to sides, palms up.

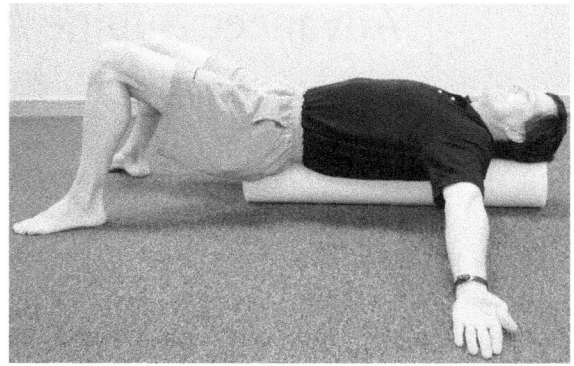

2. Keep elbows straight, press back of hands against floor.

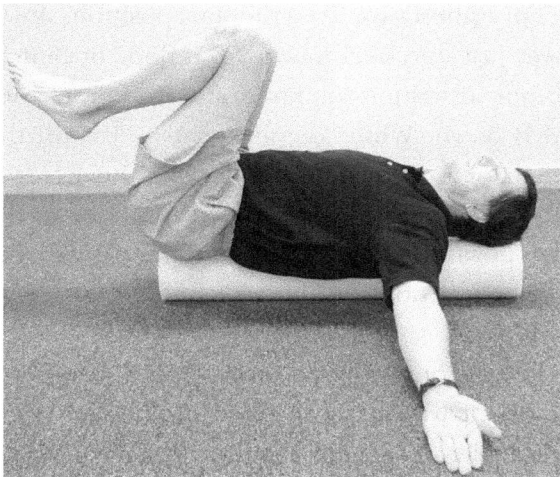

3. Tuck chin and flatten low back. Lift one leg, then the other.

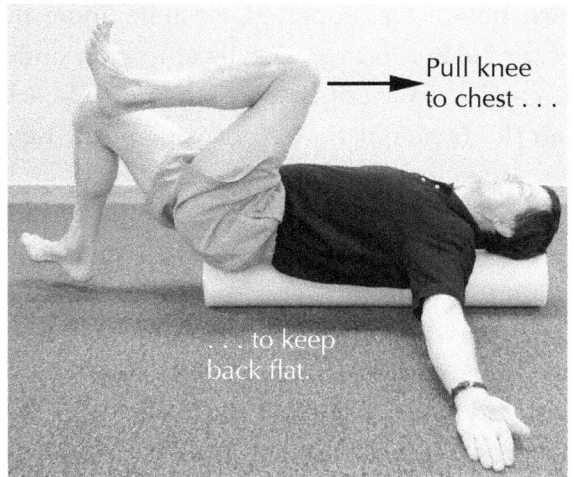

Pull knee to chest . . .

. . . to keep back flat.

4. Lower one leg to lightly touch to floor.

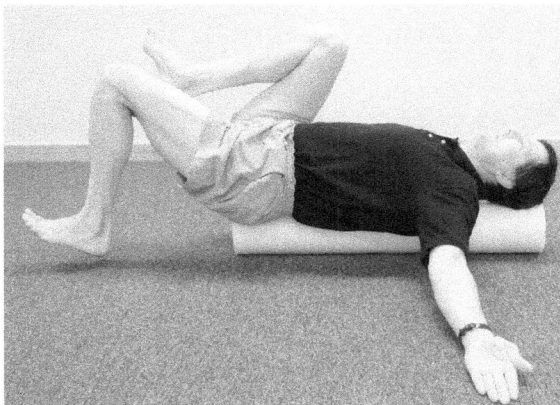

5. Slowly bring leg up, then repeat on other side. Keep low back flat.

• Do 2–3 sets of 8–10 repetitions.

AVOID PAIN!

© Brian Lambert

Advanced Supine Abdominal Work, Part 1

So, you found the other abdominal exercises too easy.

To do part one of the advanced abdominal exercises, you will lie on the floor near a heavy piece of furniture or on a weight bench. Take a bath towel and fold it so that it measures 12 inches square. Place the towel under your low back so that the lowest edge is even with your pelvic bones. The upper edge will be under the lower ribs. Reach over your head to grab under the couch, chair, or to a table leg. If on a bench, grab the bench at the top of your head. Keep your arms close to your head.

Do a 12 o'clock or posterior pelvic tilt and then slowly bring both knees toward your chest. Continue rolling the pelvis so that the hips and pelvis gently lift off of the floor or bench. Keep your knees relaxed and your thighs close to your chest and stomach. Keep your low back in contact with the towel. Your pelvis will be at least one to two inches off of the floor or bench. This is the start position for these abdominal exercises.

For **option one,** from the start position, slowly let your pelvis and legs down so that your heels and pelvis lightly touch the floor or bench, then slowly return the start position. Do not straighten your knees, and keep your low back mashed against the towel. Do 12 to 15 repetitions. Rest for 30 to 60 seconds before doing another set or proceeding to option two.

For **option two,** from the start position, slowly lower just one heel towards the floor or bench. Do not straighten the knee, and do not let your pelvis down. While keeping your pelvis off the bench or floor, lightly touch your heel to the bench or floor, and slowly return the leg to the start position. Repeat the movement with the other leg. Continue this alternating pattern to do 12 to 15 repetitions per leg.

Do one or two sets of both options. Drop your leg only part way down to make the exercise a little easier. Keep the movement slow and controlled. Keep your arms close to your head. If these options are too easy, try the ones in part two.

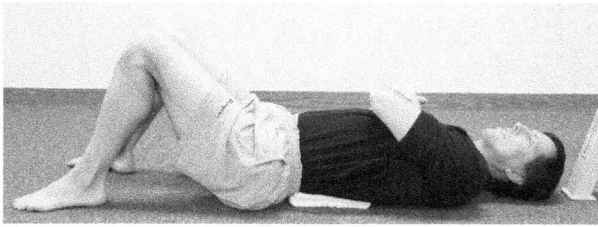

1. Lie on back with folded bath towel under low back.

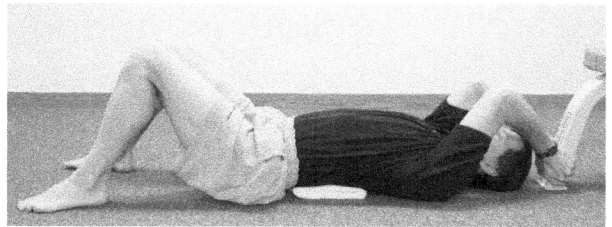

2. Reach over head and grab heavy object.

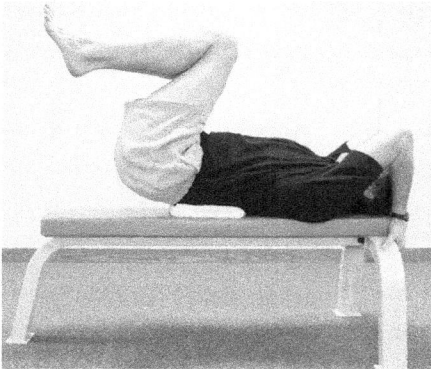

3. Or grab bench. Gently bring knees toward chest.

Option 1

Slowly lower pelvis and legs. Slowly repeat roll up.

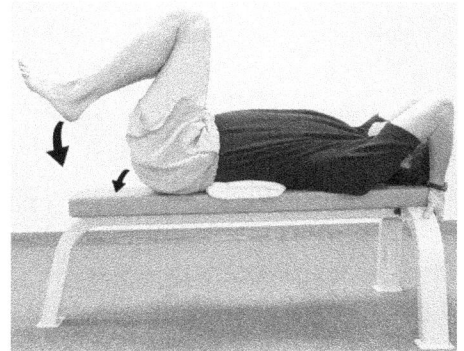

Option 2

Keep pelvis and legs up. Slowly lower one leg to lightly touch a heel. Keep pelvis up. Slowly return to start position

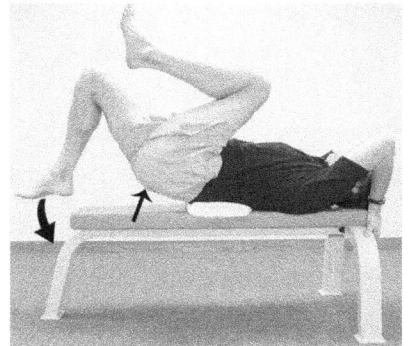

Repeat with other leg.

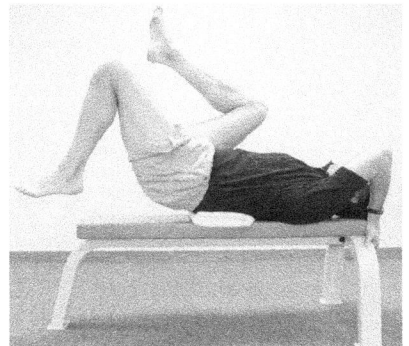

• 2 sets of 12–15 repetitions.

AVOID PAIN!

Advanced Abdominal Exercises, Part II

These exercises are for athletes who find the other stomach exercises are way too easy. They work best on a sturdy weight bench. The starting position for each of these exercises is the same as in part one. A few repetitions of the part-one options may be done as a warm-up for the part-two options.

For **option one,** from the start position, while keeping your pelvis up, slowly let your right leg down. In this option, your foot and lower leg drop off of the end of the bench. Gently force the bottom of your foot towards the floor. Keep the pelvis and hips off the bench and the left leg pulled towards your chest. Slowly return to the start position. If your bench is long or has a knee extension component, then let your leg go just off the side of the bench. Alternate legs and do 12 to 15 repetitions each leg.

For **option two,** from the start position, straighten both legs horizontally, keeping the feet together. As the legs are straightening, let your hips and pelvis down to rest on the bench, but keep your low back mashed against the towel. Keep your arms close to the sides of your head. Slowly return to the start position. Do 12 to 15 repetitions.

Option three is similar to option two except that you keep the hips and pelvis off the bench as you straighten your legs horizontally. Try to keep your legs as low as possible. Keep your arms close to the sides of your head. Return to the start position. Do 12 to 15 repetitions. Often options two and three blend together.

Option four: "The Twist." From the start position, rotate your lower body 90 degrees to the right, then lower the legs and pelvis so that the side of your right hip and right ankle touch in the center of the bench. Keep your hips and knees flexed. Keep your upper torso flat on the bench and your arms close to the sides of your head. Return to the start position, and repeat to the left. Continue alternating sides so that you do 12 to 15 repetitions in each direction.

You can do one or more sets of each option.

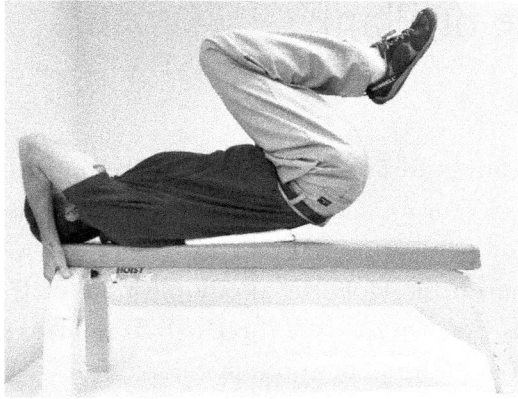

1. Start with both legs and pelvis up.

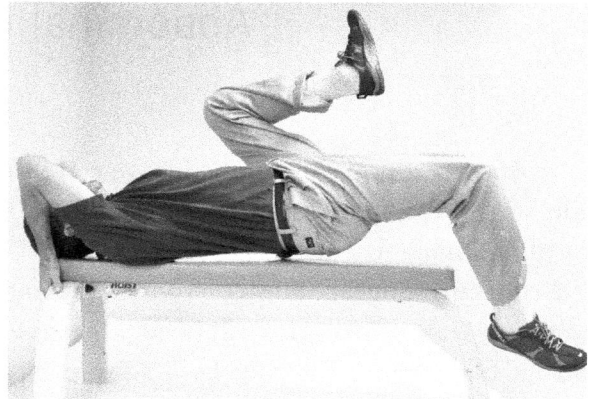

Option 1

Keep pelvis up, and let one leg drop down beside bench. Return to start position. Repeat on other side.

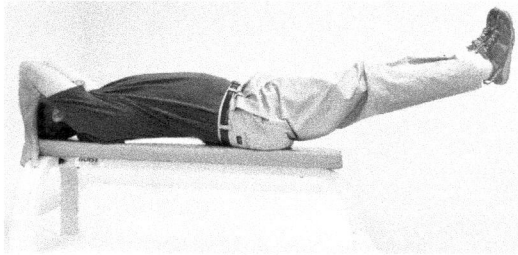

Option 2

From start position, straighten both legs. Let pelvis down, back pressed against towel. Return to start position.

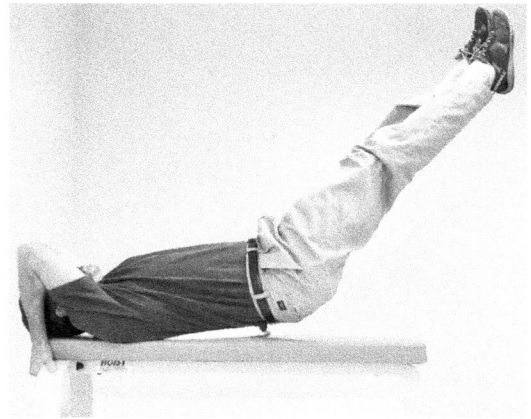

Option 3

From start position, straighten both legs. Keep pelvis up. Return to start position.

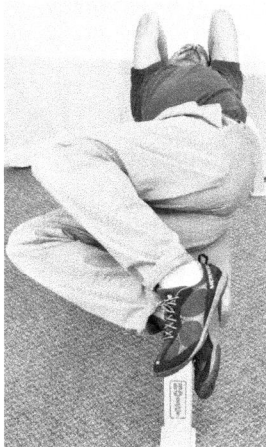

Option 4 "The Twist"

From start position, twist body so that hip bone and ankles lightly touch center of bench. Return to start position. Repeat on other side.

> • For each option do 1–2 sets of 15–20 repetitions.

AVOID PAIN!

Abdominal Bridge or Plank

With correct positioning, the bridge can provide you with a good isometric contraction of the abdominal muscles.

Begin by resting face down on your elbows and forearms. Your upper arms will be at 90 degrees to your body. Straighten your body so your hips and knees are straight, and you are resting on the tips of your toes. Tighten the abdominal muscles so the pelvis is moved into a slight 12 o'clock or posterior tilt. Hold this position for 30 to 40 seconds. You can repeat it three to four times as part of your abdominal workout.

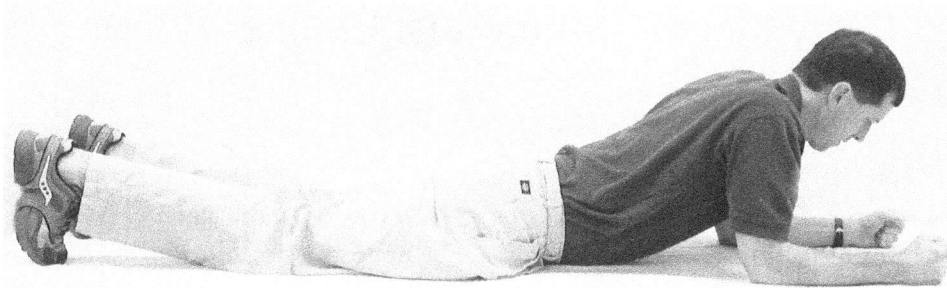

1. Prop on elbows and toes.

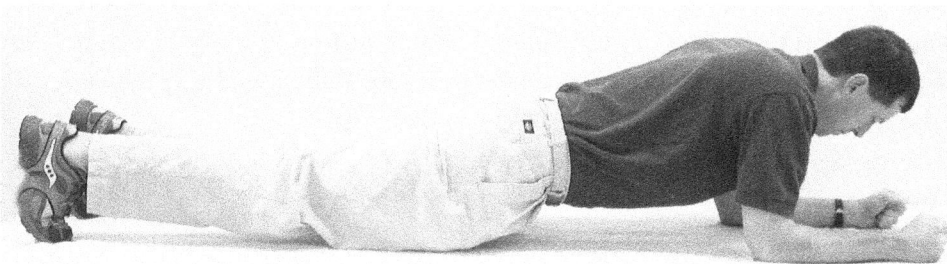

2. Lift pelvis up.

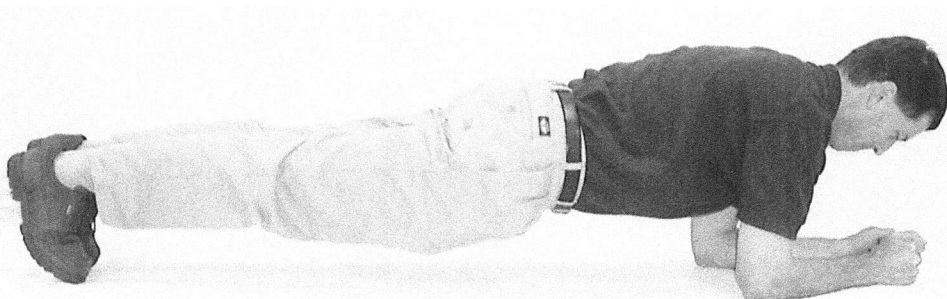

3. Align shoulders, hips, ears, and ankles. Keep tummy tight and tucked.

- Hold 30–45 seconds
- Do 3–4 repetitions.

AVOID PAIN!

Advanced Abdominals: Chair Exercise

Another option for abdominal strengthening is done with an office chair or rolling stool. It works similarly to the rolling devices advertised on TV, but better.

Begin by kneeling in front of an office chair. Place your elbows and forearms on the seat of the chair. Stabilize the upper arms at an approximate 90-degree angle to the body. Let the chair roll forward by gently pushing with the hips and knees. Keep the abdominal muscles tight so the spine does not sag downward. Keep the head aligned with the shoulders.

Roll forward as far as good control will allow, then return to the starting position.

Keep the tummy tight throughout the entire motion. Rolling at a slight angle will help recruit the oblique abdominals. A sequence of rolling straight, then back to neutral, slightly to the left (back to neutral), and then slightly to the right (back to neutral) would be considered one repetition. Repeat eight to ten repetitions in two to three sets.

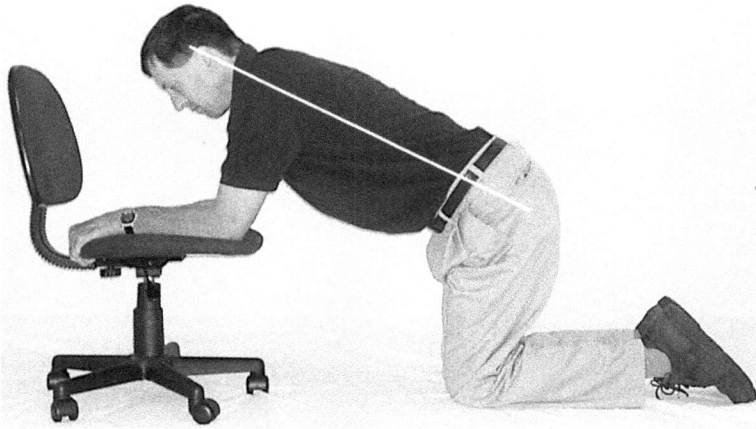

1. Starting position

- 3 sets of 8–10 repetitions
- 30 seconds of rest between sets

AVOID PAIN!

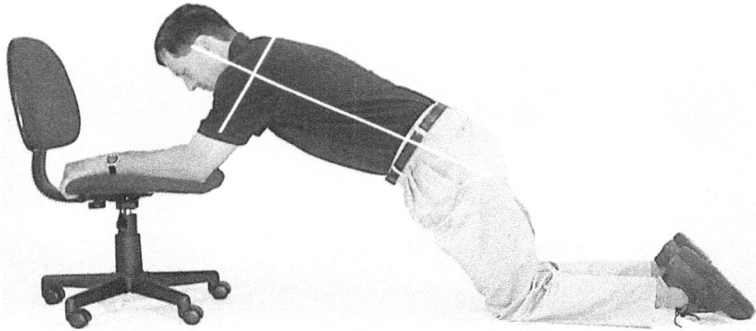

2. Push chair outward. Keep shoulders and arms stationary. Use abdominal muscles for control of out and back motion. Stay within range of control.

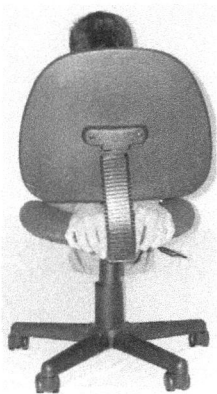

3. To center

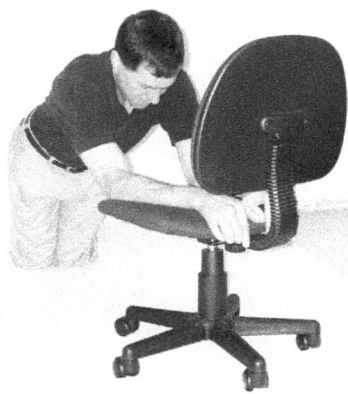

4. To one side

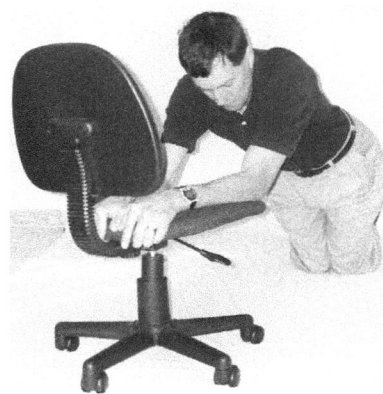

5. To other side

© Brian Lambert

Advanced Abdominal Exercises | 129

VI
Upper Body Exercises

Posture and overall function can be improved with correct execution of upper body exercises. The neck and posture exercises discussed earlier can be made almost unnecessary if a good upper body-strengthening program is followed on a regular basis.

For most people, a free-weight exercise program works best for several reasons. It is portable and can be done at home or in a gym. The exercises facilitate control of postural muscles rather than letting a machine provide control. The techniques can be modified to suit a given body type or functional restrictions. You can also design a free-weight exercise program to target a specific area or to train for a specific activity. If you are new to weight lifting or are recovering from an injury or surgery, you might want to start with some of the basic back and neck exercises before starting a weight-lifting program.

General training and conditioning can be done with a program that emphasizes high repetitions and lower weights. High repetitions generally mean 12 to 15 repetitions. These exercises are generally done in two sets of 12 to 15 repetitions with a 30 to 60 second rest between sets. Each exercise is done with sufficient weight so that the targeted muscle group is fatigued by the end of the set, and good form is maintained.

Good form means maintaining good posture and/or alignment while exercising to target a muscle group. Avoid pain! Each movement of the exercise should be slow and controlled, taking at least two to three seconds per direction of each movement. If an exercise causes pain, try to modify the exercise by decreasing the movement or decreasing the weight. If pain persists with a specific exercise, try another exercise that targets the same muscle group. A ten to fifteen minute warm-up period is recommended before starting an exercise session. This can include walking, biking, or light jogging.

The upper body free-weight exercises are divided into three groups: chest, back, and shoulders. An exercise session would consist of one or two exercises from each group. Free-weight exercises can be done every other day or three days a week. When transitioning from posture exercises to weight lifting, people will often start with just three exercises. These are usually: bench fly on the roller, doorframe lateral raises, and the seated reverse fly. Others are added as desired. Try to vary the order in which each exercise is done within each session. An exercise session can also include advanced abdominal exercise as well as advanced hip exercises. Generalized quadriceps, hamstring, and calf exercises can be included for the legs, and biceps and triceps exercises for arms.

A high repetition, low weight workout will generally increase strength, tone, and control, but not increase muscle bulk. Working with a personal trainer may help with correct execution of the exercises as well as guiding you in a general fitness program.

Typical 3-Day Workout Schedule

DAY 1	DAY 2	DAY 3
Warm-up	Warm-up	Warm-up
Reverse and side step lunges	Olympic-style squats	Reverse and side step lunges
Chest: Bench press and bench fly	Lateral shoulder: Overhead press and incline lateral raises	Back: Bent over row and frontal pull down
Lateral shoulder: Doorframe lateral raises and upright rows	Chest: Push-ups and dumbell press	Lateral shoulder: Doorframe lateral raises and frontal raises
Back: Single arm row and incline reverse fly	Back: Seated reverse fly and seated row	Chest: Dumbbell press and Bench flys
Abdominals: Supine heel touch-down and abdominal bridge	Abdominals: Chair exercise and supine heel touch downs	Abdominals: Supine heel touch-downs and bridges
Optional: Incline bicep curls and supine elbow extension	Optional: Quadriceps, hamstrings, and calf work	Optional: Upper and/or lower extremity work

Upper Body Exercises For The Back

Seated Reverse Fly

Scapular retractors include rhomboids, and lower and middle trapezius muscles.

These muscles pull the shoulder blades towards the center of the back. The seated reverse fly exercise targets these as well as the spinal extensors of the thoracic spine. Very often, this exercise is started without any weight. As the repetitions and sets get easier, you can add weight.

Sit on a bench or in a chair with knees and feet together. People who are very tall or very tight might need to sit on something higher than a normal chair or weight bench. The knees are partially extended to form a 45-degree angle. There are two ways to arrive at correct trunk positioning. The first is bending forward so that the chest is resting on the knees with your arms hanging straight down, lifting your head and shoulders away from your knees while keeping your stomach as close to the thighs as possible. Lift the upper body up to a 45-degree angle. Push the breast bone forward (Imagine the figurehead on a sailing ship). Look toward your toes. Think about aligning the ears, shoulders, and hips. This positioning can also be achieved by leaning forward from the hips to a forty-five degree angle with the breast bone pushed forward.

Once in the correct position, you should feel some isometric contraction or work in the muscles between the shoulder blades. Now raise the arms by squeezing your shoulder blades together. Let the shoulder blades pull the arms up to horizontal. The arms should now be straight out from your sides with the palms facing the floor. You should be able to see your hands with your peripheral vision. Elbows should be almost straight. Slowly relax the shoulder blades to lower the arms to the start position while maintaining the upper body position, and then repeat the arm raise. The raised position of the arms can be called the "piper cub" configuration (like the little straight wing airplane). If the muscles are very weak, there is a tendency for the arms to angle back in a "delta wing" configuration (think of a jet), which is easier but not as effective at targeting the muscles between the shoulder blades. If positioning or pain is a problem, the next exercise, the incline reverse fly may be a better choice (page 136).

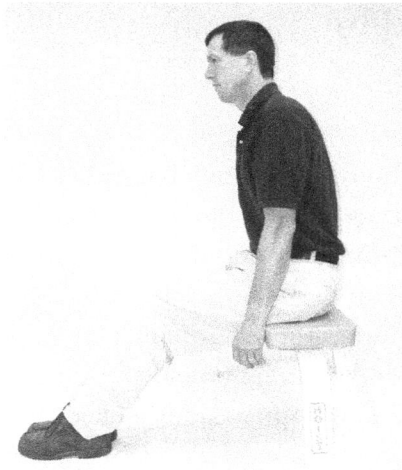

1. Knees bent at 45°

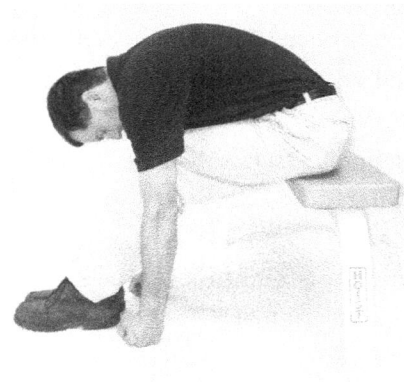

2. Rest chest on knees.

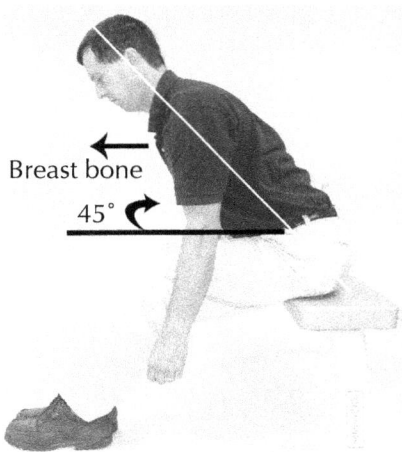

Breast bone

45°

3. Raise body to 45° angle. Look at toes with breast bone pushed forward. Hold this position.

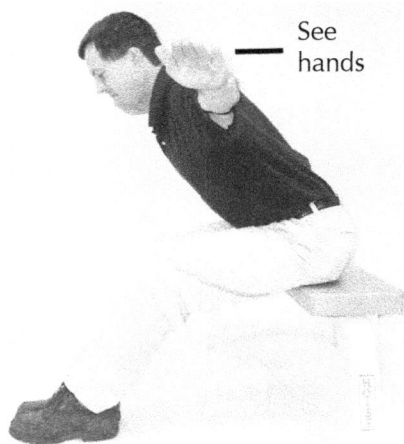

See hands

4. Raise arms to horizontal by squeezing shoulder blades together. Keep hands in peripheral vision. Lower arms slowly and repeat arm raise.

- 2 sets of 12–15 repetitions
- Beginning weight: 0 lbs

AVOID PAIN!

Incline Reverse Fly

The incline reverse fly is usually easier than the seated reverse fly for targeting the muscles between the shoulder blades, but it requires a weight bench that will incline. This exercise is generally started with two to five pounds of weight.

An adjustable incline bench should be raised to a 45-degree angle. Lie face down on the bench with your chin or forehead down. The hips should be at an approximate 90-degree angle to your body. Your arms hang down with your elbows straight, but not locked. Raise your arms by squeezing your shoulder blades together to let the shoulder blades pull your arms to horizontal. Palms should be facing the floor, and the arms should be straight out from your body, with the elbows straight but not locked. You should be able to see your hands with your peripheral vision. Lower your arms slowly and repeat.

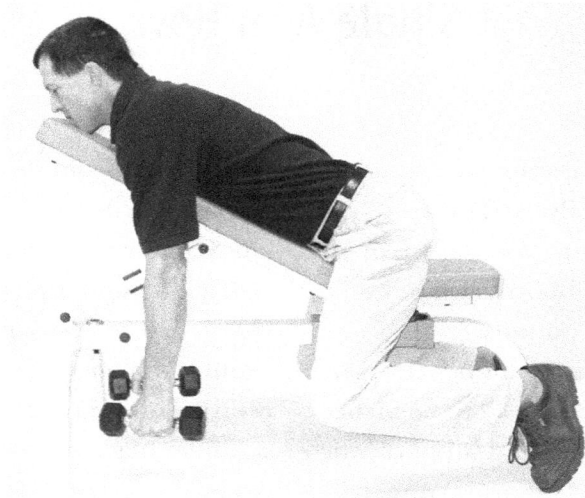

1. Incline bench to 45°. Chin or forehead down. Soft elbows.

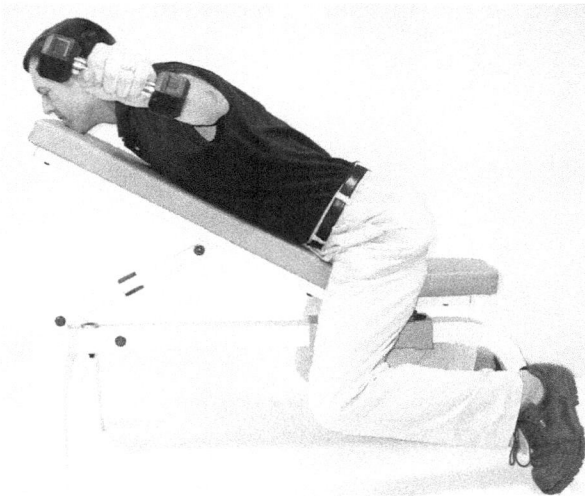

2. Raise arms by squeezing shoulder blades together. Raise to horizontal, make sure you can see hands. Lower arms slowly and repeat.

- 2 sets of 12–15 repetitions
- Beginning weight: 3–5 lbs

AVOID PAIN!

Single Arm Row

This exercise targets the scapular retractors and part of the latissimus dorsi. This is a very powerful motion for the body. We use it to open heavy doors and to start stubborn lawn mowers. You may start with 10 to 20 pounds.

Place left knee and shin on the bench. Your right foot on the floor should be 12 to 18 inches from the bench. Bend forward and support your upper body weight on your left arm. Your right arm should hang straight down. The area inside of the left arm, trunk, left thigh, and bench should almost form a square. To maintain good position of the head and neck, look down at the bench and not ahead. With a weight in your right hand, begin the row by moving your right elbow towards your right hip then, raising your elbow towards the ceiling.

Throughout the motion, your arm should remain close to your side, and your forearm should remain vertical. Let your arm slowly return downward, and let the weight pull your shoulder blade down without rotating the trunk. Now repeat the elbow raise. You should feel the work along the lower portion of your right shoulder blade. Try not to overuse the biceps by making sure that the forearm stays vertical. Letting your arm rub the side of your body will help reduce the tendency to use incorrect muscles.

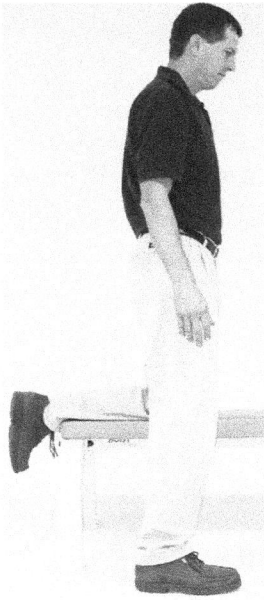

1. Kneel one leg on bench.

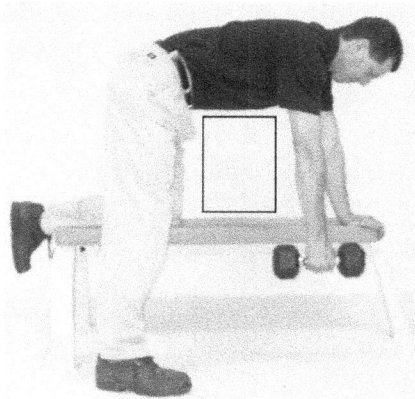

2. Bend forward and support upper body so that a rectangle is formed. Look at bench. Pickup weight.

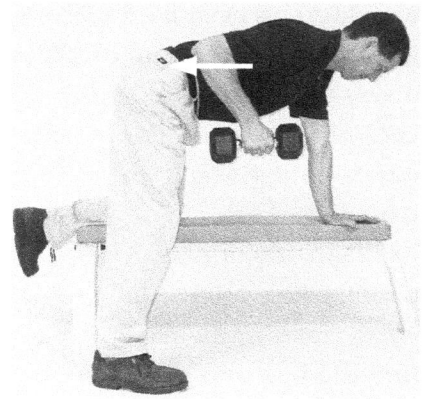

3. Begin by moving elbow toward hip.

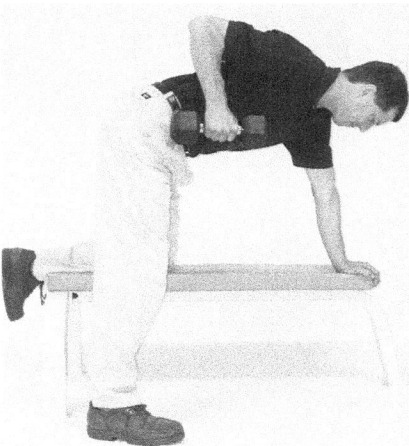

4. Then toward ceiling. Keep forearm vertical.

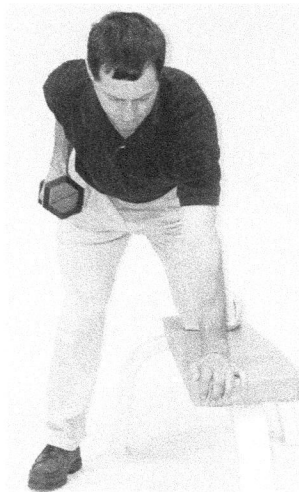

5. Keep arm close to side.

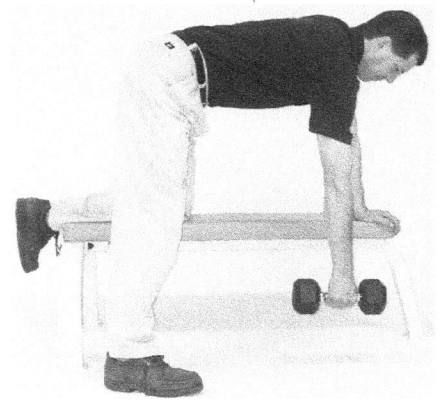

6. Lower weight toward floor. Let it stretch shoulder downward, but don't rotate trunk. Repeat.

- 2 sets of 12–15 repetitions
- Beginning weight: 10–20 lbs

AVOID PAIN!

Frontal Pull-Down

Pull-down exercises target the latissimus dorsi muscles. This exercise requires a cable machine. Frontal pull-downs are strongly encouraged. Pull-downs behind the head are strongly discouraged because you are not able to keep the ears aligned with the shoulders. Generally start with 20 to 30 pounds of weight.

Begin positioning for the exercise by grabbing the bar with the hands twice your shoulder width apart. You may need to experiment to find the best and most comfortable grip width. Sit down, pulling the bar with you. Lean back from the hips to approximately a 60-degree angle from the bench. Find neutral spine and pelvis by moving back and forth from 12 to six o'clock and finding the midpoint between the movements. Align the ears over the shoulders.

Pull the bar down to lightly touch the top of the chest to where your collar bones attach. The cable should be within one inch of your chin. You can imagine your arms sliding down a roof, pulling the bar and cable downward. The work should be felt between the shoulder blades and down to the lower back. Let the bar pull your arms back up to stretch the shoulders, but do not lose the positioning of the trunk. Repeat the pull-down. A version of this exercise can be done with a latex band (page 112).

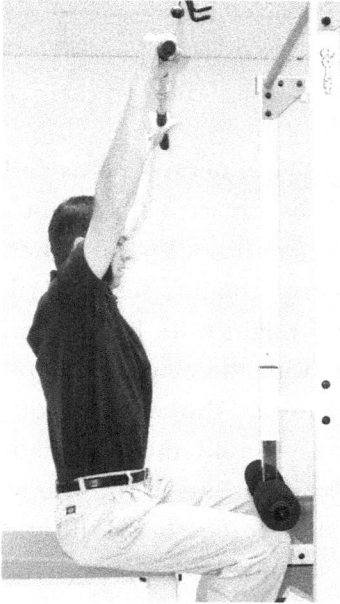

1. Grab bar so that hands are slightly wider than shoulders, then sit.

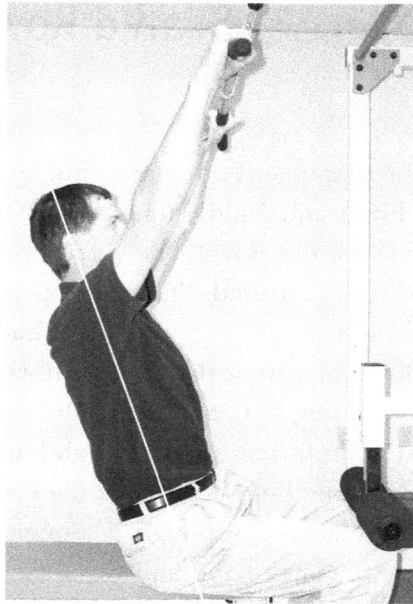

2. Lean trunk back to 60°. Neutralize spine and align ears with shoulders.

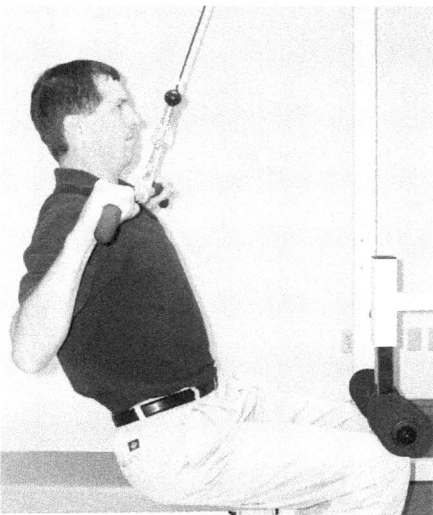

3. Pull bar downward to breast bone, just under chin.

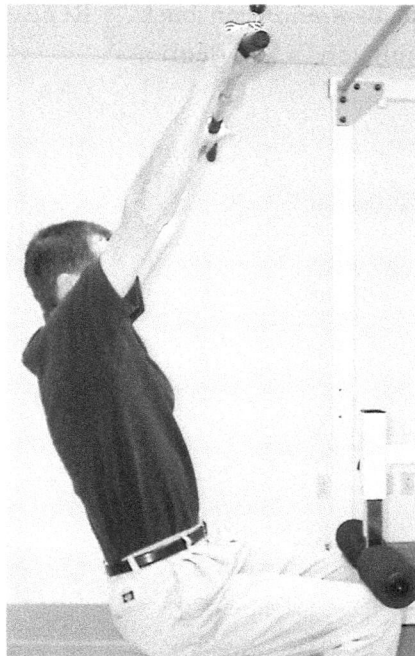

4. Slowly let bar return up and allow shoulders to stretch without losing trunk position and repeat pull down.

- 2 sets of 12–15 repetitions
- Beginning weight: 20–30 lbs

AVOID PAIN!

Lower Extremity/Back Stretches | 141

Seated Row

This exercise targets the scapular retractors including the rhomboids, lower and middle trapezius, and possibly some latissimus dorsi. The back extensors are also heavily recruited. Start with 15 to 20 pounds of resistance.

The exercise is generally done sitting flat on the floor, but if correct positioning of the spine cannot be realized because of tight hamstrings, sitting on a short stool or block may help. A cable machine with a low pull is required, although the exercise can be done with a latex band and some imagination.

Sit in front of the machine with your legs straight and your feet braced against the machine. Grab the vertical bars and lean back from the hips to approximately a 30 degree angle from the vertical. Find neutral pelvis and low back by moving between six o'clock (anterior tilt) and 12 o'clock (posterior tilt), and then stop in the middle. Look straight ahead. Vertical handles or a "rope" might work better than a horizontal bar. Start with the elbows straight. Draw the handles back toward the center of your abdomen. Your elbows should move straight back so that your arms stay close to your body. Squeeze the shoulder blades together at the end of the pull. The work should be felt through the upper back. Slowly release to the start position with the elbows straight and the shoulders protracted. Do not let your trunk slump forward. Repeat the pull.

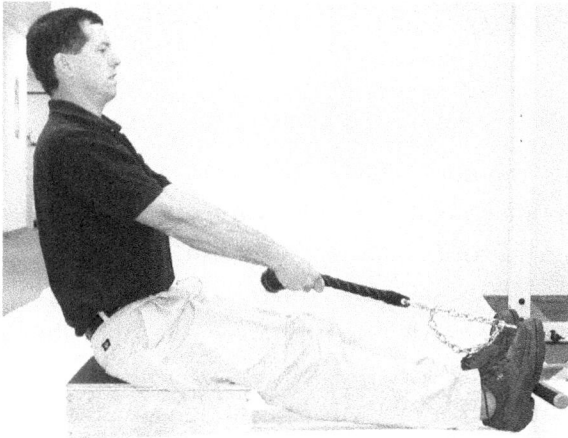

1. Sit on floor or very low box.

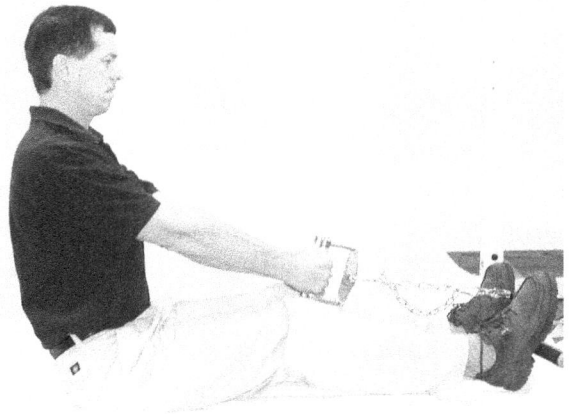

2. Knees straight as possible to achieve neutral spine/pelvis

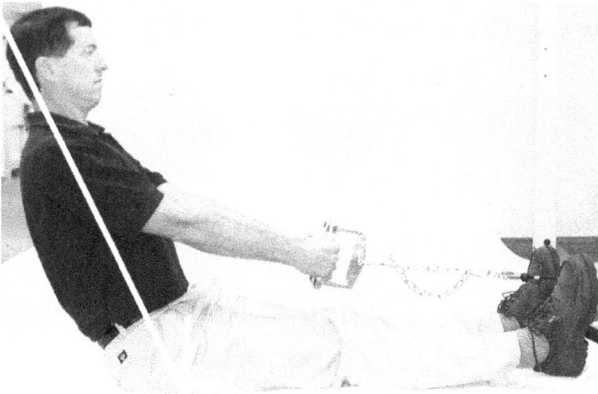

3. Lean back 30°. Grab "A" bars or rope.

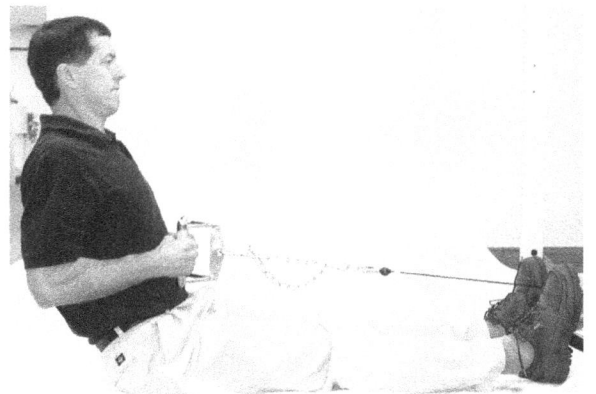

4. Pull bar to center of upper abdomen by pulling elbows straight back. Work is felt between shoulder blades.

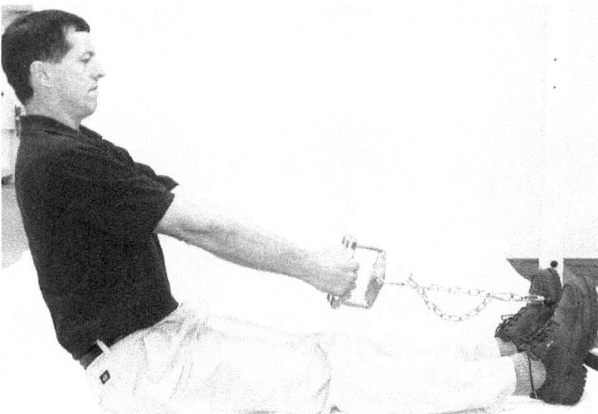

- 2 sets of 12–15 repetitions
- Beginning weight: 15–20 lbs

AVOID PAIN!

5. Let the weight pull arms back out to feel some stretch in shoulders and repeat exercise.

Bent-Over Row

This exercise requires being able to perform a reasonably good wall or Olympic-style squat (pages 32 and 24, respectively). The target area includes the scapular retractors and all of the spinal extensor muscles of the thoracic and lumbar spine. It may not be a good choice if you have low back problems. Start with 15 to 20 pounds of weight.

The bent-over row can be done with dumbbells, but is probably best done with a bar. Begin with a grip that is one and a half to two times your shoulder width. Move into a good squat position so that your thighs are 30 to 45 degrees from horizontal. Keep your shins vertical and your chest up. Look straight ahead. Now raise the bar towards your upper chest. Your elbows will move towards the ceiling, and your forearms will remain as vertical as possible. Your shoulder blades will squeeze together, and the bar should lightly touch your chest. Lower the bar slowly, letting the shoulder blades drop, but do not lose the squat positioning. Repeat the lift.

- 2 sets of 12–15 repetitions
- Beginning weight: 20–25 lbs

AVOID PAIN!

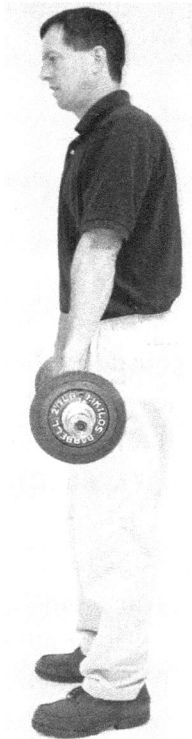

1. Start in standing position holding bar or dumbbells with wide grip.

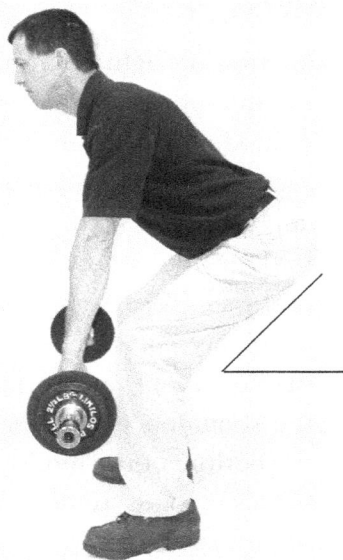

2. Sit into squat position with thighs 30–45° from horizontal. Shins vertical and chest up.

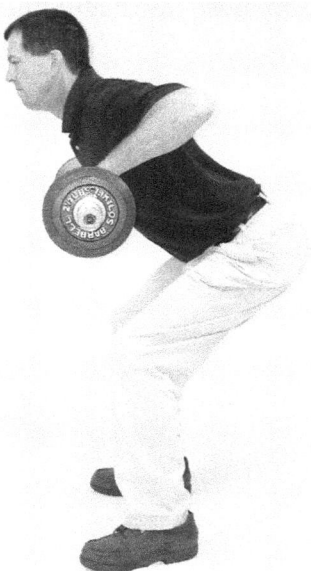

3. Bar pulled to upper chest.

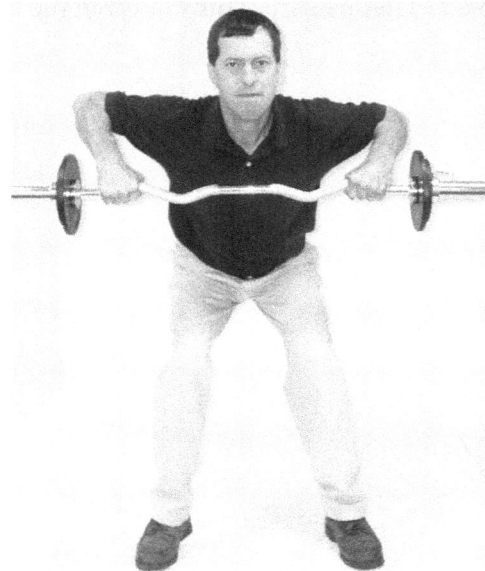

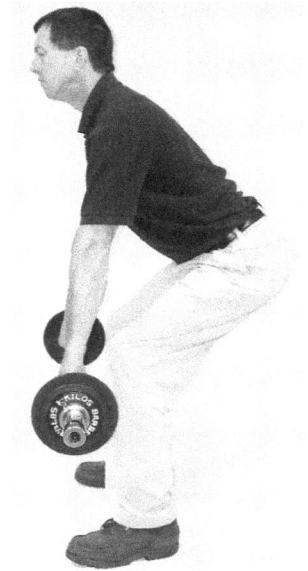

4. Slowly relax arms and repeat lift.

Upper Body Exercises for the Chest

Bench Fly

The bench fly is a fairly easy exercise that targets the pectoral or chest muscles. When done correctly you can stretch the chest muscles and straighten a flexed upper back. Begin with a three- to five-pound dumbbell in each hand.

Lie on a bench so that your feet are supported. If the bench is very short, a chair or stool can be used as a foot prop. To ensure good shoulder blade movement, have a rolled-up bath towel running from under your head to your lower back. This exercise can be done on the floor or bed using pillows to elevate the upper body. Doing a bench fly on a foam roller is extremely effective (page 155).

Once lying down, find neutral for the low back by moving the pelvis back and forth between six and 12 o'clock to find the middle position. The chin is slightly tucked. The arms are now brought up over the chest. The ends of the dumbbells should touch. Introduce a slight to moderate bend to the elbows to form a "hug a tree" position. Maintain this constant elbow angle throughout repetitions of the exercise. Let the arms fall straight apart. Avoid any rotation of the shoulders. The arms should remain in an imaginary corridor so that, when viewed from the side, they would form a straight line through the shoulders and chest. As the arms come to the bottom of the motion, squeeze the shoulder blades together under you towards the towel. A slight stretch should be felt in the chest muscles. Return to the start position and repeat. If you are having trouble with the "corridor" concept, do this exercise on a foam roller so that your armpits line up with the outside of a doorframe. This will force the arms to move in straight line.

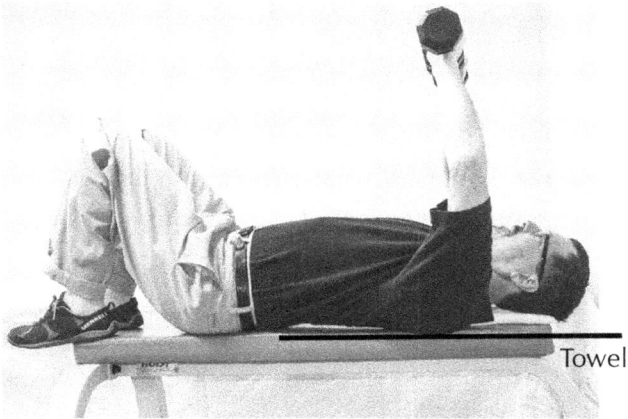

1. Lie with feet on bench on a rolled-up bath towel. Find neutral low back. Hands aligned over chest. Chin slightly tucked.

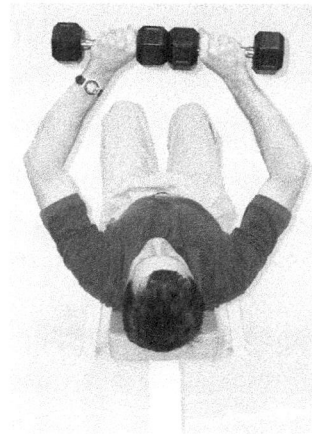

Towel

2. Arms in "Hug a Tree" position. Maintain a constant elbow angle.

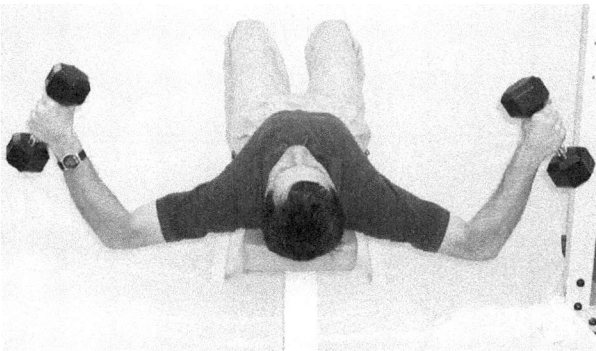

- 2 sets of 12–15 repetitions
- Beginning weight: 3–5 lbs

3. Let the arms fall apart. Arms, elbows, and hands move as solid units.

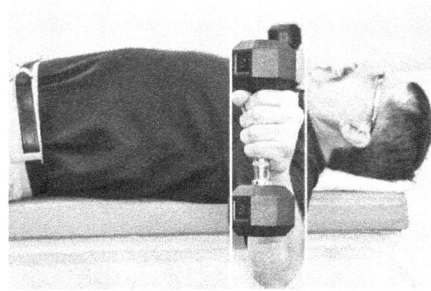

4. Maintain straight line through hands, elbows, and shoulder. Stay in corridor.

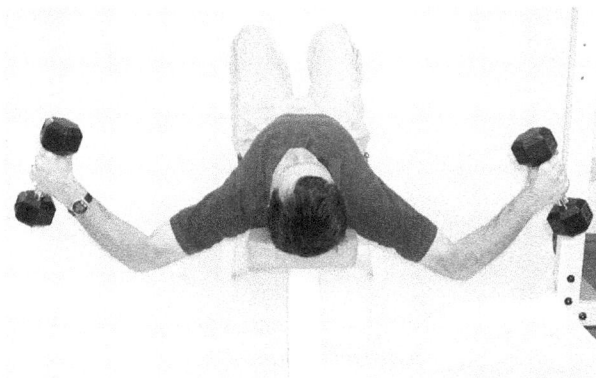

5. Squeeze shoulder blades together at bottom of movement.

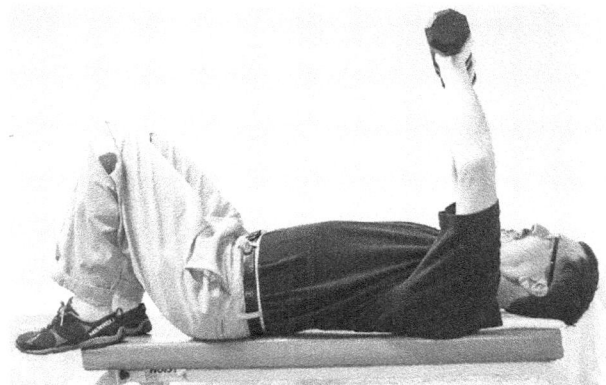

6. Return to start position and repeat.

AVOID PAIN!

Dumbbell Press

A dumbbell press has elements in common with both a bench press and a bench fly. You will use slightly more weight than with the fly, but substantially less than with the bench press. You can use a weight bench with a rolled-up bath towel running from under your head down to your low back, a foam roller, or prop yourself up on pillows. Begin with five- to eight-pound dumbbells in each hand.

Position your low back and pelvis in neutral with your chin slightly tucked. Begin with the elbows straight so that the dumbbells are over the center of your chest. The thumb end of the dumbbells should touch. To bring the dumbbells down, let your elbows move straight towards the floor, keeping forearms vertical. The thumb end of the dumbbells should rest in the crease where the shoulder and chest muscles meet. You can squeeze your shoulder blades toward the towel before pushing the weights back up to the starting position to repeat the exercise.

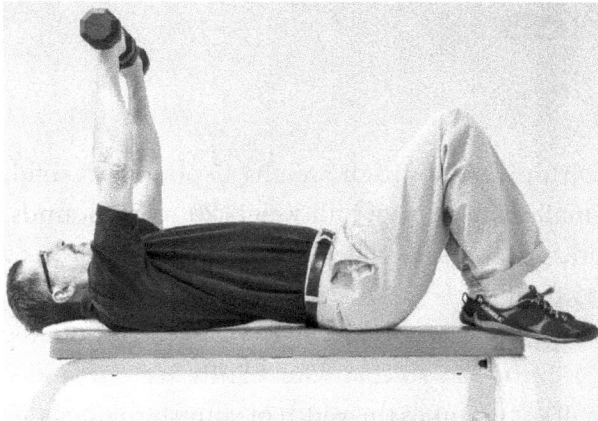

1. Lie on bench, arms straight with weights over chest. Put a bath towel under head and back.

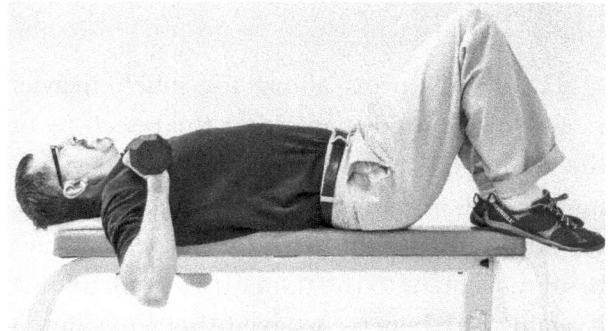

2. Bring weights down. Elbows move straight toward floor.

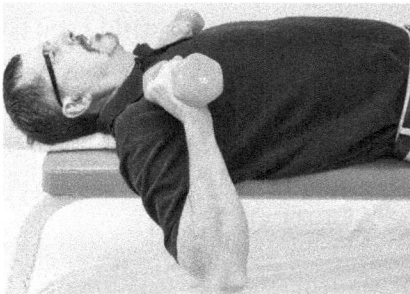

3. Weights will rest in crease between shoulder and chest.

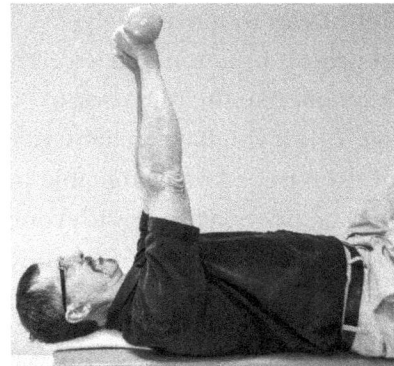

4. Push straight back up over chest and repeat.

- 2 sets of 12–15 repetitions
- Beginning weight: 5–8 lbs

AVOID PAIN!

Bench Press

The bench press allows for much heavier weights to be used than either the bench fly or the dumbbell press. In addition to providing more resistance to strengthen the chest muscles, the extra weight helps to restore backward bend movement to the upper back by flattening it against the bench. A flexed thoracic spine is generally one of the first areas of postural breakdown. A rolled bath towel placed under the head and running to the low back may relieve excess strain in the shoulder joints by allowing the shoulder blades to move freely.

A bench press is best done on a weight bench with a rack system like the one used for Olympic Squats (page 24). If you have no experience with this kind of exercise, a knowledgeable helper or "spotter" may be necessary. Lie with your feet on the bench on your towel with your spine and pelvis in neutral, with the chin slightly tucked. An Olympic bar, by itself, weighs 45 pounds. A solid, small diameter bar will weigh 20 to 25 pounds, and EZ curl bars will weigh anywhere from 15 to 25 pounds.

Begin with a total weight of 10 to 20 pounds. Grab the bar so that your hands are one and a half to two times the width of your shoulders. Lift the bar off the rack and bring it over your upper chest. Keep your wrists neutral. Do not let them bend forward or backwards. Keep the bar over your chest throughout the movement. Bring the bar down to your chest, letting the elbows move straight towards the floor. Lightly touch the bar to the breastbone before returning the bar to the start position. Check that the wrists remain in a straight or neutral position. Repeat the bench press. You can decrease the thickness of the towel if you feel unsteady.

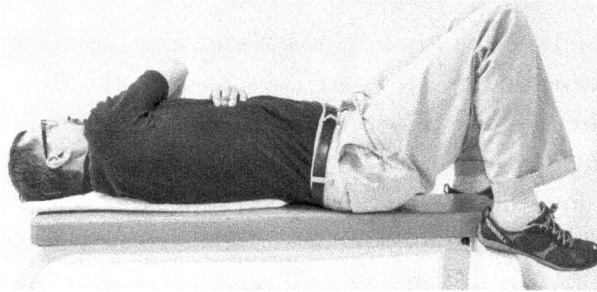

1. Lie with feet on bench with neutral back and chin slightly tucked. Place rolled bath towel under you.

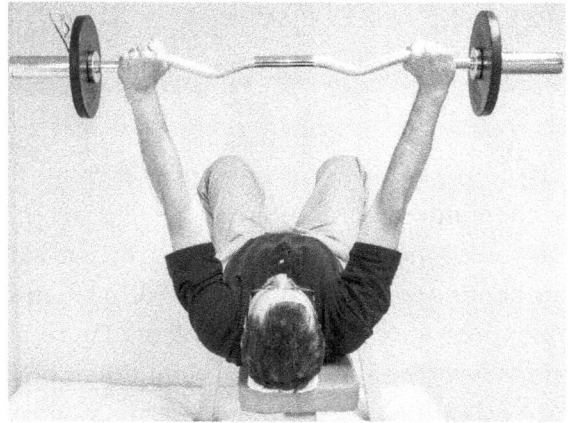

2. Lie on bench, arms straight with weights over chest.

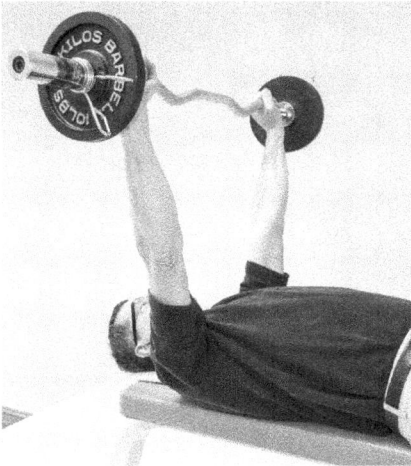

3. Bring bar over chest. Keep wrists neutral.

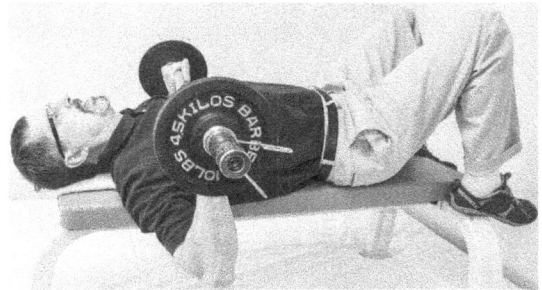

4. Slowly lower bar to lightly touch upper chest. Elbows move straight toward floor.

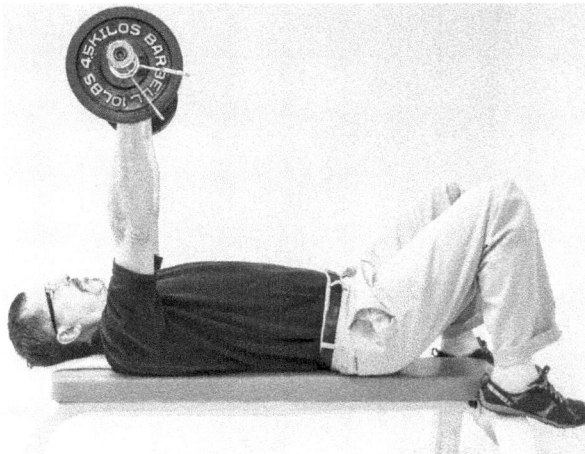

5. Return to start position.

> • 2 sets of 12–15 repetitions
> • Beginning weight: 10–20 lbs

AVOID PAIN!

Basic Push-ups

Basic push-ups are a very good exercise for the chest and upper arm muscles.

If your upper body is very weak, you can start with bent knee, chair, or even "wall push-ups." Sometimes wrist pain is a problem. There are various devices to hold on to when doing push-ups. You can try using five-pound dumbbells as a handle. On a soft surface, you might try doing push-ups on your knuckles.

For the basic floor push-up, start in the up position. Your elbows are straight but not locked, and your hands should be under your shoulders. Now slowly lower your chest towards the floor. In the down position, your upper arms will form a 45-degree angle to your body. Your chest will almost touch the floor. Keep your body straight through the movement and look towards floor. Practice the abdominal bridge or plank if you have trouble with this part. Since you cannot add resistance to this exercise, you can increase the repetitions.

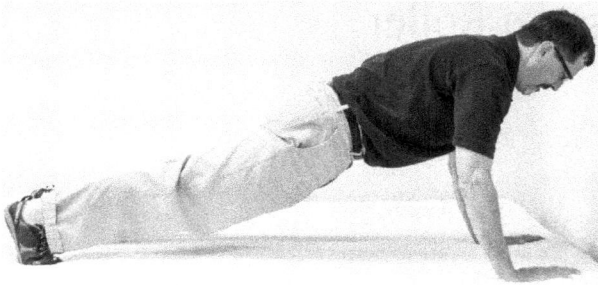

1. Up position with hands under shoulders and elbows straight. Look at floor.

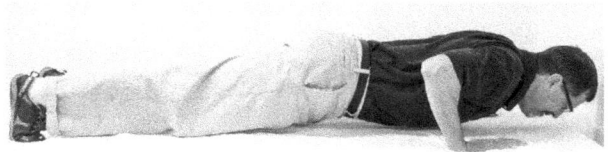

2. Down position with elbows bent and angled 45° away from body.

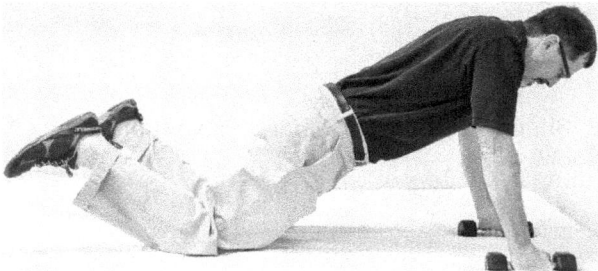

Bent knee pushup. In up position, use dumbbells if needed.

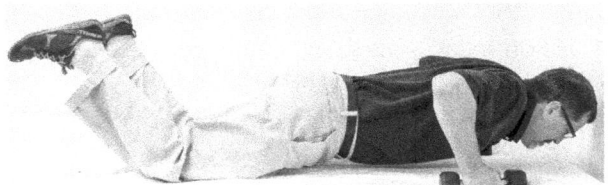

Bent knee pushup. Down position.

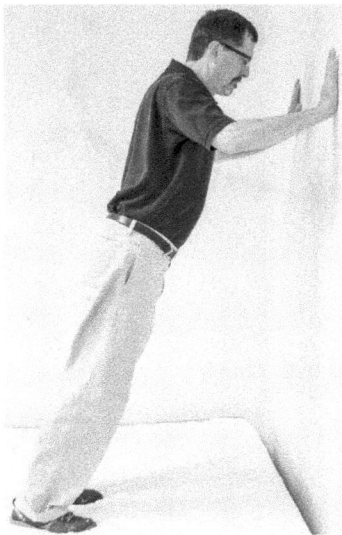

Wall pushup

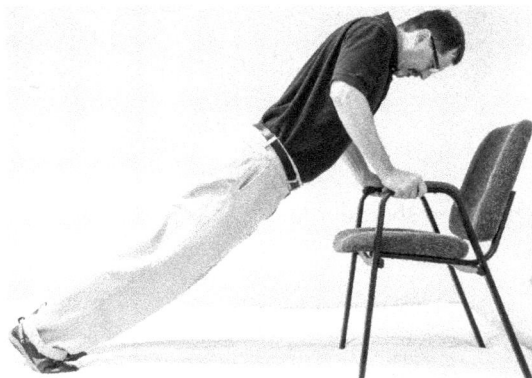

Incline pushup

- Do 2 sets of 12–15 repetitions
- Keep torso straight

AVOID PAIN!

© Brian Lambert

Dumbbell Press on Roller

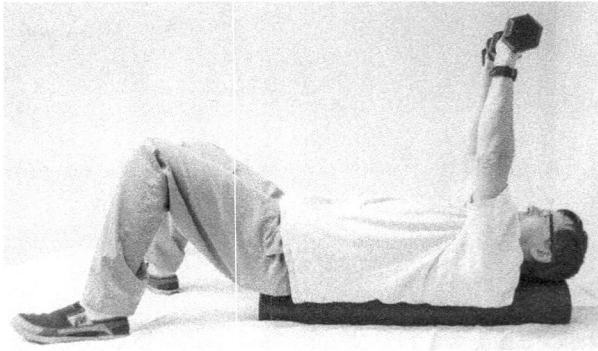

1. Lie on roller, arms straight with weights over chest. Find neutral low back.

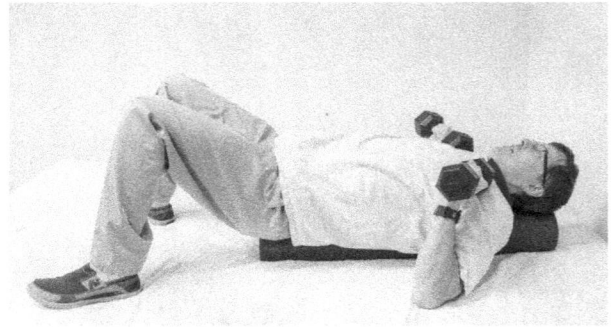

2. Bring weights down. Elbows move straight to floor.

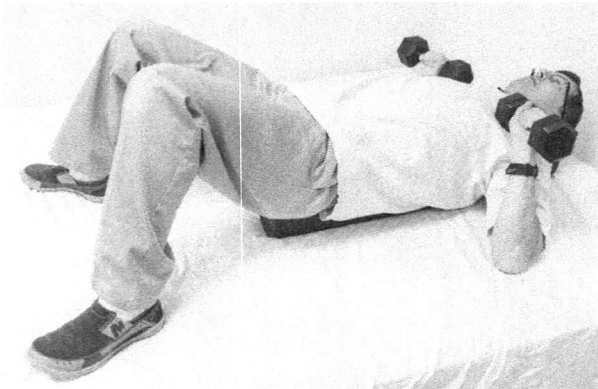

3. Weights will rest in crease between shoulder and chest muscles.

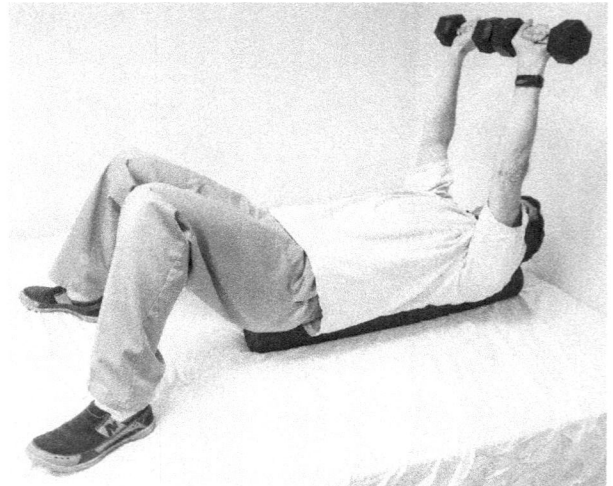

4. Push straight back up over chest.

- 2 sets of 12–15 repetitions
- Beginning weight: 5–8 lbs

AVOID PAIN!

Bench Fly on Foam Roller

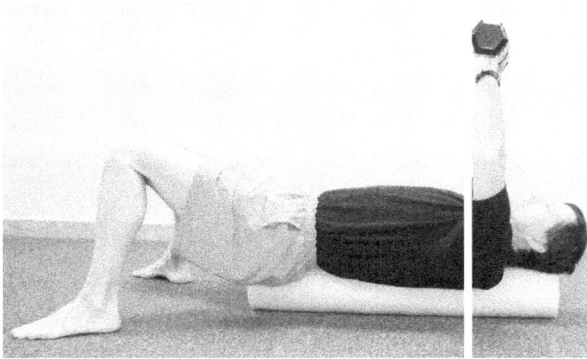

1. Lie with feet on floor. Find neutral low back. Hands aligned over chest, chin slightly tucked. Imagine the white line is a doorframe. Line up arm pits with doorframe.

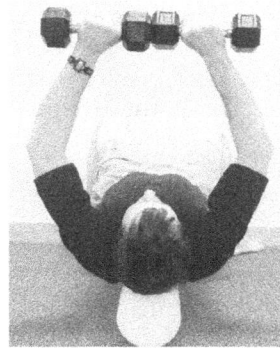

2. Arms in "Hug a Tree" position. Maintain a constant elbow angle.

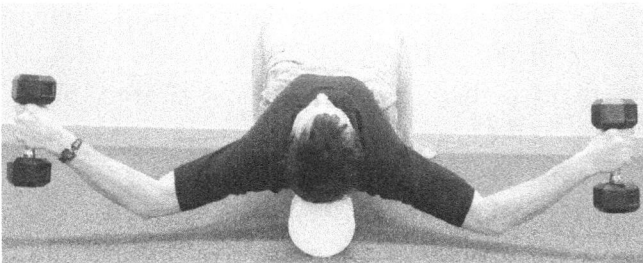

3. Let arms fall apart. Arms, elbows, and hands move as a solid unit.

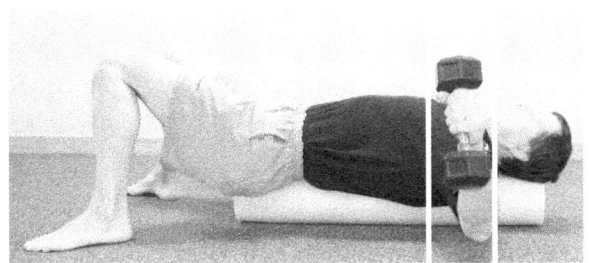

4. Maintain a straight line through hands, elbows, and shoulders. Stay in corridor.

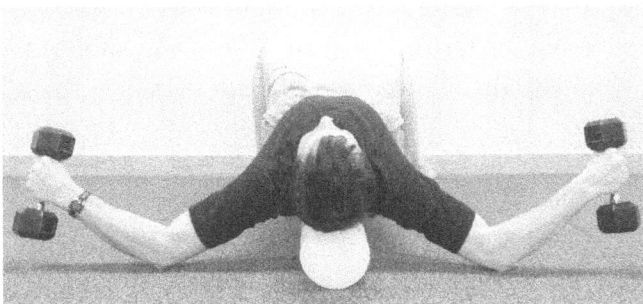

5. Squeeze shoulder blades together at bottom of movement.

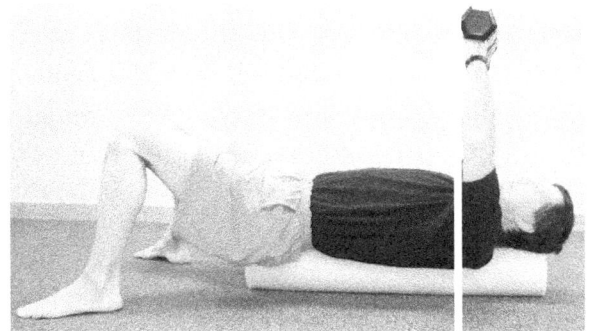

6. Return to start position and repeat.

- 2 sets of 12–15 repetitions
- Beginning weight: 3–5 lbs

AVOID PAIN!

Upper Body Exercises For The Lateral Shoulders

Doorframe Lateral Raise

This exercise targets the deltoid and rotator cuff muscles. Keep in mind that your scapular stabilizers and postural muscles are automatically engaged as soon as you pick up any object. You must try to use optimal positioning with this and any other exercise to reinforce good posture. This is especially important with exercises that you do when standing.

Begin with your back against a post or doorframe (being flat against a wall will interfere with shoulder blade movement). Your feet should be four to eight inches from the bottom of the doorframe and shoulder width apart. Find neutral spine and pelvis by moving from a 12 o'clock to a six o'clock tilt three or four times. Stop with the spine and pelvis at the midpoint of these movements. With the chin down so that you look straight ahead, push the back of your head towards the doorframe. Try to touch the back of your head to the doorframe or come as close as you can comfortably. This should position you fairly close to ideal posture. Standing against a doorframe or post will also prevent swinging, swaying, or other alterations of form that would degrade the exercise.

Generally start with three to five pounds of weight in each hand. Begin with the arms at your sides with the palms facing in. The thumb side of the hands should aim forward. Raise the arms straight out from your sides. Allow your arms to rotate so that when horizontal, the palms will face forward, and the thumb side of the hands will aim toward the ceiling. If you think of the dumbbells as flashlights, the beams would now point at the ceiling. The weights should be back far enough to be almost out of your peripheral vision. Keep the elbows soft, but do not allow them to bend to a significant degree. Slowly lower the arms, rotating them back to their starting point. Repeat the lateral raise. Raise arms only to horizontal. Remember to maintain the postural alignment throughout your 12 to 15 repetitions.

If lateral raises cause shoulder pain, raise the arms to 60 degrees instead of horizontal, or try very low-resistance upright rows (page 158). Usually after two or three weeks you should be able to do lateral raises without pain.

Hands almost out of sight.

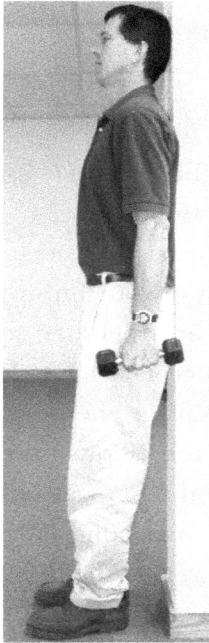

1. Stand with feet 4–8 inches from a doorframe. Look straight ahead with back of head against doorframe Start with neutral low back.

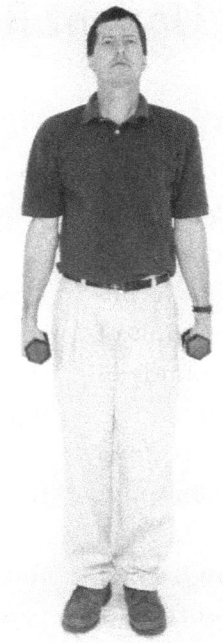

2. Start with palms facing inward.

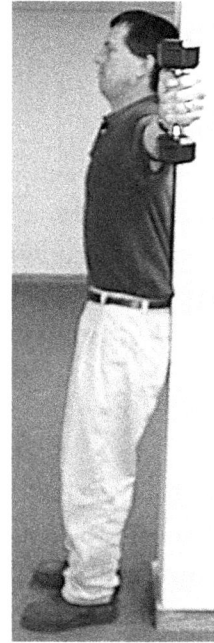

3. Raise arms straight out from sides. Rotate palms forward as arms come to horizontal.

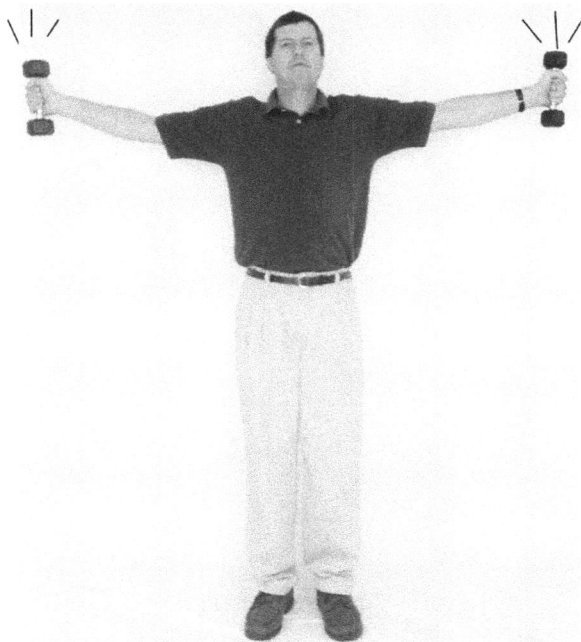

Point "flashlights" up

- 2 sets of 12–15 repetitions
- Beginning weight: 3–5 lbs

AVOID PAIN!

4. Keep elbows soft. Slowly lower to sides and derotate to starting position. Repeat.

Upright Row

This exercise targets the lateral deltoid, rotator cuff, and the upper trapezius region. The biceps may be recruited to some degree. The motion used with this exercise is similar to lifting a suitcase or groceries out of the trunk of an automobile. Begin with 15 to 20 pounds of weight.

Like the lateral raise, this exercise is done with your back against a doorframe or post. Your feet should be four to eight inches from the bottom of the doorframe, with the back of your head touching, or close to, the doorframe. Your chin is down so that your head is level and you are looking straight forward. Position your spine and pelvis in neutral.

Hold a dumbbell or bar in its center so that it hangs down in front of your hips with elbows straight. Your hands are together so that the thumb and index fingers of each hand are touching. Do the "row" by raising the weight straight up. Begin by moving the elbows upward. Keep the weight as close to the body as possible. Lift the bar or weight to collarbone height. Lower the weight slowly, and repeat the lift. If you have pain, lift within a range of motion that is comfortable and/or use a lighter weight.

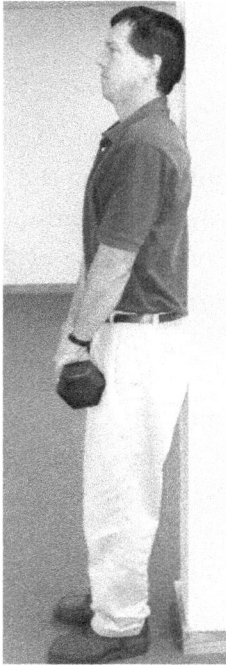

1. Stand with feet 4–8 inches from a doorframe. Look straight ahead with back of head against doorframe. Establish neutral low back.

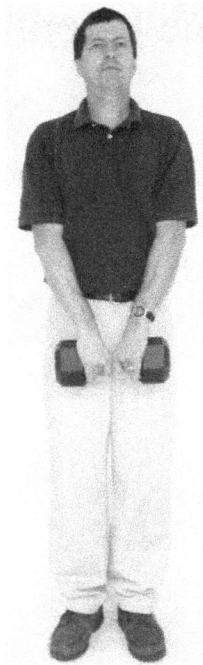

2. Grab weight or bar in center.

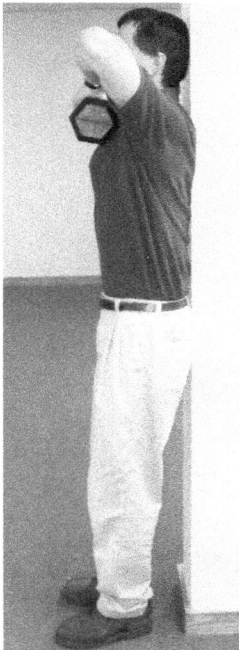

3. Lift by moving elbows up, pulling weight to collar bone.

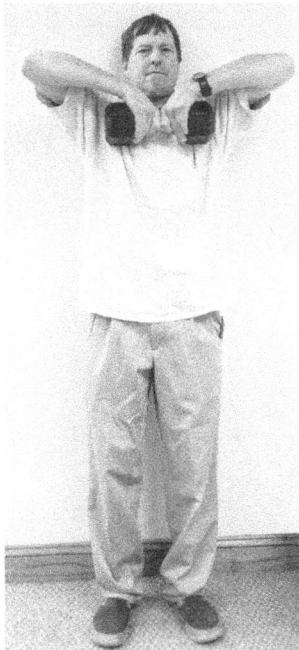

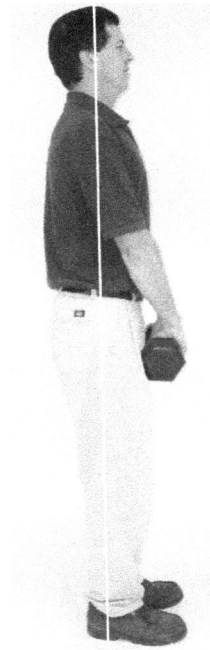

4. Lower slowly and repeat.

- 2 sets of 12–15 repetitions
- Beginning weight: 15–20 lbs

AVOID PAIN!

© Brian Lambert

Incline Lateral Raise

Another lateral shoulder exercise is done on an incline bench in a side-lying position. Start with three to five pounds. Use an incline bench set at a 30- to 45- degree angle. Position yourself on the incline bench in a side-lying position. Support your head on the downside arm. The other arm holds a weight resting palm down on the top hipbone. The pelvis and spine are generally neutral.

Raise the arm as a unit, keeping the palm facing downward and elbow soft. Maximum motion is 90 to 100 degrees from the side of the body. Try to avoid any rotation in the shoulder. Slowly lower the weight to lightly touch the hipbone, and repeat the lift. This exercise can be done without a bench by leaning over the arm of an overstuffed chair or sitting sideways in a recliner.

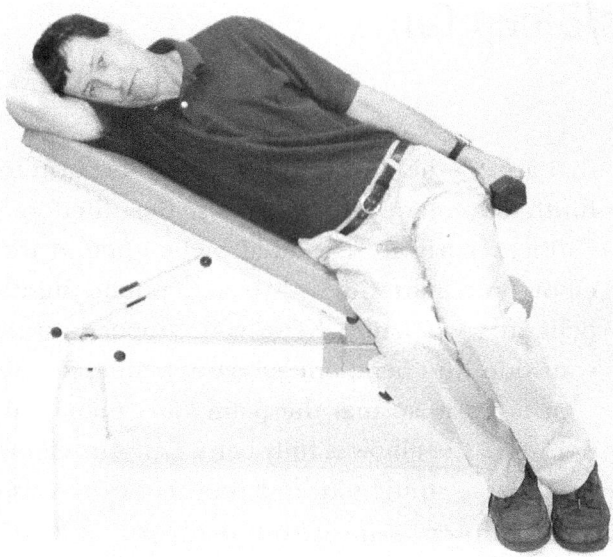

1. Lie on your side on 45° incline bench. Support head on inside arm. Neutral low back.

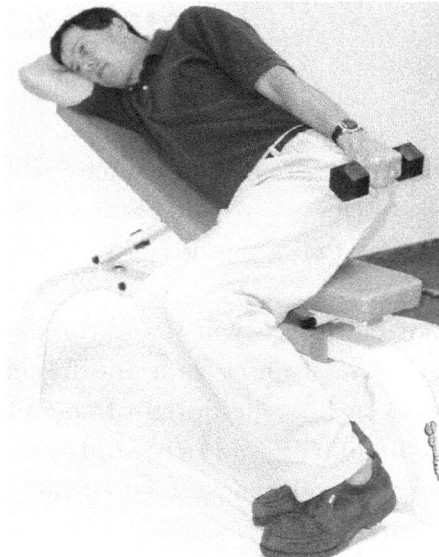

2. Weight is resting on hip with palm facing downward

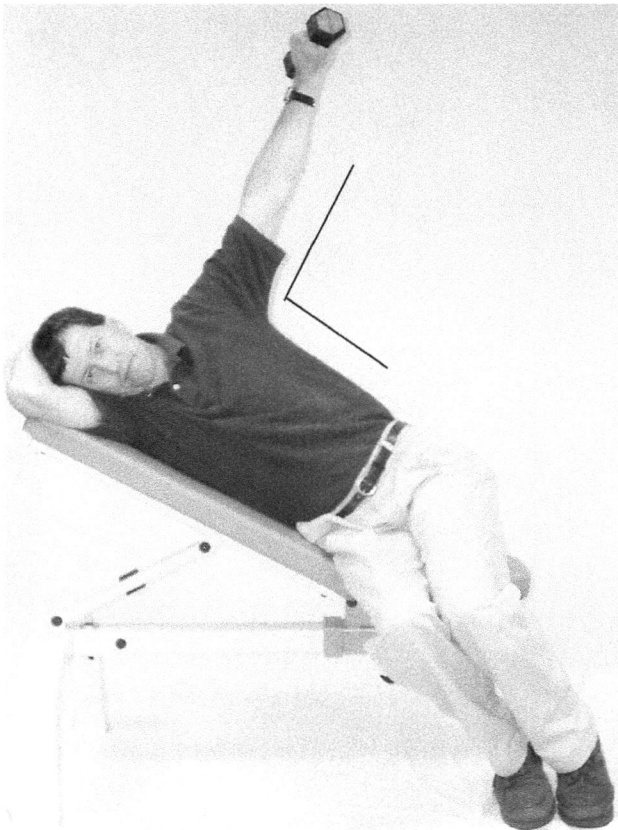

3. Raise weight to 90°–100° from body. Keep palm facing downward and elbow soft.

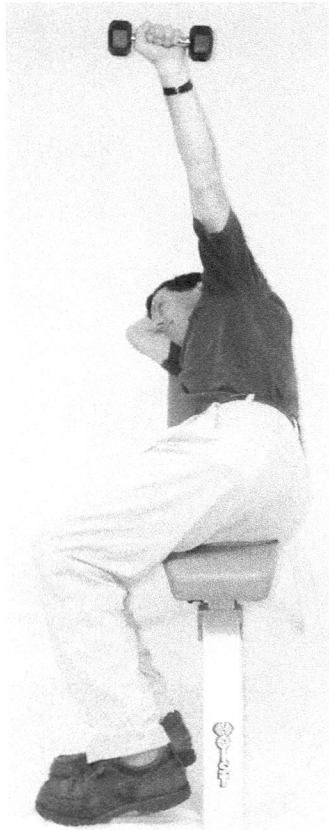

4. Keep arm aligned with hip. Lower slowly and repeat.

- 2 sets of 12–15 repetitions
- Beginning weight: 3–5 lbs

AVOID PAIN!

Frontal Raises/Bicep Curls

A variation on the doorframe exercise will strengthen the muscles in the front of the shoulder. Start with three to five pounds of weight in each hand.

Position yourself, just as you would for the upright row and lateral raises, in a doorframe or with your back against the upright frame of an exercise machine. With your pelvis and spine in neutral and your head against the doorframe with the chin down, alternately raise one arm at a time to a 90-degree position. The palms usually face downward with the elbows soft. Return that arm to the start position. Allow one arm to finish movement before you raise the other one.

Bicep curls are executed by bending at the elbow only. Start with five- to eight-pound dumbbells in each hand. Keep your upper arm at your side, and bend one elbow at a time. Rotate your forearm so that the palm faces the shoulder when the elbow is fully bent. Let your elbow completely straighten and repeat the exercise with the other arm. If you like bicep curls, try incline bicep curls (page 168).

Frontal Raises

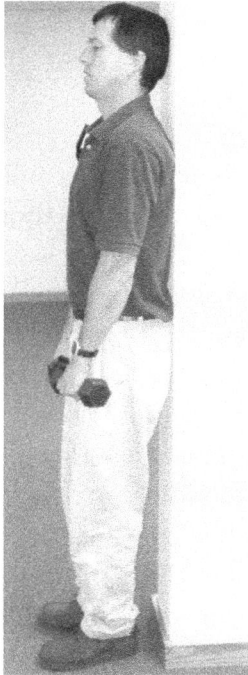

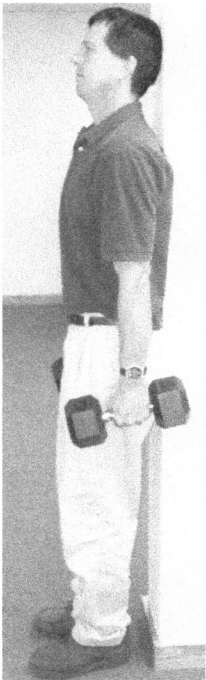

1. Neutral low back. Raise one arm at a time to 90°.

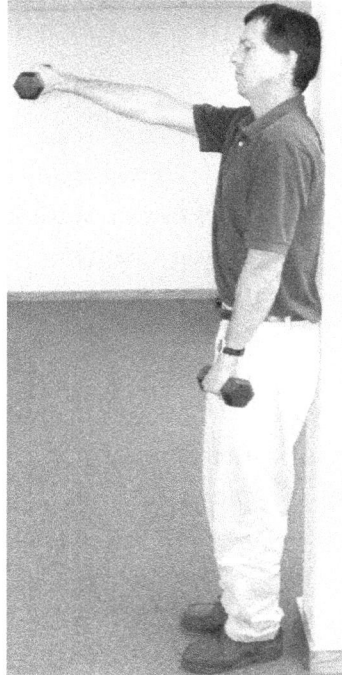

2. Keep elbows soft and palms down

Bicep Curls

Bend elbows one at a time.

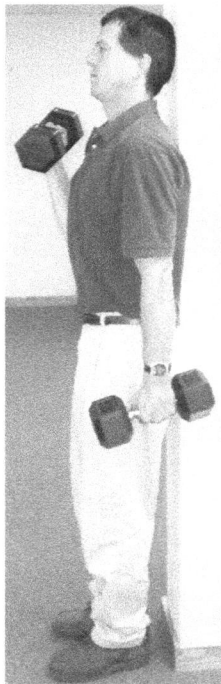

- 2 sets of 12–15 repetitions per arm
- Start with 3–5 lbs: Frontal Raises
- 5–8 lbs for Bicep Curls

AVOID PAIN!

Overhead Dumbbell Press

One more lateral shoulder exercise is also done standing in a doorframe or against a post. Begin with three to five pounds. If you have a history of shoulder pain or restrictions in shoulder movement, you may want to skip this exercise.

Stand in a doorframe or with your back against the outside corner where two walls meet. Your feet should be four to eight inches from the wall. Find the neutral position for your low back and pelvis by moving them from a six o'clock tilt to the 12 o'clock and stopping midway between the extremes of the motions. Look straight ahead with your head pushed back as far as it will comfortably go.

Start with your elbows bent and your upper arms by your sides. The ends of dumbbells should almost touch your shoulders. This exercise can be done as a double-arm, or single-arm raise.

For the single-arm raise, slowly push one dumbbell straight up overhead and then return to the start position. Repeat the movement with the other arm. Continue so that each arm completes 12 to 15 repetitions. Rest thirty to sixty seconds and do another set.

For the double arm raise, slowly push both dumbbells towards the ceiling, then slowly return them to the start position. Again, complete 12 to 15 repetitions. Rest and do a second set.

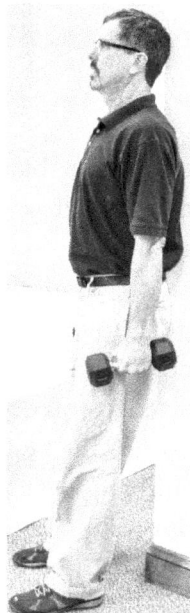

1. Stand with feet 4–8 inches from doorframe. Look straight ahead. Find neutral lower back.

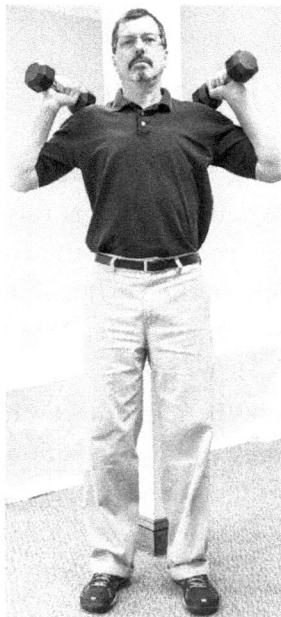

2. Start with elbows bent so that weights almost touch shoulders.

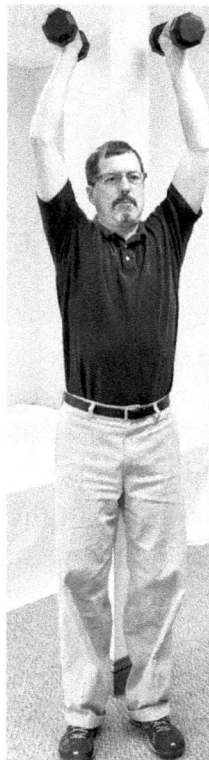

3. Either push both weights straight up overhead.

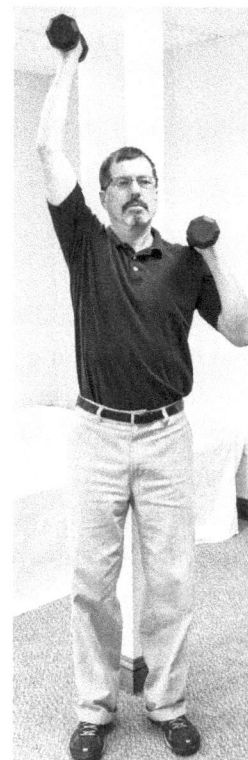

4. Or do one arm at a time. Alternate sides.

- Keep low back neutral
- Do not do this exercise if it causes pain
- 12–15 repetitions
- Beginning weight: 3–5 lbs

AVOID PAIN!

Exercises for the Serratus Anterior, Triceps, and Biceps

Supine Elbow Extension

The serratus anterior is a large flat muscle that attaches along the side of the rib cage below the arm pit and runs around the back of the rib cage, under the shoulder blade, to attach along the front inside edge of the shoulder blade. This muscle holds the shoulder blade against the rib cage and tilts it upward to angle the ball and socket with its attending rotator cuff and deltoid muscles upward as the arm is raised. Poor functioning of the serratus anterior means that the rotator cuff has to work harder every time you move your arm.

A poorly functioning serratus anterior is generally the result of faulty posture and all its accompanying mechanical problems in the neck, upper back, and rib cage. The serratus anterior muscle is one of the most neglected muscles in the upper body. Insufficient functioning of this muscle is probably responsible for many rotator cuff tears and inflammation of the tendons (tendonitis) and bursa (bursitis) of the shoulder.

The supine elbow extension exercise will help retrain poorly operating serratus anterior and tricep muscles. Common tricep exercises such as "kick backs" and "push downs" only work two parts of the triceps, the short and lateral heads that attach to the upper arm. When done correctly, the supine elbow extension exercise will recruit the serratus anterior and all three parts of the triceps. The third part of the triceps is the long head that attaches to the shoulder blade. When the arm is raised, the third head works in synergy with the rotator cuff muscles, and it assists the serratus anterior muscle by pulling the shoulder blade to help angle it upward.

Start with two to three pounds of weight. Lie on a bench with your feet supported. If you don't have a bench, position yourself across the bed or on a couch so that your arm will hang over the edge. Bring one upper arm to a position beside your head even with your eye. Bend the elbow, letting the lower arm hang straight down over the edge of the bench or bed.

Stabilize the upper arm in this position by monitoring and/or holding it with the opposite hand. Slowly straighten the elbow to a gently locked position, and then slowly let it bend to return to its start position. Work should be felt along the triceps into the outside edge of the shoulder blade below the armpit.

If pain or a pinching sensation occurs in the top of the shoulder, move the upper arm to a more vertical position even with your chin and repeat the exercise. Keep the upper arm absolutely stationary while the elbow is moving. The upper arm should be kept close to your head.

As the exercise gets easier, the upper arm will be positioned more horizontally to provide more activation of the serratus anterior and triceps. Do two sets of 12 to 15 repetitions.

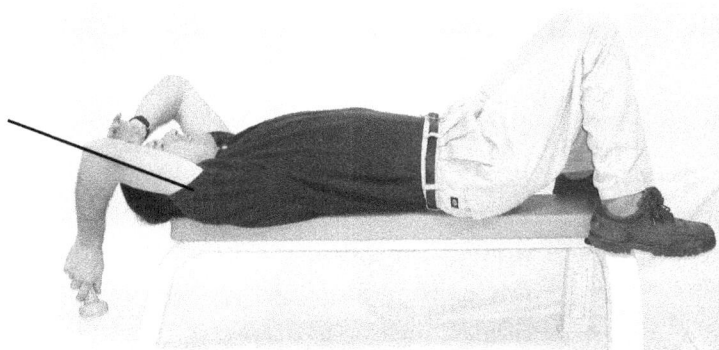

1. Lie on bench, bed, or couch so that arm can hang over head. Upper arm beside head and next to eye.

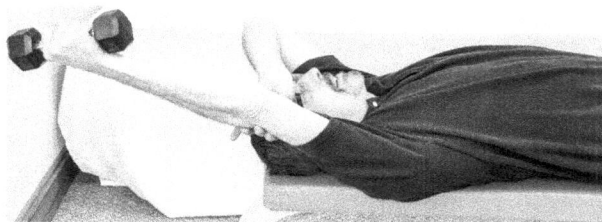

2. Straighten and gently lock elbow. Do not let upper arm move. Relax to start position. If comfortable, do repetitions in this position.

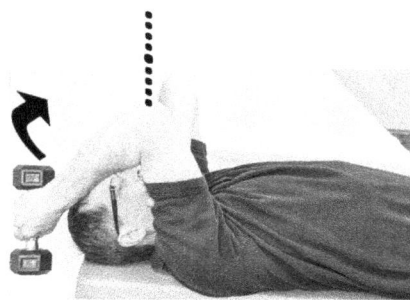

3. If there is pain, stabilize upper arm vertically, and repeat elbow extension.

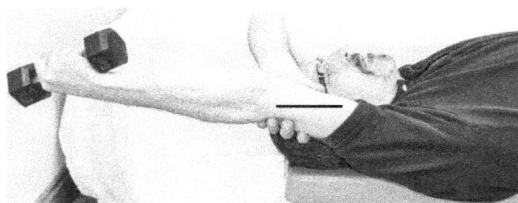

4. If tricep is working well, position upper arm horizontally, and repeat elbow extension.

- Keep upper arm stationary
- Find best position for upper arm to best work tricep
- 2 sets of 12–15 repetitions
- Beginning weight: 2–3 lbs

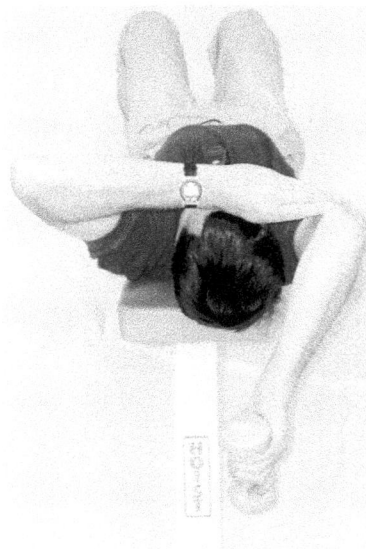

5. Keep upper arm close to head. Monitor with opposite hand.

Incline Bicep Curl

Incline biceps curls work to strengthen the biceps, as well as provide a stretch for the chest and shoulders. Generally start with five to eight pounds.

Lie on your back on a 45 degree incline bench with the low back and pelvis in neutral and the chin slightly tucked. Your arms will hang straight down beside the bench with elbows straight. Alternately bend each elbow. Keep the upper arm stationary. Bring the weight all the way to your shoulder. Move only one arm at a time. Continue to do two sets of 12 to 15 repetitions for each arm.

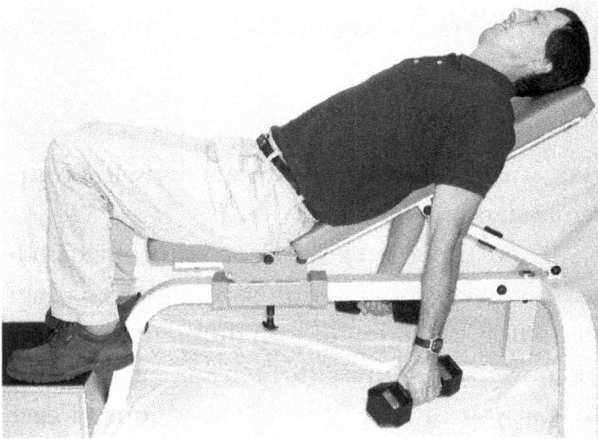

1. Lie on 45° incline bench with low back neutral, chin slightly tucked, and arms hanging down.

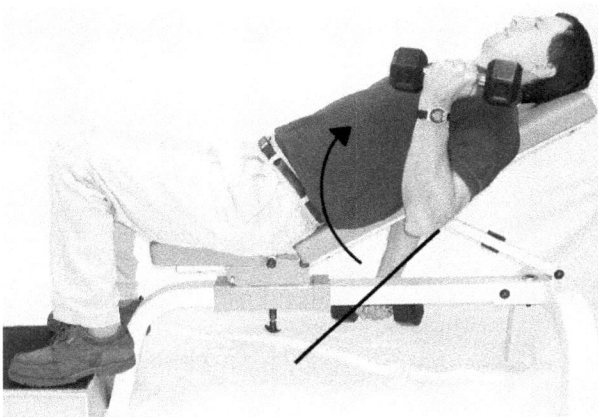

2. Alternately bend at the elbows. Keep upper arm stationary.

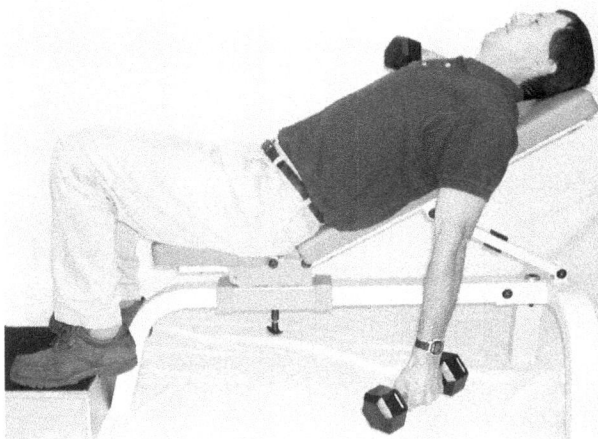

3. Repeat on other side.

- 2 sets of 12–15 repetitions
- Beginning weight: 5–8 lbs

AVOID PAIN!

Latex Band Exercises for the Shoulders

Since dumbbells are heavy, they are not the ideal piece of exercise equipment to take on out of town trips. Latex band (or tubing) is lightweight and portable, and can be a very good substitute for free weights. A disadvantage of exercising with latex bands is that it may be harder to correctly use your postural muscles. An advantage to exercising with latex bands is that you can work on different muscle groups while standing or sitting.

When using latex band or even old bicycle tubing, always work within your pain-free range of motion. Experiment with different directions of movement. Adjust the tension of the band so that you can do 12 to 15 repetitions in each direction.

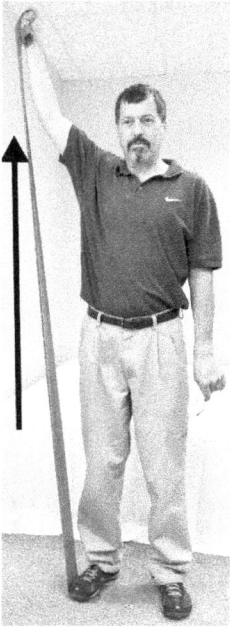

To side

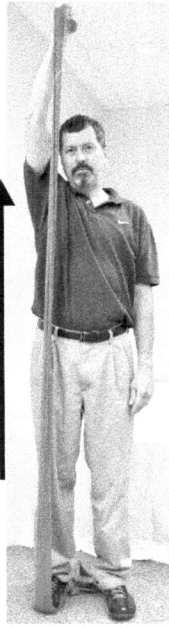

To front

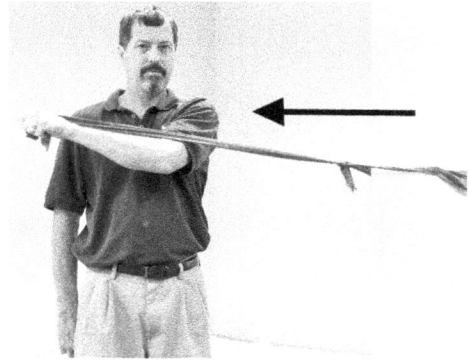

Across body

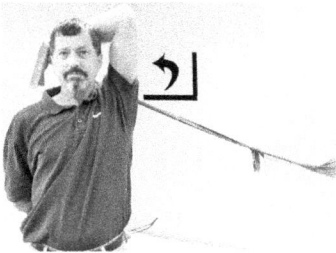

Behind head

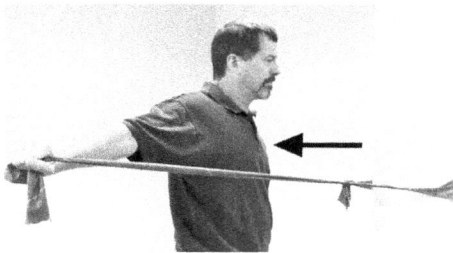

Abduction

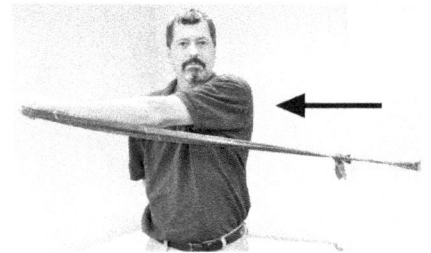

Adduction

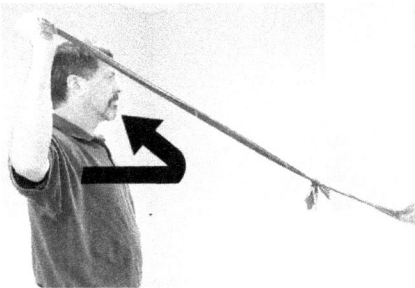

External rotation

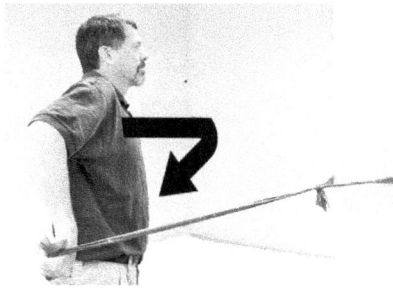

Internal rotation

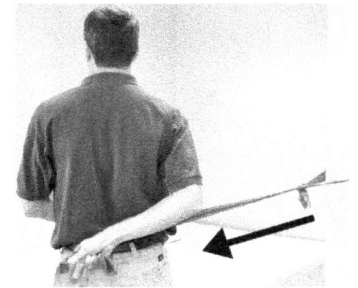

Behind back

- 2 sets of 12–15 repetitions
- Use comfortable resistance

AVOID PAIN!

VII

Foam Roller Exercises

The use of foam rollers (or logs) has become commonplace in many physical therapy clinics and fitness centers. They come in different sizes but the six by thirty-six inch version seems to be the most useful. You can purchase foam rollers through online vendors or directly from physical therapy clinics.

Rumor has it that foam rollers were used as packing material for a piece of equipment that was delivered to a physical therapy office. Physical therapists tend to be imaginative people. They figured out various exercises that could be done on the rollers and the rest is history. Physical therapists, however, don't have a monopoly on imagination. Once there was a plumber who was given a foam roller to use for his very tight thoracic spine. He said that the exercises on the roller felt great but he returned it during his follow-up visit. He explained that he had glued some carpet on a piece of plastic pipe and was able to do his exercises on his homemade roller. If you can't take a roller with you when you travel, use your imagination. Improvise with rolled up towels or blankets. Clients have reported that some hotels have rollers in their fitness centers.

In the following pages are various foam roller exercises. These exercises should feel good and/or cause "good pain." To avoid injury, do not push on the side of the lower rib cage and do not push on your neck. Techniques on the roller include; rolling back and forth, stretching or draping over the roller, and massaging by moving side to side or in a circular motion on a small area. Generally, anything that feels good is probably a good exercise.

Foam Roller Technique
Lengthwise Version

A 36- by 6-inch foam roller is a wonderful tool for loosening the spine and for massaging the back muscles. There are several basic techniques that can be modified to suit individual needs. The lengthwise version is a good starting point for most people.

The lengthwise version is started by lying on a foam roller so you that are supported from your tailbone to your head. Bend your knees so your feet are flat and 12 to 24 inches apart. If just lying on the roller feels good, you can relax on it for eight to ten minutes, and/or gently move a little from side to side.

Relax for a few seconds centered on the roller with your arms resting on the floor at your sides. Now perform a moderate 12 o'clock tilt, slightly tuck your chin, and raise your arms over your head, keeping your elbows almost straight. You should feel a comfortable stretch through the arms and sides of the rib cage. Limit your motion if pain occurs in the top of the shoulders. Moving the arms farther apart may also alleviate discomfort, as will pointing the thumbs towards the floor. Hold the stretch for 15 to 20 seconds then return your arms to the floor.

To position for a diagonal stretch, first stabilize your trunk on the roller by resting your arms on the floor at your sides. Shift your hips to the left so that the left side of your pelvis is only one inch off center. Straighten your left hip and knee. Keep your heel on the floor. For better balance, move your leg six to eight inches to the left. Move your upper body to the right so that your head and shoulders are shifted no more than one inch to the right. Rest your head against the side of the roller just behind your left ear. Raise your arms over your head. Adjust your right, left, and diagonal positioning so that you are perfectly balanced and draped across the roller. Do not do a 12 o'clock tilt.

Hold this position for 15 to 20 seconds. Bring your arms back, move to the center position, and repeat the stretch on the opposite diagonal. If these stretches feel good, they can be repeated several times per session and several times per day. The main objective of these stretches is to restore mobility in the rib cage and thoracic spine. Many of the muscles in this area run at oblique angles so they are ideally stretched with twisting movements. If you want more aggressive stretches, try the thoracic spine technique (page 186) and the techniques that use the end of the roller (pages 182 and 184). If the roller is too uncomfortable or awkward, try the towel roll (page 78).

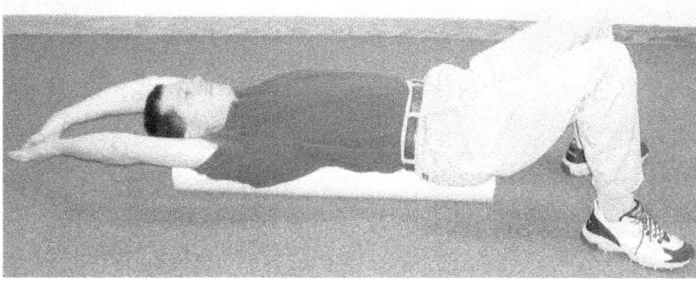

Lengthwise Version

1. Chin tucked and tummy tight with flat back

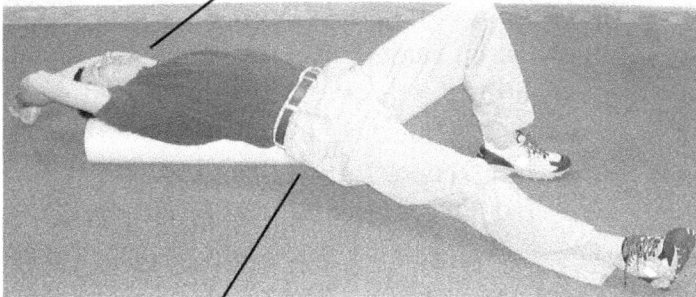

Diagonal Version

2a. Move head beside roller, 1 inch off center.

2b. Move opposite hip 1 inch off center with knee straight.

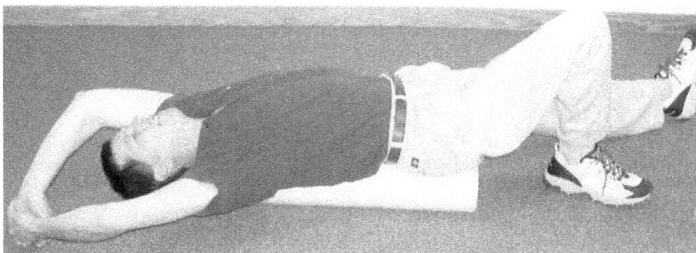

3. Drape body over roller. Find relaxed position.

- Repeat each posiiton 1–3 times
- 15–20 seconds per position

AVOID PAIN!

Foam Roller
Bottom-Down Technique

Our upper back or the thoracic spine has some degree of natural forward bend or kyphosis. Because almost all of our normal activities keep us bent, the kyphosis tends to increase. And it's not just the back that is bent. It's the whole upper torso: spine, rib cage, and all of the attendant muscles. This is why we become stooped as we get older. Age by itself doesn't bend people over. It's what we do that bends us over. Foam roller exercises can help you restore backward-bend mobility to the upper torso.

For a beginning backward-bend exercise, sit on the floor with your knees bent. Place the roller behind and perpendicular to your body so that when you lean back, you will contact the roller at the bottom of your shoulder blades. Start farther up your back if the pressure from the roller is too much. Put your laced fingers behind, and hold your head keeping your forearms close to your head. Look towards the ceiling. Gently lean back about five degrees and hold. Individual vertebrae will only bend backward about five degrees, so do not try to touch the back of your head to the floor. After 20 seconds, move the roller one inch up your back, and again lean back for 20 seconds. Continue up your back in one-inch increments, holding 20 seconds/inch. Work your way up to the base of your neck or as high as you can get with the roller sliding out. You can make two to three trips up and down your back. If one direction is easier, then only go in that direction. If the roller is too hard, then use a flat pillow, towel, or blanket over the roller. For more aggressive work, look at some of the other foam roller exercises.

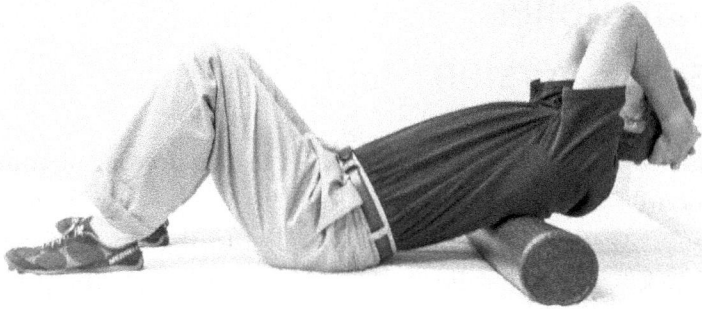

1. Lean against roller so it is even with bottom of shoulder blades. Support head with arms close to head.

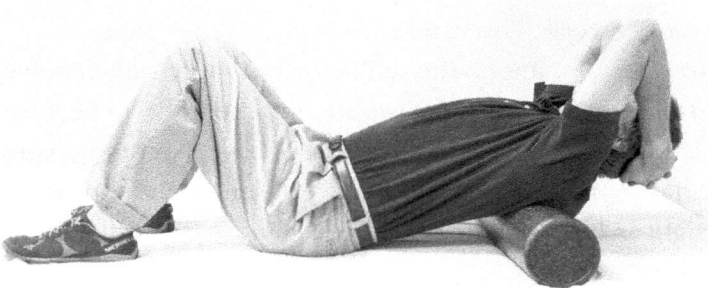

2. Look at ceiling, and lean back 5°. Hold for 20 seconds, then move roller one inch up back. Hold for 20 seconds.

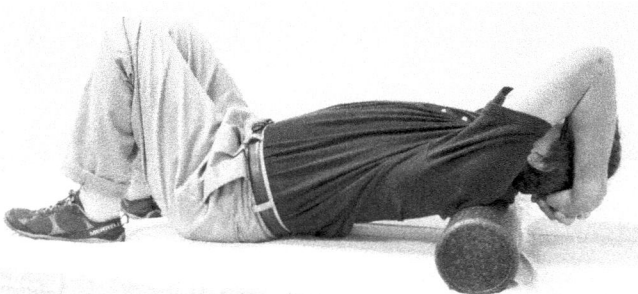

3. Work up to base of neck in one-inch increments. Keep elbows pointed up and look at ceiling.

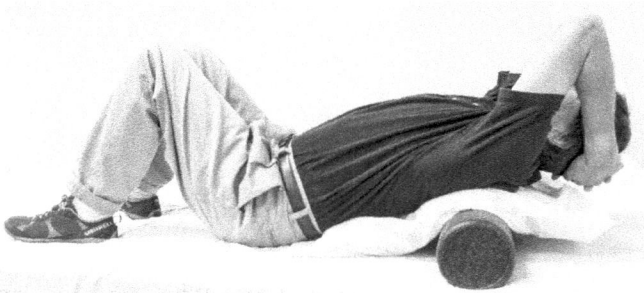

4. Pillow option

- Return to start position
- Do 2–3 repetitions

AVOID PAIN!

Foam Roller
Crosswise Version

This version of the foam-roller exercise is generally good for improving backward-bend mobility of the thoracic spine.

Start by sitting on the floor and leaning back over a 36- by 6-inch foam roller so that it's positioned across the lower part of your shoulder blades. Lace your fingers behind your head and point your elbows toward the ceiling so your forearms are touching the sides of your head. Bend your knees and position your feet flat on the floor 12 to 18 inches apart.

Lift your bottom off the floor into a bridge position. Let your head back so you look straight at the ceiling. Now pull with your legs to move the roller slowly to the top of your shoulder blades. You may need to lift your bottom up a little higher, or you will feel the roller sliding out from under you. Now slowly push with your legs to move the roller down to the bottom of your rib cage. You may need to lower your bottom to keep your trunk parallel to the floor. If you get the roller too far down your back, the pressure may be uncomfortable. Generally do not go below ribcage level. Repeat the rolling motion, and return the roller to the top of your shoulders. This can be done eight to ten times.

Now do the rolling technique at slight angles. Move your feet two steps to the right. Repeat the rolling motion described above. Now move your feet two steps to the left of center and repeat the movement. Try to keep your torso parallel to the floor.

If you find that the roller is too uncomfortable or too hard, place a folded towel or long flat pillow between you and the roller.

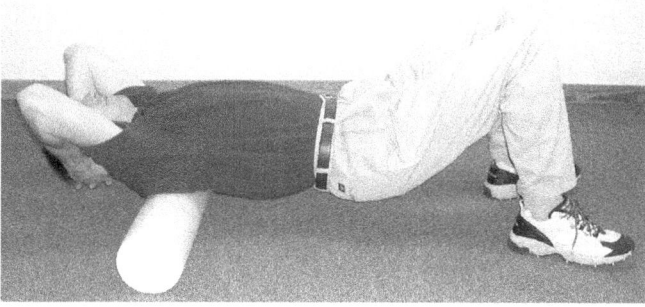

1. Support head. Body parallel to floor.

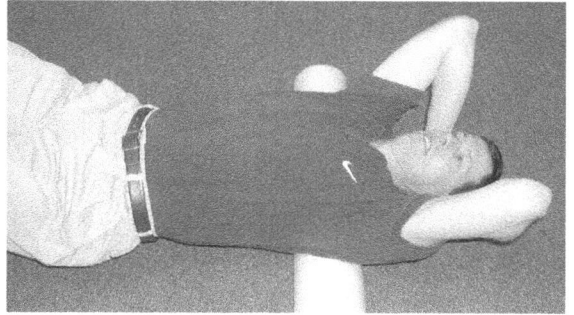

2. Look at ceiling. Roll from bottom of shoulder blades to base of neck.

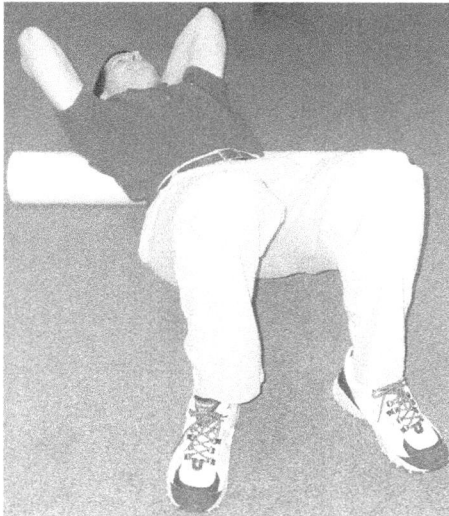

3. Slight angle of body

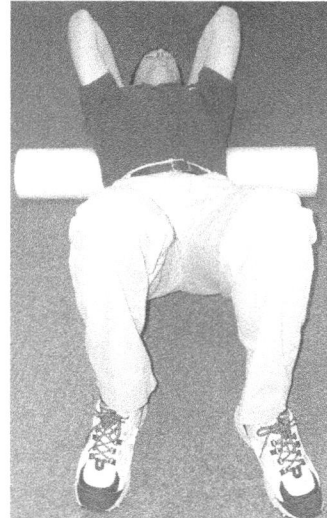

4. Do not go below bottom of rib cage.

• 8–10 rolls each direction

AVOID PAIN!

Foam Roller
Lumbar Spine Technique

This technique may be good for you if there are extension or backward-bending restrictions in the low back, or if you tend to have a very flat spine. Do not use this exercise if you have a sway back or any lower back instability.

Sit on the floor. Pull the roller against the back of your pelvis and base of your spine. Hold the roller against your pelvis as you lean backwards over it, then rest the forearms on the roller. Lean backwards only five degrees. Hold this position for 20 seconds, then move the roller one inch up your back. Hold for another 20 seconds. Repeat this process to work your way to the bottom of the shoulder blades. From here, either work back down your back or put your hands behind your head and continue as described in the "bottom down technique" (page 176). As with other foam roller techniques, if needed, use a flat pillow, folded blanket, or towel between you and the roller.

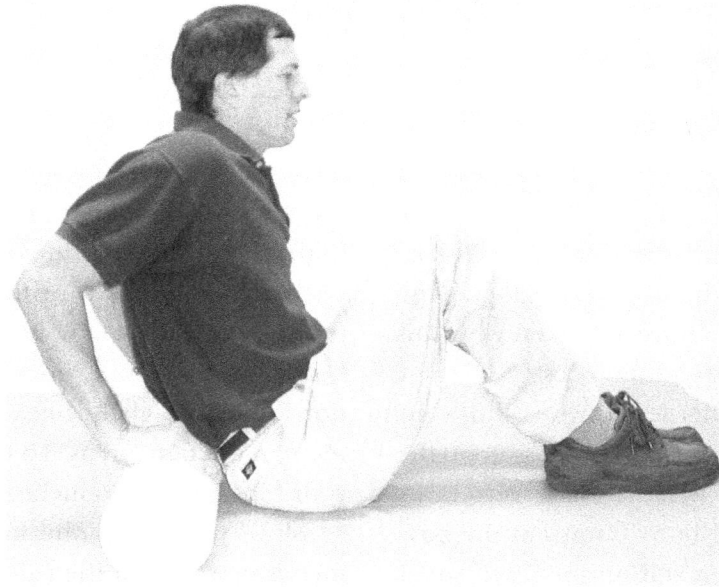

1. Pull roller tight against pelvis.

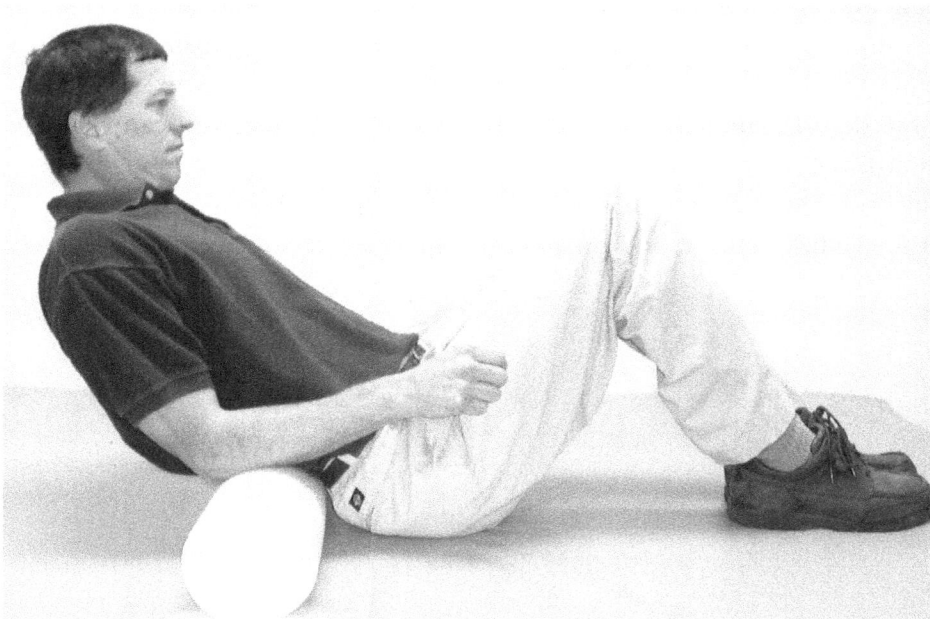

2. Rest forearms on roller. Lean back 5°. Hold for 20 seconds. Move roller 1 inch up back and hold again. Work way up to shoulder blades.

AVOID PAIN!

Foam Roller
Head Off End Technique

This technique is helpful if backward-bend movement is restricted at the very top of the thoracic spine. Long-term restrictions in backward bending will cause a "hump" to develop at the base of the neck. Care must be taken with this exercise not to over-extend the neck.

Lie on the foam roller lengthwise. With your finger tips, find the spinous processes of the seventh cervical and first thoracic vertebrae. These are the first big bony bumps at the base of your neck. Move yourself on the foam roller until the edge of the roller is one half to three quarters of an inch below the first thoracic vertebra. Do not push directly on your neck. Lace your fingers together and hold your head. Move the pelvis and lumbar spine into a 12 o'clock or posterior tilt.

Tuck the chin slightly, and let your head and neck move towards the floor. Keep the head in a retracted position and level. You should be looking straight at the ceiling. This should provide a feeling of pressure or stretch in the spine near the edge of the roller. Try turning your head slightly to one side or the other to find the most restricted spot. Hold this position for fifteen to twenty seconds. It may be helpful to pull your head away from your shoulders to provide a traction force through the neck to enhance the movement in the tight areas. To increase the force, lift your hips one to two inches off the roller.

Move your body one half to three quarters inches upwards on the roller. The roller should now be one half to three quarters of an inch lower on your spine than where it was started. Retighten the 12 o'clock tilt, re-tuck the chin, and let your head and neck down again. Play with positioning from one side to the other. Try combining this exercise with the thoracic spine technique. You can repeat the technique through the top six to eight inches of the thoracic spine. The next technique may provide a more aggressive approach.

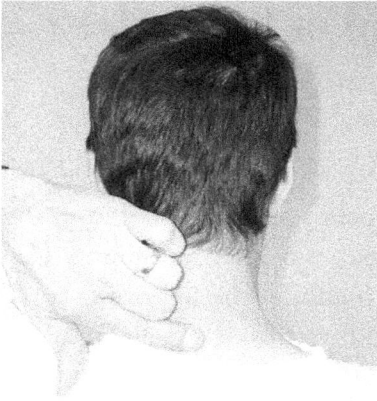

Find largest "bumps" at base of neck. These are spinous processes of C7 and T1.

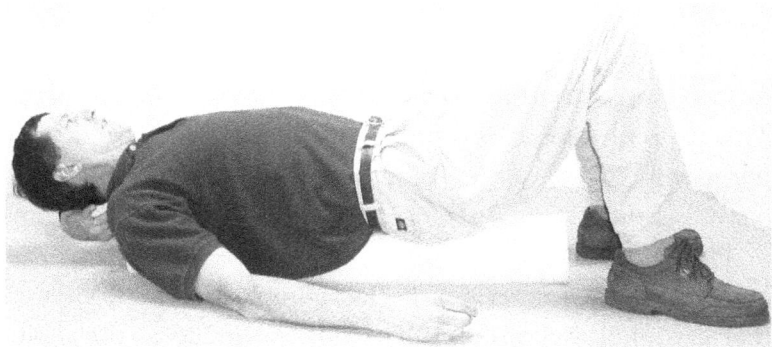

1. Lie on roller. Slide up roller so that edge of roller is ½ inch–¾ inch below the "bumps." Support head.

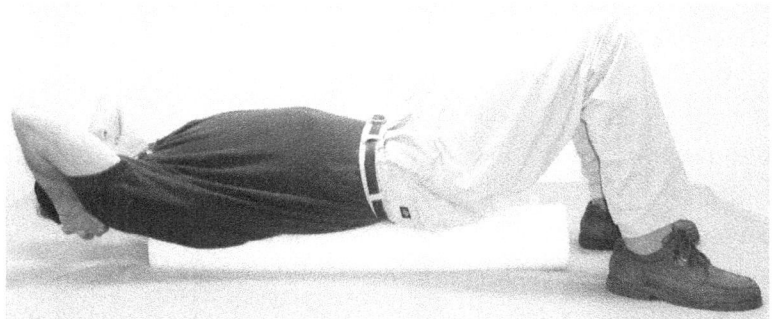

2. Do a 12:00 posterior tilt. While keeping head level, let your head sink to floor. Keep head level.

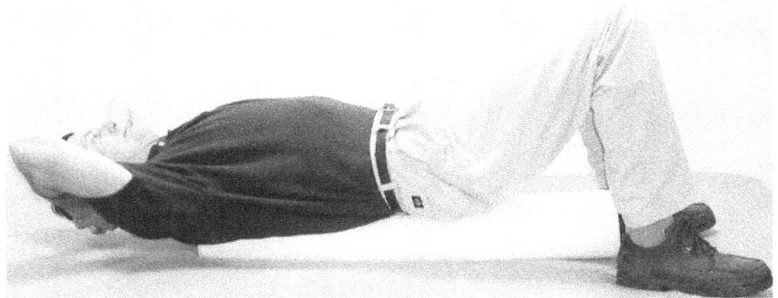

3. Hold position for 15–20 seconds. Stretch should be felt in space at edge of roller. Move slightly to right or left and hold again. Move ½ inch–¾ inch below the C7/T1 "bump."

AVOID PAIN!

Upper Thoracic Extension with the Edge of the Roller

A hump at the base of the neck begins when two or more vertebrae are stuck bent forward. This exercise works to restore backward-bending mobility to these flexed vertebrae to eliminate the hump.

Place the roller on the floor so that one end is against a wall. Lie on your back on the floor so that the other end of the roller contacts the big bumps at the base of your neck. Do not push directly on your neck. Let the back of your head rest on the roller. Your arms are at your sides and knees are bent.

You should feel comfortable pressure on the upper thoracic vertebrae (*i.e.,* the hump). Use padding on the end of the roller and a pillow under your head if needed. For at least 20 seconds, gently rock back and forth by pushing with your legs. If rocking is uncomfortable, then relax and take a few slow deep breaths. Move one inch down your back, away from your neck, and repeat 20 seconds of gentle rocking or deep breaths. Continue this process to work your way six to eight inches down your spine.

To loosen the back part of the rib cage and the deep back muscles, position the end of the roller one to two inches below the "bumps," and then two to three inches to the left of the spine (*i.e.,* move your body to the right). Put your left hand on your right shoulder. Push against the floor with your right arm to keep the back of the right shoulder five to six inches off the floor. Again, gently push with the feet to cause a rocking motion to massage the deep muscles and to push the back of the rib cage in the direction of the pelvis. Massage tender/tight areas for at least 20 seconds. Move down an inch and repeat. Move to the other side of the spine and look for tender and tight areas. Remember to switch your arms. Work your way six to eight inches down your rib cage. This is a great exercise to simultaneously push the ribs back down towards the pelvis and to loosen tight muscle tissue.

Some people can do this exercise twice every day. Other people get too sore and will skip a day or two between their sessions.

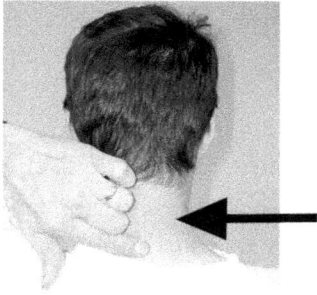

Do not push on neck.

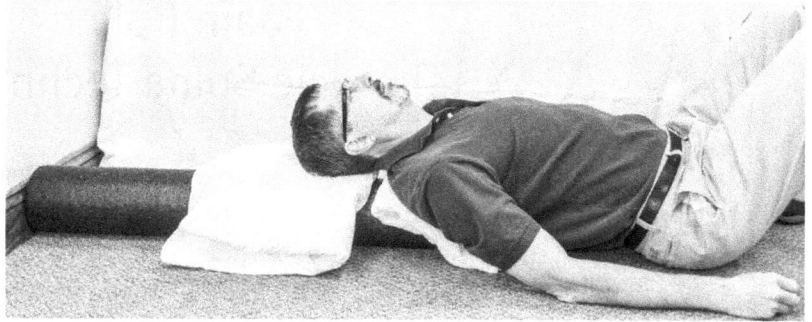

1. Place one end of foam roller against a wall. Lie with edge of roller contacting the largest "bumps" at base of neck. Pad end of roller and use pillow under head if necessary.

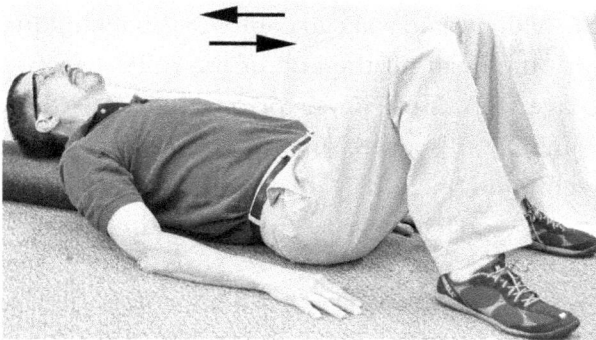

2. Gently rock back and forth on vertebrae or ribs.

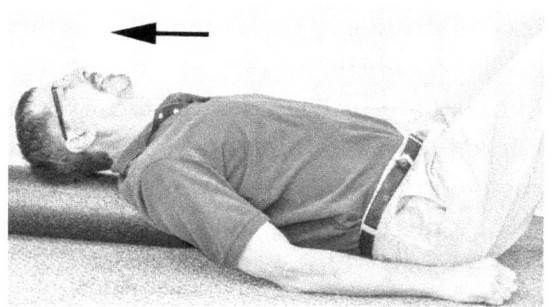

3. Move 1 inch up and repeat. Move again and repeat. Focus on tight areas. Work 6–8 inches down, back from bumps.

AVOID PAIN!

4. To work on ribs and muscles, cross arm and shift to position with roller between spine and shoulder blade. Spend at least 15 seconds on each position or tender area.

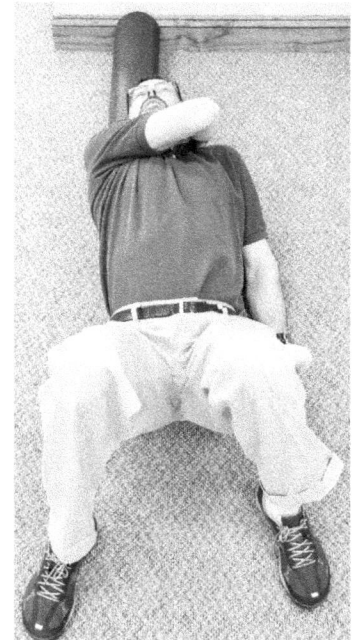

Foam Roller
Thoracic Spine Technique

Persistent stiffness and mobility restrictions in upper torso can be addressed with this technique. Not all of the muscles in the upper body run strictly length-wise. Quite a few run obliquely. To aggressively stretch these oblique muscles, you must twist and drape your upper torso over the roller.

Begin by lying with the roller across your back so that it is at the bottom of your shoulder blades. Lace your fingers and hold your head with your forearms close to the side of your head. Lift your hips and shift your body to a 45-degree angle on the roller by walking your feet to the side. At this point, the roller should be between your shoulder blades. Gently lower your head and shoulders and then your hips. Relax and let your body drape around the roller. Take one or two deep breaths. Increase or decrease your angle on the roller. Shift more to one side or the other. Find sections of your spine and rib cage that feel restricted, and try to coerce them into moving. Small rocking movements may help. Spend no less than 20 seconds working on areas that feel tight. Extra time may be needed on very stubborn parts. Remember to work on the opposite angle. If the upper thoracic vertebrae are the main target, you can combine this technique with the head off the end of the roller exercise (page 182). If the lower torso is the target, then combine this exercise with the lumbar spine technique (page 180). Bear in mind that you are trying to get your torso to bend and twist backwards. It has probably been years since it has gone in that direction. Take your time. Relax. Resist the temptation to curl forward. Use padding if needed.

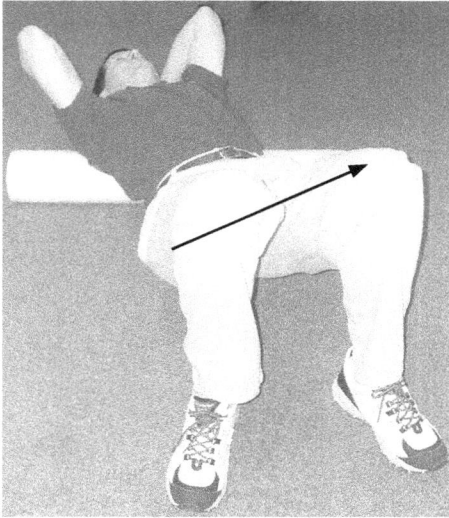

1. Lie with roller across back. Shift to angle by walking sideways.

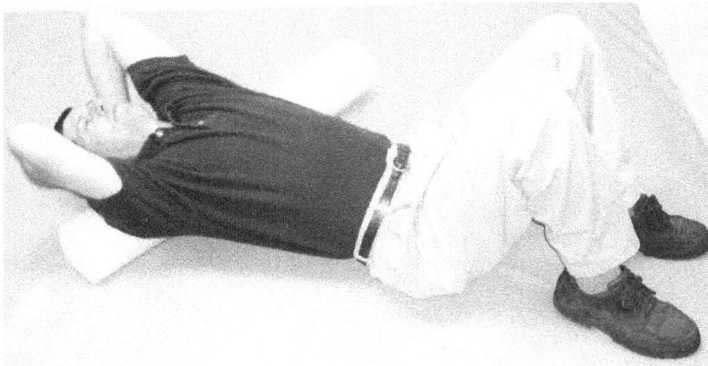

2. Position roller between shoulder blades. Let your body drape and relax over roller.

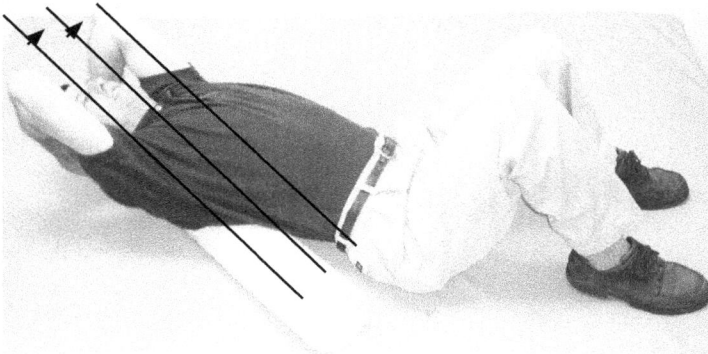

3. Adjust angle and/or position on roller to address tight areas of spine.

- Look at ceiling.
- Keep forearms close to head, and keep shoulder blades protracted.
- Drape. Relax. Breathe deeply.
- Hold positions for 15–20 seconds.

AVOID PAIN!

Other Uses for the Foam Roller

With a little imagination, you can roll and massage almost any part of the body. Just rolling over a muscle will help loosen tight tissue. However, movement on the roller does not have to be restricted to rolling. If you find a localized tight spot, you can move side to side or in a small circular massaging movement to help break up fibrotic tissue.

Over the following pages are foam roller exercises for the arms and legs.

Upper Rib Cage Mobilization with a Foam Roller

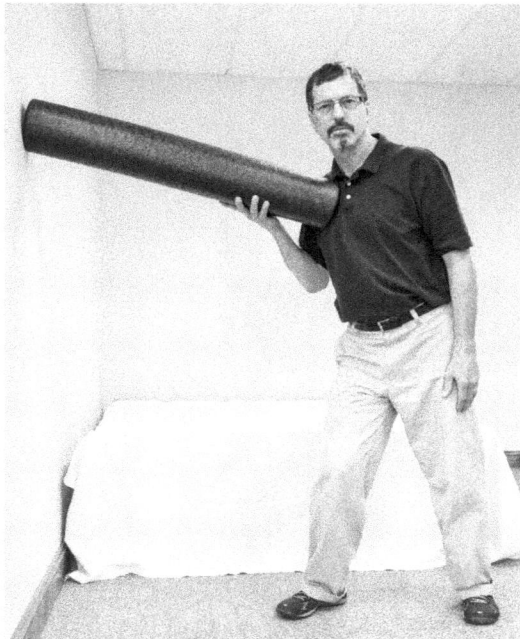

1. Lean forward so that top edge of roller is just below collar bone.

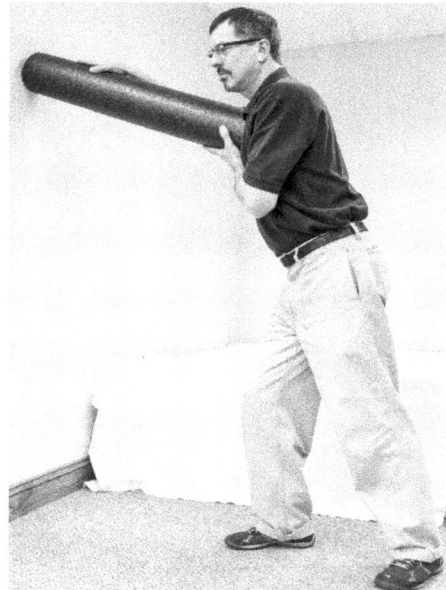

2. Fully exhale and let rib cage relax. Take a slow, deep breath. Don't let ribs move. Hold 15 seconds and relax.

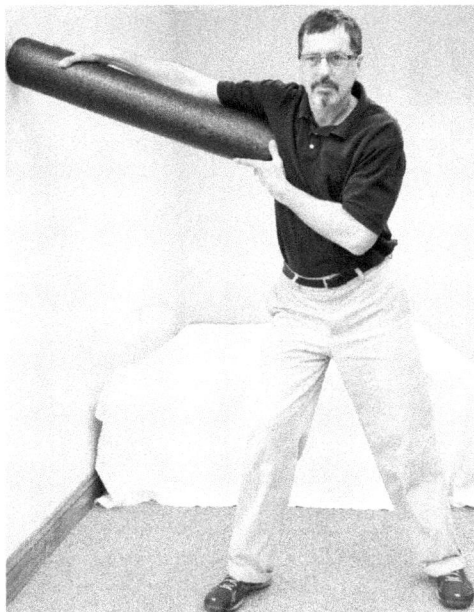

3. Place top edge of roller high in armpit. Repeat exhale/inhale cycles.

- Use comfortable pressure
- Repeat each position 3–4 times

AVOID PAIN!

Foam Roller Arm Pit Technique

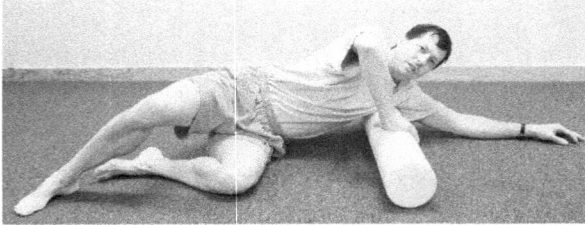

1. Foam roller on floor. Lie on side with roller in armpit

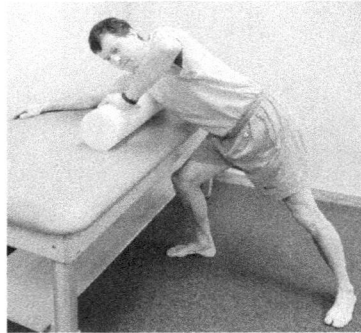

2. On counter or table, lean over with roller in armpit.

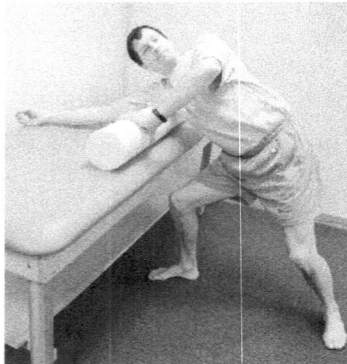

3. Roll back and forth across back portion of armpit by resting over roller sideways.

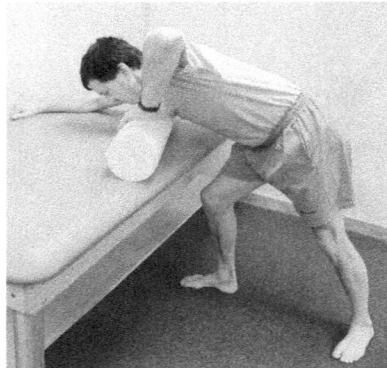

4. Turn more face down to roll front of armpit.

• Do 2–3 times per side

AVOID PAIN!

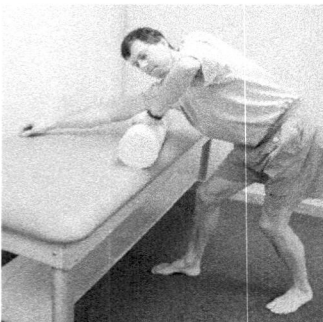

5. Roll back and forth 8–10 times. Use smaller oscillation over very tight areas.

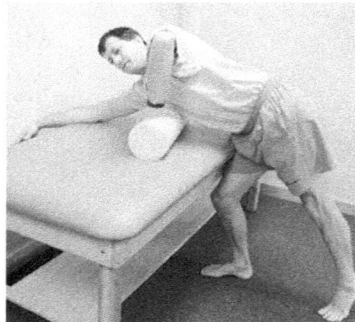

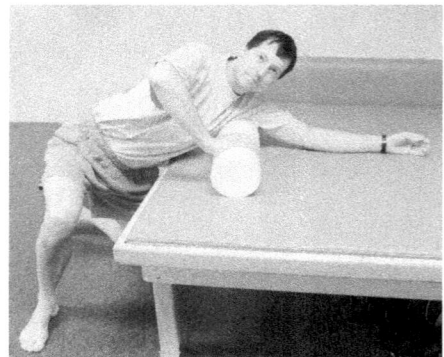

6. Technique on low table.

Foam Roller Lower Leg Technique

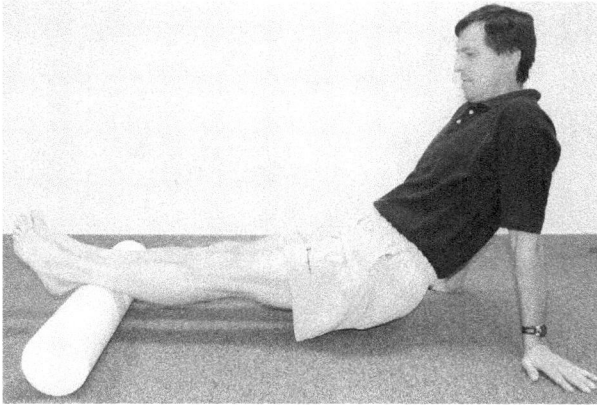

1. Sit on floor with roller under calves.

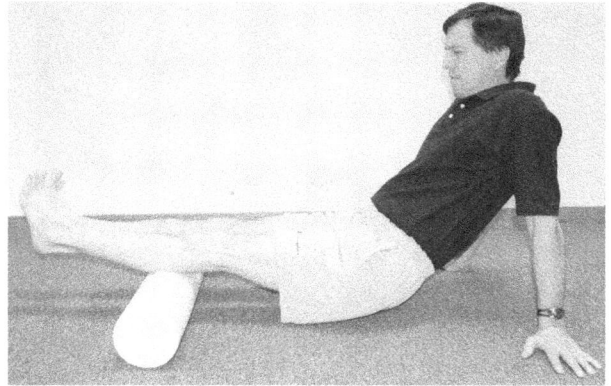

2. Roll up and down length of calf muscles. Point toes toward nose. Cross one leg over other for more pressure.

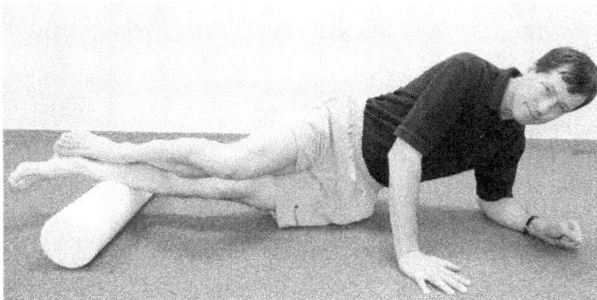

3. Lie with roller contacting front and outside of one leg.

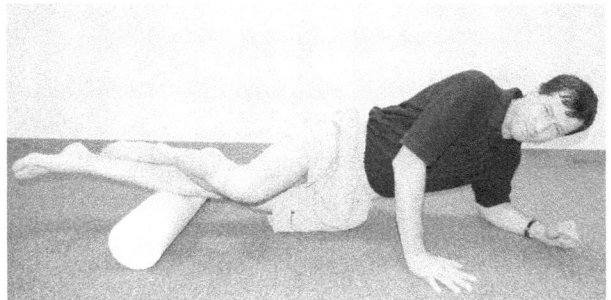

4. Roll up and down length of lower leg from ankle to knee.

- Do one leg, then other
- Do 8–10 times per leg

AVOID PAIN!

Foam Roller Inner and Outer Thigh Technique

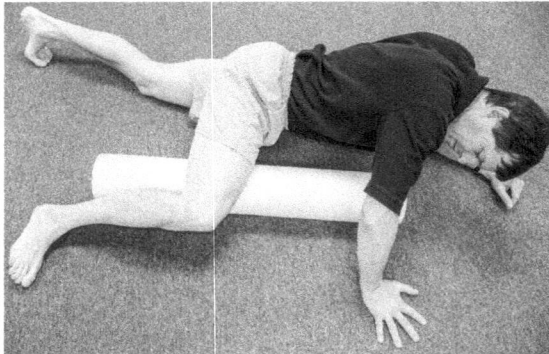

1. Straddle roller so inside of upper leg is on roller.

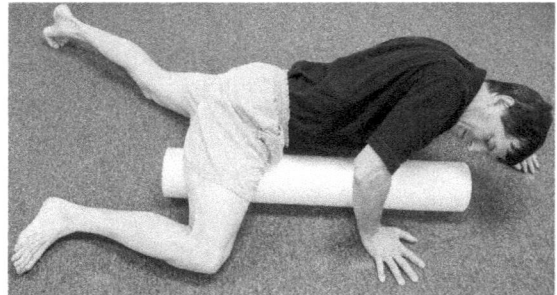

2. Move torso side to side to move roller from hip to knee.

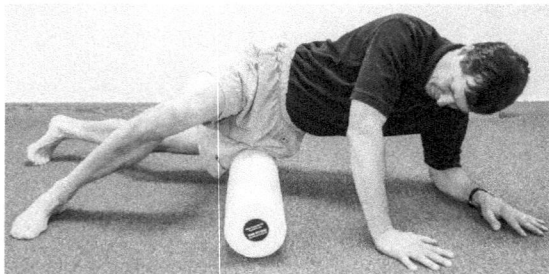

3. Lie sideways across roller so outside of thigh rests on roller.

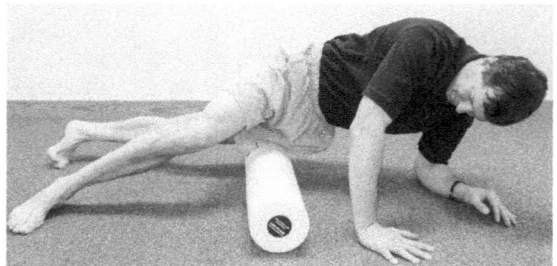

4. Stay below hip bone and above knee.

- Roll slightly forward or backward to find hot spots
- Do 8–10 rolls per leg

AVOID PAIN!

Foam Roller Thigh Technique

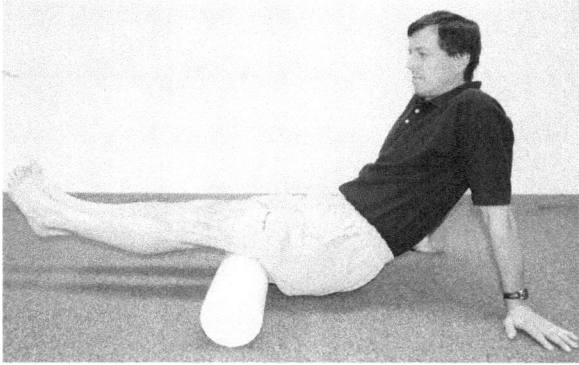

1. Roll back and forth over entire length of hamstrings.

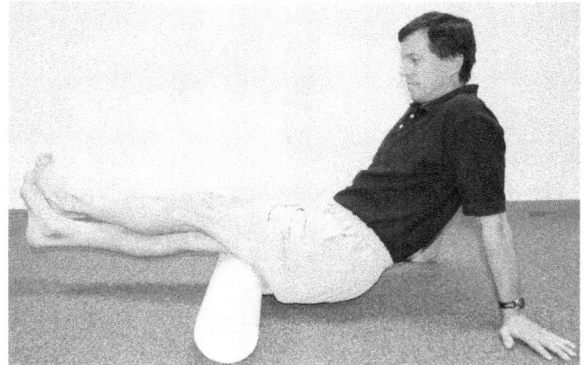

2. Cross a leg over for single leg verison.

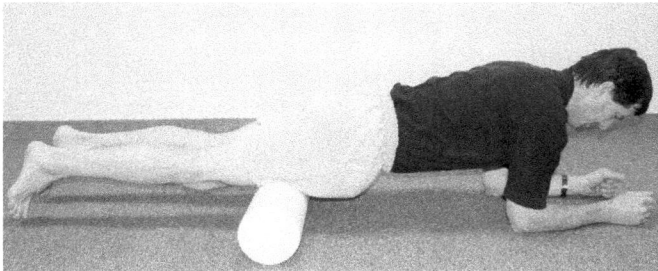

3. Roll back and forth over entire length of quadricep.

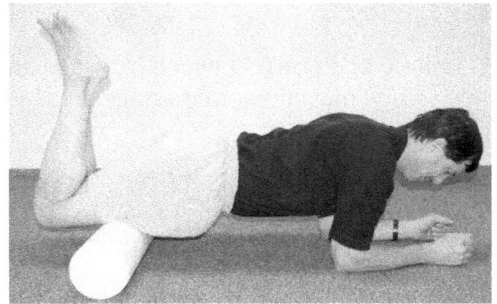

4. Bend knees or lift one leg for more pressure.

- Do 8–10 rolls per muscle group
- Roll slightly to left and right to change position of legs on roller

AVOID PAIN!

Self-Mobilization of the Anterior Hip

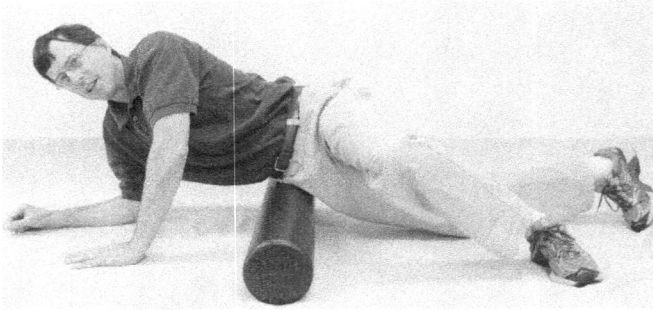

1. Lie with roller positioned just below pelvic bone.

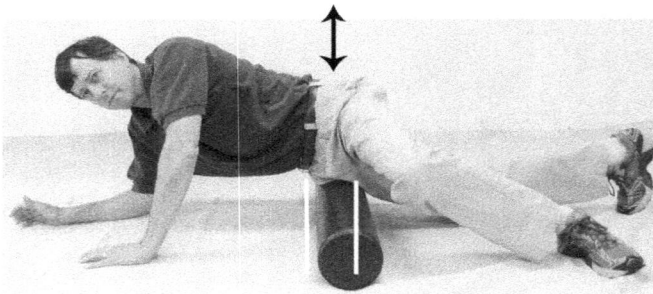

2. Roll up and down between hip bone and pelvis. Try side to side movement to massage area.

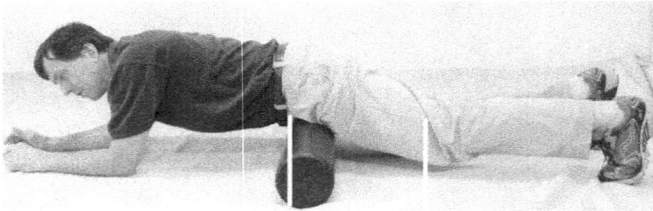

3. In a more prone position, roll further down leg.

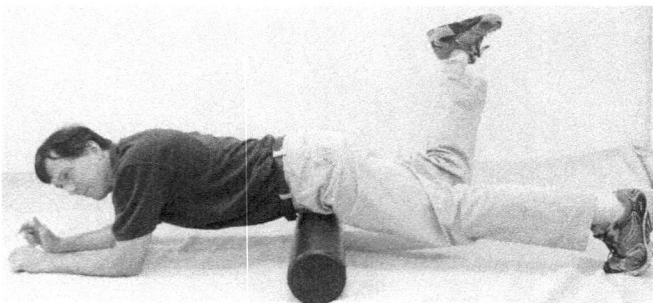

4. Lift and/or bend knee to add pressure.

- Roll 12–18 times per leg
- 1–2 times per day

AVOID PAIN!

VIII

Key Knee Exercises

There can be multiple factors that contribute to knee pain. Having weak and tight thigh muscles (especially the quadriceps) can play a big part. Poor control of gluteal and stomach muscles can add extra load to the knees. If your knee won't fully straighten, you end up walking (or running) on a bent knee. This can cause pain.

Even if you have a very arthritic knee, these exercises can help you be more comfortable. In addition to the following exercises, a comprehensive exercise program for the knees should include gluteal and abdominal retraining as well as strengthening and stretching of thigh, hip, and hamstring muscles.

Quad Set/Straight Leg Raise

When you completely straighten your knee, the last eight to ten degrees of movement is called "terminal extension". It is critical that the thigh or quadriceps muscle function well in terminal extension to help the knee control the forces encountered in walking and running. Even a mild injury to the knee can cause some weakness in the quadriceps. The weakness may initially go unnoticed because our body may adapt by keeping the knee stiffer when the foot hits the ground, which means the joint surfaces absorb more force. Some of the extra force may also then be transmitted to the foot and up into the hip and pelvis.

The quad set/straight leg raise is a good starting point for knee rehab. Lie on your back with the uninvolved leg bent so the bottom of the foot is flat on the floor. The involved leg is straight with a rolled-up bath towel under the knee. Tighten the thigh muscle by pushing the back of the knee down against the towel. The knee should straighten, and the heel will lift slightly. This is the "quad set." Lift the leg while maintaining the quad set to keep the knee as straight as possible. Slowly raise the leg so that the heel is eight to 12 inches off the floor then slowly lower the leg. Once it is down, relax the quad. All of this should take about ten seconds. Rest for three to five seconds then repeat the quad set/leg raise. Keep the exercise slow and controlled. Generally do three sets of ten repetitions.

If lifting the leg is painful, do quad sets only. Hold for five seconds, rest five to ten seconds and repeat. Do three sets of ten repetitions. You can hold a "12 o'clock tilt" while raising the leg to take strain off the low back. If your knee won't straighten, see "How to straighten a bent knee" (page 202). You can add ankle weights to further strengthen the muscle. For a very weak quad, you can do this exercise three to four times per day. If this exercise is too easy, try a quad machine (page 198) at your local fitness center or a knee extension set up on your home machine.

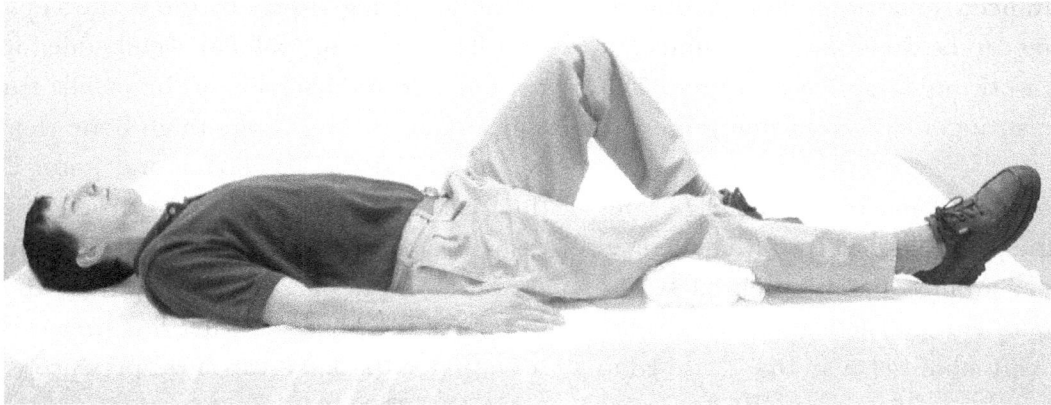

1. On back with folded towel under knee. The uninvolved leg is bent with foot flat on floor. Tighten thigh muscle of straight leg by "shrugging" knee cap, then raise leg, keeping knee as straight as comfortable.

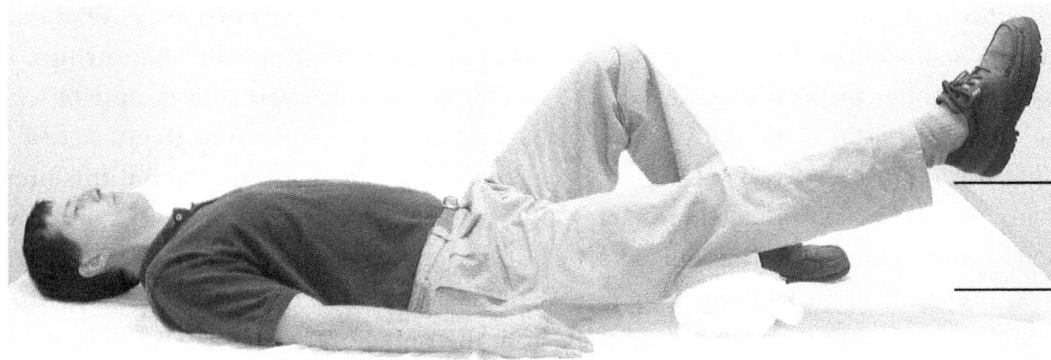

8–12 inches

2. Lower leg slowly and relax. Retighten quad muscle and repeat. A slight 12:00 tilt can be added before lifting leg.

• Do 3 sets of 10 repetitions

AVOID PAIN!

Quad and Hamstring Machine

More advanced quadriceps and hamstring strengthening can be done with a machine. For best results, work only one leg at a time. This prevents the stronger side from doing most of the work.

Sit on your quad machine, and align your knees with the pivot shaft. Vertically challenged folks may need a pillow behind their back. The knees start out bent at a 90-degree angle. If the machine is adjustable, set it so that there is no resistance from 90 to 45 degrees, otherwise use both legs to extend the knees to 45 degrees. Next relax the uninvolved leg while keeping the involved leg at 45 degrees. Now slowly straighten the involved leg, and very gently lock it straight (zero degrees) for a second or two before letting it return to a 45-degree bend. The only sensation that you should feel is the quadriceps working. Use enough resistance so that you can do two sets of 15 repetitions. If you have pain, grinding, or any "noises" in your knee, do not let your knee bend quite so far. Try working from a 30, 20, or even 10-degree angle of bend to gently locked straight. Work with in a range that is quiet and comfortable. You may also reduce the resistance and do two sets of 20 to 25 repetitions.

Why work from forty five degrees to zero? The quadriceps muscle is connected to the top of the lower leg (tibia) by the quadriceps tendon. The knee cap (patella) is embedded in the tendon, and the backside of the patella runs in a groove at the end of the thigh bone (femur). This is called the patello-femoral joint. Using the quad to move the lower leg from 90 to 45 degrees against resistance, creates tremendous pressure on the backside of the knee cap. The straighter the knee gets, the less pressure you have under the knee cap. Less pressure is better, especially if you have some wear (arthritis) in the knee.

For most people with knee pain, strength of hamstrings is not usually an issue. If you are recovering from a knee injury, then you may need to strengthen them as part of a knee rehabilitation program. To strengthen the hamstrings, some machines will have you sitting, and others will have you facedown or prone. In either case, only exercise one leg at a time. Again, this prevents the stronger side from doing most of the work, but also greatly reduces strain in the low back. Unlike the quad exercise, there is no reason to limit the range of motion. Do two sets of 15 repetitions, using sufficient resistance so that the muscles are fatigued.

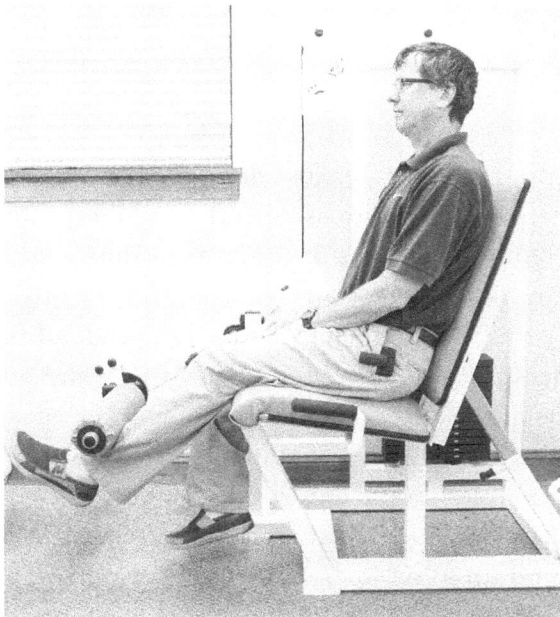

1. Single leg only quadriceps

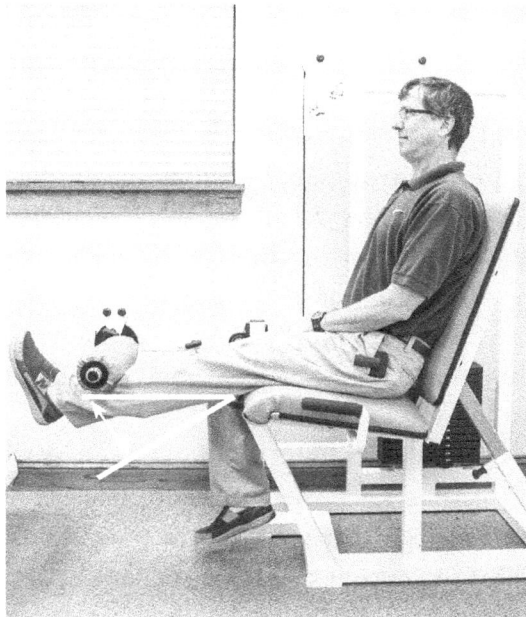

2. Extend through the last half of the movement. Return to halfway down and repeat the movement.

1. Lie on machine for hamstring.

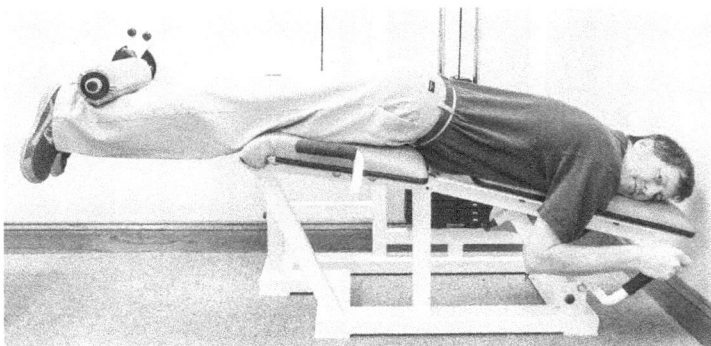

2. Flex single leg only. Lower slowly. Repeat.

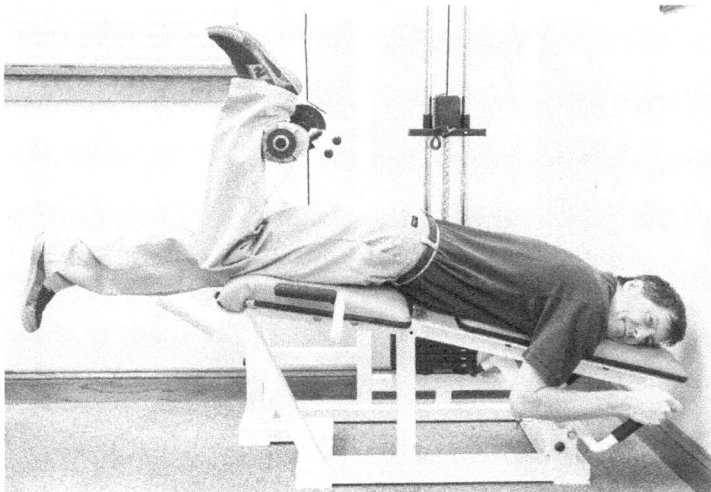

• 2 sets of 15 repetitions

AVOID PAIN!

Quad Massage

Tight soft tissues in a small muscle under the lower quadriceps just above the knee cap can contribute to knee pain. The articularis genu pulls soft tissue out of the way of the knee cap as the knee is straightened. When inflamed and dysfunctional, it causes pain that feels like it is coming from the knee joint.

To loosen this tight tissue in the right knee, sit with your knees bent to 90 degrees and 10 to 12 inches apart. Lean forward and brace or support the outside of your right knee with your right hand. Rest your left elbow or forearm on your left thigh, and use the knuckles of your left hand to massage the muscles on the inside of the right lower thigh just above the knee. Search for tight/tender areas. Spend 30 to 60 seconds on these areas, pushing almost to the point of pain. To massage the muscles on the outside of the thigh, switch hands, brace the inside of the knee with your left hand, and massage the outside of the lower thigh with the knuckles of the right hand. Use your knuckles or the point of your elbow on the muscles on top of the thigh.

Tight tissues are usually tender, and can be found up to six to eight inches above the knee. You can work on these areas three to four times a day until they resolve.

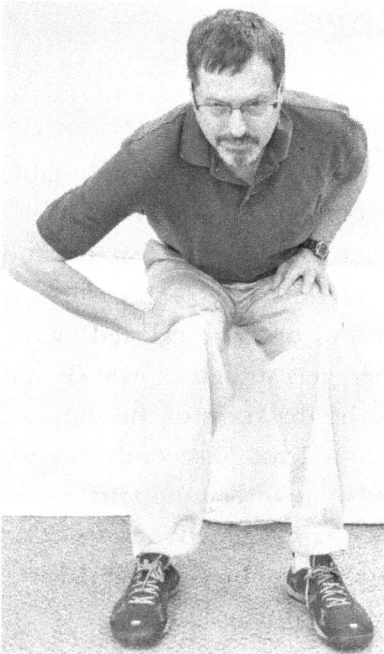

1. Sit in chair. Use hand to brace outside of knee.

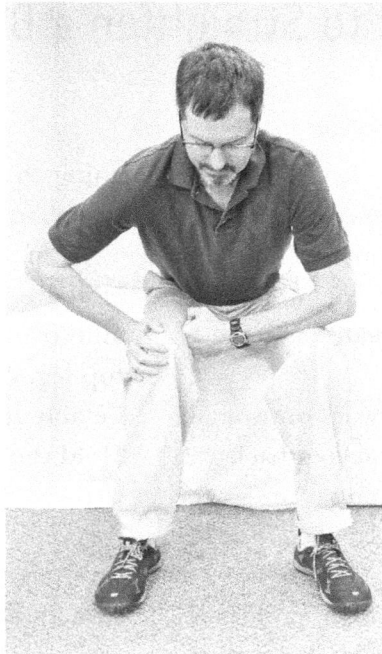

2. Deep massage muscles 1–4 inches above knee with knuckles.

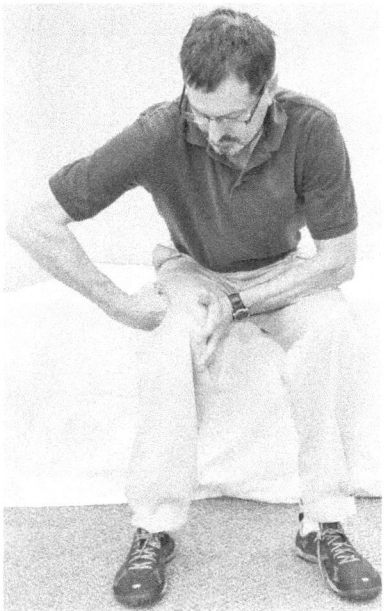

3. Then brace inside of knee, and massage outside muscles.

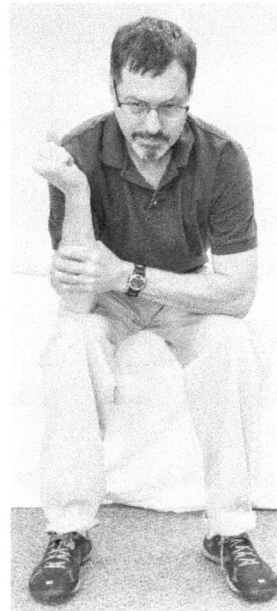

4. Massage top with elbow or knuckles.

- Search for and massage tender areas for 30–60 seconds
- Push almost to the point of pain

AVOID PAIN!

© Brian Lambert

How to Straighten a Bent Knee

When you lie flat on your back, if you notice that your knee does not straighten, you might be walking on a bent knee. Injury and swelling may cause you to lose the last few degrees of motion. Walking on a bent knee will create or worsen a knee problem.

A simple but effective way to work on straightening the knee is done by lying on your back with a rolled-up bath towel or small pillow under the involved knee. Cross the uninvolved leg over the involved one ,and gently press the knee down against the towel or pillow. Having support under the knee allows the muscles to relax and straightening to occur. You should feel a comfortable stretch in the back of the involved knee.

To make the exercise more comfortable and effective, adjust the thickness of the support and/or the amount of pressure exerted by the top leg. As the knee gets straighter, you should be able to reduce the thickness of the support. Hold the stretch for at least 20 seconds. Do two to three repetitions up to three to four times per day until your knee is straight. When working on straightening the knee, also do the quad-set/straight leg raise exercise (page 196).

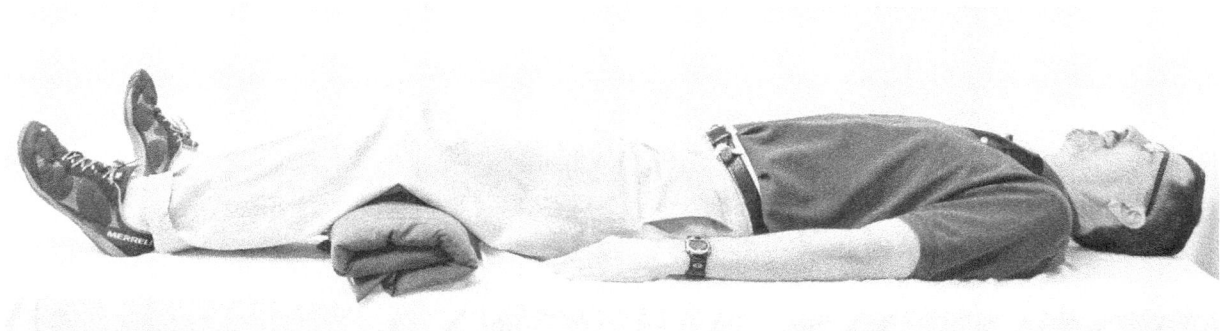

1. Lie on back with rolled towel under knee.

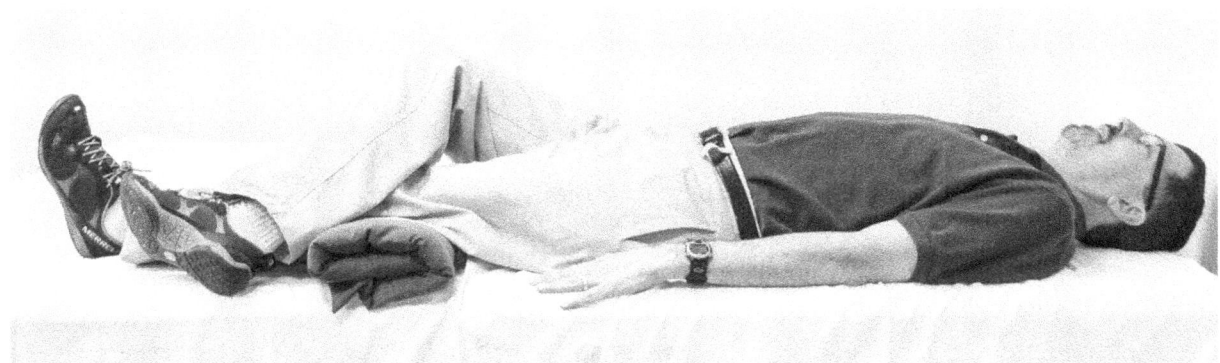

2. Cross opposite leg over bent knee, and gently press down to feel stretch behind knee. Reduce size or remove towel to increase stretch.

- Hold at least 20 seconds
- Relax and repeat 3–4 times

AVOID PAIN!

IX

Case Studies

The patients depicted in these summaries represent people who had problems associated with breakdown of the musculoskeletal system. Manual therapy and other pain relievers (*i.e.,* ultrasound, hot and cold packs, and electrical stimulation) were used with some of the patients. All of the patients were instructed to avoid "bad" pain with all of their activities, including their exercises. Patients one through eight were treated between 2001 and 2004. Patients nine through fourteen were seen between 2010 and 2013.

Patient No. 1
Neck and Shoulder Pain

A 65-year-old man described a two- to three-month history of neck and shoulder pain. The problems had not resolved with rest and medication. He said that pain was now starting in his upper arm.

He had extremely poor posture. He had a bent and rigid upper back that placed his head in a very protracted position in front of his shoulders. He could not lie flat on his back on a firm treatment table and have his head touch the table. The muscles in the front of his chest were extremely tight, restricting overall shoulder motion. Motion of the head and neck was limited and painful in almost all directions. Mechanical dysfunction was found and treated in the thoracic spine and rib cage. The patient began a home exercise program. Because of the severity

of the patient's postural problems, the exercises were modified for comfort and effectiveness. The Play Dead and Supine Attention exercises were done with his head on a folded bath towel. The towel was thick enough to allow his head to stay level when he was lying flat on his back. The towel roll exercise was started with a single towel placed under the center of the spine and enough support under the head to allow the head to stay level. The upper arm would only flex to 135 degrees (180 degrees is considered optimal). The wall angel was done sitting and without the arm component. The patient could not move his head within two inches of the wall. The patient was also given the arm stretch to improve mobility across the chest musculature.

On subsequent visits, manual therapy techniques were used with good success. But their benefit would have been extremely limited if the patient did not continue his home exercises. No changes were made with the home program on the second visit. By the third visit, we were able to reduce the thickness of the towels under the head with the attention, play dead, and towel roll exercises. A significant reduction in pain was noted. The fifth and final visit was three weeks after the patient's initial session. Even though his posture was not perfect, military, ramrod straight, it was much better than what he started with. The patient could lie flat on his back comfortably without any support under his head. He could raise his arms to approximately 160 degrees when doing the towel roll stretch. He was doing this exercise with two towels placed under the center of his back. He could do the wall angel standing (with knees bent) with the head on the wall and the arms raised to 140 degrees.

The patient was discharged with the recommendation that he continue with his exercises on a daily basis.

Patient No. 2
Neck and Arm Pain

A 55-year-old University professor described a one-year history of neck, right shoulder, and arm pain. The arm pain would radiate down to the elbow.

She had extremely poor posture, with the mid and upper portion of the thoracic spine very flexed, causing fairly severe protraction of the head and neck or forward head posture. The low back was fairly flat. A moderate amount of mechanical dysfunction was found in the thoracic spine and rib cage. Mild problems were found in the neck. Movement of the head and neck caused mild pain in the neck. There was radiation of pain down the right arm with right rotation and/or side bending. There was essentially no motion of the upper back with movement of the head and neck, indicating a "kink" in the system.

There was very poor strength and recruitment in the postural muscles throughout the neck and upper back. The muscles that control the shoulder blade were very weak. She had substantial difficulty isolating the pelvic clock muscles in both the six and 12 o'clock directions.

The patient began a home exercise program. The play dead was begun with the patient flat (no towel under the shoulders). She was given the supine attention exercise. Lying on the towel roll felt good, but the patient could only use a single towel. She could flex the shoulders to only 140 degrees (180 degrees is considered optimal). Her thumbs were pointed down to the floor to alleviate shoulder discomfort with this exercise. The wall angel was done sitting with the arms raised 45 degrees above the horizontal. Five days later, the patient noted substantial improvement. Her home exercise program was reviewed and upgraded to include using a folded bath towel under her shoulders with the play dead exercise. She could also add another towel with the towel roll exercise.

A week later, the patient reported continued improvements. She was instructed in the basic techniques for using a foam roller. The wall angel was upgraded to the standing version. The other exercises were still challenging, and we left them as they were. The patient's next visit was three weeks after her initial session. She noted discomfort only after walking her dog (who pulled on the leash) and working out on the same day. That session included an overview of upper body exercises. We included the supine elbow extension exercise to specifically target the serratus anterior. Good activation of the muscle was noted with the upper arm positioned at a 135-degree angle. Impingement in the shoulders would occur with increased flexion. The foam roller exercise was modified to add a flat pillow over the foam roller because of tenderness in the spine. The following week, the patient was doing extremely well. We made minor corrections to her upper body exercises and added reverse and side step lunges. She also learned supine heel touch downs for abdominal strengthening. All of the areas were recruited well, but fatigued very rapidly.

The patient's final visit was five weeks after her initial session. She reported complete resolution of her original pain. She had occasional upper back and shoulder fatigue with sustained kitchen activities. A review of her exercises showed good technique. We added a narrow-based wall squat to further improve the mobility in her spine. The patient was discharged after this visit.

Patient No. 3
Low Back Pain

A 49-year-old woman described a 12-month history of worsening back pain. At the time of the evaluation, she rated her pain as severe. The pain was generally localized to the left lower back area. Bending or prolonged standing would worsen her problems. She would be uncomfortable after lying in bed for more than six hours. She was very uncomfortable when first getting out of bed in the morning.

Her posture was not too bad, with only mild protraction of the head and neck over a mildly increased forward bend in the upper back. Major mechanical dysfunction was found and treated in the pelvic region. Her hip abductors and extensors were extremely weak and very poorly recruited. The 12 o'clock portion of the pelvic clock was very weak and poorly isolated. The piriformis musculature was very tight bilaterally. Overall trunk range of motion was only mildly limited. There was too much movement in the lower lumbar spine with backward bending, indicating poor backward bend movement through the pelvis and upper back.

We began her home program with Supine Gluteal Retraining, Clam, Pelvic Clock, Piriformis Stretch, and the Wall Angel. The Wall Angel was fairly easy, but the other exercises required a great deal of concentration and effort.

One week later, the patient was able to upgrade the home exercise program to include prone gluteal retraining instead of the supine version. We also added the doorframe backward bend exercise to help improve motion of the sacrum. The patient was instructed in the basic techniques for the foam roller to help improve backward bend through the thoracic spine.

By the fourth week, the patient had sufficient strength and recruitment in the gluteal musculature that we were able to add the reverse and side step lunges. We deleted the Clam and Gluteal Retraining. The Wall Squat was also added to further promote active control of extension through the thoracic spine. The patient reported a mild improvement in her back pain.

Good overall progress was being made by the fifth visit. The thoracic spine was somewhat tender after a weekend trip, and she learned how to use a pillow over the foam roller to make the exercise more comfortable.

By the seventh week, the patient reported that she had been pain-free for ten days. Her exercises were reviewed and upgraded to include supine heel touch downs for abdominal strengthening.

The patient's final visit came nine weeks after her initial session. She reported only very mild intermittent problems with pain, and these occurred only after strenuous physical activity. With this session, we reviewed her current exercises, which included reverse and side step lunges, advanced abdominal exercises, piriformis stretching, and the wall angel. At the patient's request, she was shown a basic upper body exercise program that she could follow at home. She was advised to continue with all of her exercises on a three day per week maintenance schedule.

Patient No. 4
Low Back Pain

A 35-year-old man had been suffering with low back pain for several years. He was usually better in the morning than in the evening. Three to four hours of sitting would give him severe pain. He was beginning to have intermittent leg pain. Yard and housework would trigger severe bouts of back pain that would last for several days. He had been through other conservative treatments including anti-inflammatory medication, muscle relaxants, extension exercises, and even an epidural injection.

His initial assessment revealed fairly poor posture with protraction of the head and shoulders, and a moderate increase in the thoracic kyphosis. His low back tended to be flat despite his continued good compliance with his extension exercises. Trunk range of motion was fairly good, with mild pain elicited at the end ranges of movement. Shallow single leg wall squats were very unsteady, indicating weakness in the hip musculature. Moderate mechanical dysfunction was found in the spine and pelvis. Very poor strength and recruitment were found in the hip abductors and extensors. The left side was worse than the right. He had reasonably good control of the abdominal musculature. Hip mobility was fairly good except for moderately tight piriformis musculature.

During the initial session, the patient was instructed in the pelvic clock, wall angel, prone gluteal retraining, clam exercise, and piriformis

stretch. The clock was fairly easy. Some difficulty was found with the clam and gluteal retraining. The wall angel was very difficult. The piriformis stretch felt good.

One week later, substantial improvement was noted by the patient with his second visit. We were able to upgrade his home program to include the supine heel touch down for abdominal strengthening. We attempted the side step lunge for closed chain recruitment of the hip abductors, but he was unable to hit the target. He was able to do a single-leg doorframe squat with good recruitment of the muscle behind the hip bone (hip abductors). The gluteus maximus was activated well with the reverse step lunge. A narrow- based wall squat was used to promote improved backward bending through the upper lumbar and thoracic spine. Slight abdominal tension relieved discomfort in the low back with this exercise.

The patient's third visit came three weeks after his initial session. He noted mild soreness in the gluteal musculature. We reviewed his exercises, and he demonstrated difficulty with the single-leg doorframe squat. We tried the ball on the wall exercise, which worked fairly well. Once the hip abductors were found with this exercise, the patient was then able to do the side step lunge accurately. A correction was made to the reverse step lunge that involved stabilizing the lower portion of the stance leg to reduce unnecessary motion. He was instructed in the basic foam roller exercises for improving motion in the thoracic spine.

The patient's final visit was four weeks after his initial session. He was happy to report complete resolution of his back pain. His posture had substantially improved, and he demonstrated very good recruitment and strength in the supportive musculature in the trunk and the pelvis. We concluded our session with an overview of upper body exercises, and the patient was discharged.

I have spoken with this patient several times in the past year, and he continues to do well. He notes that if he slacks off on his exercises, he experiences some return of his pain. The pain will go away when he resumes his exercises.

Patient No. 5
Knee Pain

A 40-year-old woman told of several months of worsening knee pain. Kneeling and descending stairs had become painful. This pain had forced her to curtail her weekly volleyball games. Her medical history included arthroscopic surgery on this knee for torn cartilage five years earlier.

An inspection of the knee revealed very little swelling. Tests for loose or lax ligaments and cartilage tears revealed no problems. Kneecap stability and tracking were good. She had full knee range of motion, and the strength in the quadriceps and hamstrings was very good. Flexibility in the lateral thigh, hamstrings, and quadriceps was reasonably good. Moderate tightness was found in the piriformis musculature. She had moderately poor posture. Strength and isolated recruitment in the hip abductors and extensors were very poor. The abdominal muscles were very poorly controlled and weak. There was a strong tendency to push with the legs when attempting the 12:00 tilt. Shallow single leg squats were very unsteady and mildly painful in the right knee.

A home program began with prone gluteal retraining, clam, pelvic clock, piriformis stretch-

ing, and the seated wall angel. The patient was unable to do the standing version of the wall angel. The lie down exercises were to be done twice a day, and the wall angel was to be done five or six times during the day.

Ten days after her initial session, she reported mild improvement in her knee pain. Her exercises were reviewed, and only minor corrections were needed. She was able to graduate to the standing version of the wall angel.

Three weeks after her initial session, the patient noted continued gradual improvement. She noted that the exercises had become fairly easy. She was instructed in the reverse and side step lunges as well as a narrow-based wall squat. She was able to do these well and without knee pain. The clam and prone gluteal retraining were deleted from her program.

Five weeks after her initial session, the patient noted knee pain only if the knee was pushed into hyperextension. The exercises were going extremely well. She was given the supine heel touch down for advanced abdominal strengthening. We looked at the bench fly, seated reverse fly, and doorframe lateral raises for upper body exercises.

The patient's final visit came eight weeks after her initial session. She reported almost complete resolution of her knee pain. She was shown bench press, frontal pull down, and incline reverse fly exercises. She was to add weight to the reverse and side step lunges, and continue with all of the exercises on a three-day-per-week basis.

The patient was seen informally three months after her last treatment session, and she reported her knee pain had completely resolved and not returned.

Patient No. 6
Plantar Fasciitis

The plantar fascia is a structure on the bottom of the foot that attaches from the heel bone, and fans out to attach to the base of the toes to help maintain the arches in the bottom of the foot. If it becomes overloaded, pain and inflammation can result. This patient had been dealing with worsening plantar fasciitis for several years.

The patient was a 45-year-old female secretary who experienced severe pain in the bottom of both feet, especially first thing in the morning. The pain would improve as she walked about, but would worsen if she stood or walked for more than 20 minutes. Oral medication, splints, taping, and orthotics seemed to provide only marginal benefit.

An evaluation revealed that the plantar surface of the foot was fairly tender. Her posture was not too bad except for a tendency to stand with her body tipped forward so that her body weight shifted to the balls of the feet. Shallow single leg squats were extremely unsteady. The hips were fairly restricted in the piriformis musculature. There was moderate tightness through the front of the thigh including the hip flexors. Internal rotation was very limited in the left hip, but not so much in the right. The supportive musculature in the trunk and the pelvis was very weak and very poorly recruited.

The patient's home exercise program consisted of the standard wall angel, postural cueing, pelvic clock, clam, prone gluteal retraining, and the piriformis stretch. Prone gluteal retraining, clam, and pelvic clock were difficult to recruit. The wall angel was done standing, but the arms could only be rotated to 45 degrees upward because of poor abdominal control. She felt very awkward with the postural cueing exercise.

The following week, she reported less morning pain. Minor corrections were made to the exercises. Manual therapy was used to improve mobility in the left hip, and stretching was applied to the piriformis musculature.

Two weeks after her initial session, the patient reported substantial improvement. She was able to stand and walk in the morning without extreme pain. The reverse and side step lunges were added to her home program to replace the clam and gluteal retraining. Rapid fatigue of the musculature was noted in the closed chain mode. The patient was also shown the standing hip flexor stretch.

During the third week after the initial session, the foot pain continued to lessen. Minor corrections were made to the reverse and side step lunges. Deep massage and ultrasound were used over the plantar surfaces of both feet. This significantly reduced the tenderness over the plantar fascia.

The patient's final visit came four weeks after the initial session. She reported minimal pain through the morning and drastic improvements in her comfort with walking.

Now when standing, most of her weight was carried over the ankles instead of over the balls of the feet. The patient's exercise program was reviewed, and she was discharged.

Patient No. 7
Knee Pain

Knee pain is often addressed with strengthening and stretching of the quadriceps and hamstrings. Sometimes the pain will be alleviated. If problems persist when strength and mobility of the hamstrings and quadriceps are optimized, then the problem must lie elsewhere.

A 16-year-old female soccer player described a one-year history of bilateral knee pain. The right side tended to be worse than the left. MRIs and X-ray studies were negative. Previous physical therapy aimed at the quadriceps and hamstrings was ineffective. She rated her knee pain at 8/10 after her soccer games.

Her initial evaluation revealed good strength and mobility in the hamstrings and quadriceps. There was very mild swelling along the joint line of both knees. Tests for loose and lax ligaments and cartilage tears revealed no problem. She had mild postural deficits with some protraction of the head and neck, some increase in the bend in the upper back, and a mild increase in sway to the lower back. The piriformis muscles were moderately tight on both sides. Recruitment and strength were extremely poor throughout the trunk and the pelvis. With instruction in her home exercises, we found that there was almost no isolated recruitment of the gluteus maximus. Retraining began with the supine version of gluteal retraining. Hip abduction was extremely weak and difficult to isolate with the clam exercise. The pelvic clock exercise was started. Six o'clock was fairly easy. The abdominal musculature was extremely difficult to isolate in the twelve o'clock direction. The wall angel was moderately difficult.

On the patient's second visit, very mild improvement was reported in knee pain. The exercise program was reviewed, and the supine gluteal retraining exercise was upgraded to the prone version.

The third visit came two weeks after the patient's initial session. We attempted to upgrade to the closed chain exercises, but found that recruitment was not yet adequate. The patient continued with the clam and prone gluteal retraining. We were able to add the supine heel touch down for abdominal strengthening.

On her fourth visit three weeks after her initial session, she reported continuing lessening of her knee pain. At this time, she was able to recruit the hip abductors with the side step lunge, and the hip extensors with the reverse step lunge. Rapid fatigue was reported once the musculature was isolated. She was to continue with the wall angel, piriformis stretch, and abdominal strengthening.

The patient's final visit came five weeks after her initial session. She had experienced only very mild knee discomfort after playing soccer in a weekend tournament. We reviewed her exercises and made only minor corrections to the reverse step lunge. We added the standing hip flexor stretch because of mild tightness through the front of the thigh musculature. The patient was then discharged from physical therapy.

The patient's mother stopped by our office three weeks after the patient's last session. She reported that the knee pain had not re-occurred, and that the patient was able to play soccer without problems.

Case No. 8
Knee Pain

Ms. R is semi-retired professor in her mid to late sixties. Recently, she has had severe right knee pain. Before having a steroid shot, the knee was so painful that she was using a walker. She arrived in our clinic using a straight cane, but still had a very bad limp. An MRI of her knee showed moderate to severe arthritis with some areas that were bone on bone.

She had full range of motion in both knees and very good strength in the quadriceps and hamstrings. Both knees tended to angle inward and she was wearing supportive shoes with "arch supports." We found very poor strength and recruitment in the buttock and abdominal muscles. The piriformis, hip flexors, and long thigh muscles were very tight. Her home program was started with: prone gluteal retraining (without actually lifting the foot), pelvic clock, quad/thigh stretch in sidelying, and the piriformis stretch.

A week later, the knee was a little bit better. Ms. R had discontinued the sidelying quad stretch that tended to cause more right knee pain. Stretching felt good on the left side. The other exercises were going well. We stretched both hips and aggressive deep tissue massage was used on the quadriceps just above the knee. This area started out very tight and tender, and loosened up during the session. Ms. R said that her knee felt much better afterward. We added Quad Massage to her home program.

Ms. R's third PT visit was almost four weeks after her initial session. She reported that her knee was much better, but that she would still have episodes of very sharp pain when she "stepped wrong." She still used a cane, and went up and down stairs one at a time. We again stretched the hip and thigh muscles and massaged the quad. We added the side step lunge without the knee bend component. The pelvic clock was replaced with supine heel touch downs (flat on the floor, not on the roller). With good control, she could move her foot only about halfway to the floor. She continued with gluteal retraining, quad massage, and piriformis stretching.

Two weeks later Ms. R was seen for her fourth session. She was walking comfortably without the cane, and had been able to a little bit of work in her garden. The episodes of sharp pain were diminishing. The buttock muscles were getting stronger, and she was now able to lift her foot with prone gluteal retraining. We looked at the sidelying quad/thigh stretch, but this time using a belt around the ankle so the knee did not have to bend as much. This time, Ms. R felt good stretch in the thigh without knee pain. The stomach strengthening exercise was going well, and she could now touch her heel to the floor. We stretched her hips and thigh muscles and worked on loosening the quad muscles above the knee.

Ms. R's final visit was ten weeks after her initial session. At this point, she had only mild intermittent knee pain. She could go up and down stairs normally, and take long walks with her dogs. She was doing her exercises once a day, at least, six days a week. She was instructed to do her exercises "forever" and was then discharged from PT.

Nine months later, Ms. R was back. She had stopped her exercises, explaining that she thought that walking and gardening would be enough exercise. Once we got her knee calmed down and restarted her exercise program, she felt much better.

Case No. 9
Neck and Low Back Pain

Ms. A is a professional in her late fifties with a long history of neck and low back problems. Over the years, she has had numerous sessions with physical therapists and other professionals for her back and neck. In the early nineties, she had low back surgery to decompress a nerve, and three years ago, she had surgery on her neck that fused two levels. When seen for her first PT session she complained of moderate to severe neck and right shoulder pain, and low back pain with "numbness" in both legs. Stair negotiation increased her back and leg pain, and the neck and back pain interrupted her sleep. Her daily activities were all affected by the pain. Steroid injections in her neck did not help, and pain medicine only dulled the pain. She was very worried that, to get some pain relief, she might need more surgery.

We found very poor posture. Ms. A's upper back was very forward bent with her head in front of her shoulders. She had a "sway back" to compensate for the upper back. Her neck motion was limited by 50 per cent in all directions, and shoulder motion was not limited. Lower back motion was not too bad. The piriformis and hip flexor muscles were very tight. We found very poor recruitment and strength in the supportive muscles in the neck, torso, and hips. She had mechanical dysfunction in multiple areas of her spine, rib cage, and sacroiliac joints. Although, she reported pain and "numbness" in her legs, there were no indications of spinal nerve compression.

Some manual therapy was used to start loosening tight areas. Ms. A was shown: Play dead (tuck only), supine attention and gluteal retraining, pelvic clock, piriformis stretching, and the length-wise and bottom-down techniques on the foam roller.

A week later, there was not much change. We went through her exercise program, made several corrections (keep the thighs relaxed with supine gluteal retraining, "drag" the belly button and stomach muscle towards your nose with the clock, and mainly to follow the exercise instructions explicitly). We added side lying upper body rotation stretching. Manual therapy was again used on her neck, upper back, and hips. When seen two weeks later, Ms. A was much more comfortable. She was doing the exercises only once a day, but she was doing them correctly.

Ms. A's fourth visit was four weeks after her initial session. She reported substantial improvements in her neck, back, and leg pain. We added doorframe lateral raises and bench flies on the foam roller with three pound dumbbells. With seated reverse flies (zero weight), Ms A sat on a bench that was 24 inches high. We tried the exercise on a standard 18-inch bench. But it was too low, and she had difficulty correctly positioning her upper body. These upper body exercises were to be done every other day, and on those days, she could skip her other postural exercises. For her stomach muscles, we replaced the pelvic clock with "supine heel touch downs" on the foam roller. She could move her foot only half way to the floor with good control. Her other exercises were going well.

On her fifth visit, Ms A reported almost complete resolution of her neck and shoulder pain, but she still had occasional "numbness" and a sense of weakness in her legs. She was shown prone gluteal retraining. When doing the piriformis stretch, she needed to be more precise in the "preload" part of the stretch, where the thigh is at 90 degrees as the leg is brought to the center of the body, and the foot is crossed over the other leg. This is all done before the leg is pulled towards the center of the chest.

With visit number six, Ms. A's neck and shoulder continued to do well. Her legs felt better, but she complained of some stiffness in her back below her shoulder blades and above her pelvis.

She still had some backward bending restrictions in that area. She was shown lumbar and thoracic spine techniques on the foam roller, and the upper body rotation stretch II, and we replaced prone gluteal retraining with a shallow reverse step lunge.

Ms. A's final visit was eight weeks after her initial session, and she was pain free. She had returned to all of her normal activities. Her posture, mobility, and strength had all dramatically improved, and she was doing very well with her exercise program. She was discharged from PT.

Case No. 10
Knee Pain

Ms. T came to physical therapy with a several-month history of worsening left knee pain. She is in her early sixties, and stated that the pain started after a yoga class, but she did not remember any pose or position that caused her knee to start hurting. She felt the pain in the back of her left knee when she went up or down stairs, and when she walked for more than ten minutes. An X-ray showed mild arthritis. A knee sleeve and a course of oral steroids provided only temporary relief.

Ms. T was able to walk without a limp, and there was a little bit of swelling at the knee joint, but the left knee was no warmer than the right one. She had full range of motion, and the left quadriceps was not quite as strong as it should have been. There were no signs of tears in the ligaments or cartilage. The buttock and stomach muscles were poorly recruited and very weak. Her posture was very poor, there was mechanical dysfunction in her sacroiliac joints, and her hip

and thigh muscles were very tight. She was very unsteady on each leg when asked to do shallow single leg squats.

We started Ms. T on a home exercise program that included prone gluteal retraining, pelvic clock, self-mobilization of the sacrum with a towel, and piriformis stretching. She was shown how to use a quad machine. On the foam roller, she was shown the thoracic spine and edge of the roller techniques.

Ms. T's second visit came, because of inclement weather and other scheduling issues, almost three weeks after her initial session. She had done her exercises on a reasonably consistent basis, and reported that her knee pain was almost gone. We discontinued the pelvic clock and replaced it with supine heel touch downs on the foam roller where, while keeping her lower back flat against the roller, she could only move her foot halfway to the floor, and very few repetitions were required to fatigue her stomach muscles. Her difficulty with this exercise was very surprising to Ms. T because she had been using an "ab machine" regularly at a local fitness center. She was shown the reverse step lunge to replace prone gluteal retraining. She did well when standing on her left leg, but had difficulty getting the correct positioning to ideally recruit the right buttock muscles. Once isolated, the muscles rapidly fatigued. Again, Ms. T was surprised because she had been doing a leg press exercise, and she had been told that this machine would strengthen the buttock muscles. She was also shown doorframe lateral raises, bench flies on the foam roller, and seated reverse flies.

Two weeks later, Ms. T was seen for her third and final session. Her knee was pain free, and she had returned to all of her normal activities. She was having trouble with the reverse step lunge.

When standing on her right leg, she needed to have her left leg more to the left and back. This gave her better alignment of the right leg and required a tighter grip on the doorframe. As the buttock muscle gets stronger, she will be able to decrease the amount of force on the doorframe. With her stomach exercise, she could let her foot about three quarters of the way to the floor. She was shown several more upper body exercises from the first edition of *Precision Exercises,* and then discharged from physical therapy.

Case No. 11
Neck, Back, and Leg Pain

Ms. S is an office worker in her mid-fifties. She came to physical therapy because of lower back and neck pain, and pain and "numbness" in both legs. She had the neck pain for about a month, but has had back and leg issues for many years. In the late nineties, she had fusion surgery on her lower back. A recent X-ray showed two of the screws were broken, but that the fusion appeared stable. At the end of most days, she had back and leg pain that she rated at seven out of ten, and that her feet were usually numb. She complained of stiffness in her neck, and occasional aching in her left shoulder. Her surgeon was considering fusing two additional levels in her lower back.

Trunk range of motion was 60 percent limited in all directions. Neck range of motion was limited by forty percent. Her posture was moderately poor. She had moderate to severe mechanical dysfunction in her spine, rib cage, and pelvis. She had very poor control of the supportive muscles from her neck down to her pelvis. Muscles around her hips were very tight, and

the piriformis muscles were extremely knotted. She was desperate for some pain relief and, if possible, to avoid further surgery.

Ms. S was willing to take on an extensive home exercise program. She was shown play dead, pelvic clock, self-mobilization of the sacrum with a very small towel, supine gluteal retraining, supine attention, towel roll (to loosen the thoracic spine), and piriformis stretching. She reported feeling some pain relief after instruction in her exercises.

Twelve days later, Ms. S reported that she had improvements in pain and mobility. When we reviewed the pelvic clock, we found that she was using her upper thigh muscles for the 12 o'clock portion instead of her stomach muscles. We had her use both hands as claws to help pull the stomach muscles and pelvis towards 12 o'clock. She was shown prone gluteal retraining, but, because of over-activation of her back muscles, was instructed not to do the lift portion of the exercise. She was shown the supine hip flexor stretch. Gentle manual therapy was used to improve mobility in her spine and pelvis.

On the third visit, Ms. S was doing well and we added the length-wise and bottom down cross-wise techniques on the foam roller to replace the towel roll exercise. Her other exercises were going well and were left unchanged.

Ms. S's fourth visit came almost one month after her first session. She still had some pain, but was feeling better and reported that each exercise session gave her temporary but immediate pain relief. She had returned to doing supine gluteal retraining because the prone version had become uncomfortable. She was shown how to use a tennis ball for sacral mobilization, and the lumbar and thoracic spine techniques on the foam roller. She was able to transition from the pelvic clock exercise to supine heel touch downs. She could only move her foot half way to the floor. She felt good work in her stomach muscles, and she was able to keep her lower back pressed against her fingers.

During sessions five through nine, Ms. S continued to make good progress. She had a minor setback after taking a trip where she rode in the back seat of a small car, and was also not ideally compliant with her exercise program. Once she got back to her regular routine, she felt much better. We start massaging the muscle in the front of her hip with the foam roller. She was shown piriformis massage and how to use the edge of the foam roller on the upper thoracic spine and rib cage.

With visits ten through twelve, Ms. S had some "ups" and "downs," but continued to improve. We added doorframe lateral raises and bench flies on the foam roller with three pound dumbbells and seated reverse flies with no weight. She was able to do the standing hip flexor stretch, but would continue using the supine version. She was also shown the upper body rotation stretch I. Because she was feeling good, three days a week, Ms. S had started walking one mile.

Visit thirteen was four months after Ms. S's initial session. She was maintaining reasonably good spinal, pelvic, and rib cage mechanics, and her posture looked good. She was very diligent with her exercises on a once-per-day basis. She reported feeling noticeably worse if she missed a session. She was shown single arm and upright rows with eight pounds, dumbbell presses on the foam roller with five pounds, and we replaced prone gluteal retraining with the reverse step lunge exercise.

Ms. S was seen later for her final PT session. She reported that she was symptom-free as long as she did her exercises on a regular basis. She was walking four miles three times per week. We

reviewed her exercise program, and she was discharged from physical therapy.

Case No. 12
Low Back Pain

An elite high school athlete was referred to physical therapy after two episodes of severe lower back pain that he rated at nine on a zero to ten scale. These episodes occurred over the course of a month, and he had constant pain that he rated a three. The pain was in the left side of the lower back, and did not radiate into his legs. It was worse after games and practices. X-rays did not show any problems.

Mr. E had very good posture and minimal guarding in his lower back muscles. He had good trunk range of motion, but said that he felt stiff. He had severe sacroiliac dysfunction and moderate backward bending in the upper lumbar vertebrae. He had almost no ability to activate his buttock muscles, and they were very weak. He had very poor control of his stomach muscles as well. The piriformis muscles were very tight, but the hip flexors were not an issue.

When Mr. E tried prone gluteal retraining, he tended to contract his back and leg muscles, but had absolutely no activation of his buttock muscles. With the supine version, he was able to generate only a slight gluteal contraction without activation of the back and leg muscles. He had moderate problems with the 12 o'clock portion of the pelvic clock. He was shown piriformis stretching and self-mobilization of the sacrum with a tennis ball. He was instructed to always sit with lumbar support. Mr. E reported feeling much better after going through his exercises.

A week later, Mr. E reported that he had less pain, and that he felt looser. He had done some running, but did not practice or play soccer. We found good spinal and pelvic mechanics. He was able to start prone gluteal retraining, and was shown supine heel touch downs on the foam roller to replace the pelvic clock and the quadruped piriformis stretch. We found that Mr. E's upper body was very tight, and he was subsequently shown the upper body rotation stretch II.

On his third visit, Mr. E continued to improve. His lumbar and pelvic mechanics were good and he was able to resume technical drills and had increased his running. Because of complaints of stiffness in his upper back we added cross-wise and thoracic spine techniques on the foam roller. When we reviewed prone gluteal retraining we found that he was doing the exercise too fast. He was not "lengthening" before lifting and he was allowing his knee to bend when he did lift. He was instructed spend two to three seconds on each step of the exercise and to focus on doing each step correctly.

Mr. E's fourth visit was three weeks after his initial session. He reported some transient tightness in his lower back after he played a full, 90-minute, soccer game; otherwise he felt good. He was shown reverse step lunges. He reported severe fatigue in the buttock muscles after only four or five repetitions, with the left side being worse than the right. He was probably going to continue prone gluteal retraining while learning the reverse step lunge. We also added bench flies on the foam roller with ten-pound dumbbells, doorframe lateral raises with five-pound dumbbells, and seated reverse flies without weights.

Progress was still good with the fifth session. We felt that Mr. E could reduce the frequency of sacral self-mobilization to four times a week. Corrections were made to the reverse step lunge. These included keeping the trailing leg back and more to the side, and keeping the front shin stationary. He was shown advanced abdominal exercises (Part I), which he found to be very challenging.

Two weeks later, Mr. E reported that his low back would get tight with long car rides, but it loosened up once he was out of the car and moving around; otherwise he was doing well. We added the side step lunge where, again, the exercise was more difficult on the left side.

Mr. E had to cancel a two-week follow-up appointment because of a sprained ankle, but he reported that his back was doing well. He was seen the next week, which was eight weeks after his initial session. His lower back "felt stiff," and we found mechanical dysfunction in his pelvis. We reviewed self-mobilization of the sacrum and had him place the ball closer the center of his sacrum. We had him try Version Two where he propped up on his elbows to increase the pressure on the sacrum.

Mr. E's eighth and final appointment was ten weeks after his first session, and he was pain free. As an added benefit, he felt that his kicks were stronger and more accurate than when he started PT, and that he had more speed. We found good spinal and pelvic mechanics, made only minor corrections to his exercise program, and discharged him from PT.

Case No. 13
Hip Pain

Ms. Z was sent to physical therapy for chronic hip and groin pain. Her activities had become limited by pain and lack of mobility in her left hip and groin, and now plantar fasciitis in her left foot. Her right hip has recently started giving problems as well. For many years, she could some relief by "popping" her pubic symphysis. This no longer worked, and things seemed to be getting worse.

When evaluated, we found moderately poor posture with increased curves in the neck, thoracic spine, and lower back. There was moderate to severe mechanical dysfunction in the spine and pelvis. The stomach and buttock muscles were not working very well. She had good trunk range of motion, but her hips were very tight, and her single leg balance was very poor. She was shown prone gluteal retraining and the pelvic clock, where the buttock and stomach muscles were hard to activate. She was shown the bottom down cross-wise and length-wise techniques on the foam roller. Finally, we looked at stretching very tight piriformis muscles and using a towel for self-mobilization of her stuck sacrum. She reported feeling looser after going through the exercises.

A week later, Ms. Z reported that she had less pain. In her zumba class, she had better movement in her hips and better balance. We made corrections to prone gluteal retraining asking her to be more precise with each step of the exercise and to slow down. With the piriformis stretch, she was pulling the leg directly towards her chest instead of "preloading" at 90 degrees, then pulling to the center of the chest. With the pelvic clock, she was instructed to use both hands as "claws" to pull on the belly button and lower stomach muscles to help them draw the pelvis towards 12 'o clock. We looked at using the edge of the roller to work on her "dowagers hump."

On her third visit, Ms. Z was having only mild intermittent problems. We again corrected prone gluteal retraining. This time, Ms. Z was reminded to keep her knee straight when lifting the leg. We replaced the pelvic clock with supine heel touch downs on the foam roller. With good control, she could only let her foot go half way to the floor. Because the muscle was still knotted and tender, we added the piriformis massage to her home program. She was shown how to use the foam roller on the front muscles of her hip and the thoracic spine technique.

Four weeks after her initial session, Ms. Z was doing well when seen for her fourth visit. She reported, that for the most part, she was pain free, and was doing her exercises on a regular basis. She could, with the stomach exercise, let her foot touch the floor, while keeping her lower back flat against the roller. Prone gluteal retraining was replaced with reverse step lunges. She recruited her gluteous maximus well, and each muscle fatigued after only four to five repetitions.

The final visit was eight weeks after the initial session. Ms. Z was essentially pain free. We made a minor correction to the reverse step lunge, which involved letting the shin of the support leg angle a little bit forward to take work away from the hamstrings on the back of the thigh. She was cautioned not to let it go too far forward, which would overload the quad and knee. For many people, there seems to be a "happy" position of the shin, where the quads and hamstrings are relatively inactive, and they get good recruitment of the buttock muscle. We added doorframe lateral raises with three-pound dumbbells, bench flies on the foam roller with five-pound dumbbells, and seated reverse flies without weight. She had moderate difficulty getting the upper body positioned correctly with the reverse fly. She attempted part I of the advanced abdominal exercises, but found them too hard. She will continue doing the stomach exercise on the foam roller.

Two weeks later, Ms. Z cancelled a follow-up appointment, reporting that she was doing very well, and she felt that she could progress independently.

Case No. 14
Back and Shoulder Pain

Mr. M was in his late sixties and came to physical therapy with severe left shoulder pain and weakness. He is right handed, and the pain started one evening. Earlier that day, he and his wife had carried four sheets of three-quarter-inch plywood into his woodworking shop located in his basement. He did not recall having any problem carrying the wood. Over a two month period, he tried rest, ice, heat, and various medications, and the pain was getting worse.

Mr. M could raise his left arm only to 90 degrees, and he could not reach his wallet in his left back pocket. He rated his pain at seven out of ten, and he could not find a comfortable sleeping position. His posture was very poor, with severe mechanical dysfunction in his upper back and rib cage. Some manual therapy was used on the dysfunction in his upper back and rib cage. His home program consisted of play dead and supine attention exercises. The muscles were poorly recruited and very weak. Instruction in scalene and upper body rotation stretches revealed very tight muscles. With the foam roller, Mr. M was shown how to use the edge of the roller on his upper thoracic spine and the thoracic spine technique. By the conclusion of the session, Mr. M could reach his wallet and raise his arm to 160 degrees.

Eight days later, Mr. M was seen for his second session. He had worked on his exercises twice per day, and reported being 50 to 60 percent better. He was shown the head off end and upper rib cage techniques with the foam roller, and more manual therapy was used on his upper back area.

The following week, Mr. M was seen for severe lower back pain from "pulling a few weeds" in his yard. He could not stand up straight, but reported no leg symptoms. He had severe backward bending restrictions in his lower back and pelvis. This was treated with manual therapy, and he was instructed in self mobilization of the sacrum with a tennis ball and the prone press-up exercise. Both prone gluteal retraining and the pelvic clock were very hard because of poor muscle activation in those respective areas. Lastly, he was to stretch very tight piriformis muscles.

Mr. M was seen the next day, and reported that his back and shoulder were 70 percent improved. Corrections were made to several exercises. He needed to keep the knees straight when lifting the leg with prone gluteal retraining, more pull on his stomach muscles with the pelvic clock, more tuck with play dead, and he needed to shift farther off center when using the edge of the roller on his rib cage.

A week later, Mr. M reported that his back and shoulder were both at least 85 percent better. His low back and sacroiliac joints were much more flexible. His shoulder and rib cage had improved flexibility as well. We replaced the pelvic clock with supine heel touch downs where he could move his foot half way to the floor while keeping his back flat. He did well with reverse step lunges to replace prone gluteal retraining. He had good activation of the buttock muscles, and he fatigued after four to five repetitions. Mr. M was shown doorframe lateral raises and bench flies on the foam roller with five pounds. He had some difficulty positioning his upper body with seated reverse flies.

Mr. M's sixth and final visit was one month after his first session. He was very excited about how his exercises made him feel when he did them. His back and shoulder were improving, and were now 95 percent better than when he started his physical therapy treatments. He needed minor corrections to his reverse step lunge. He was instructed to slow down the movement. He was then able to keep the front shin stationary, and feel where the trailing leg needed to be positioned for the best activation of the buttock muscles. We added upright rows with 15 pounds, single arm rows with 10 pounds, and dumbbell press with 10 pounds. He had access to weights at his neighborhood fitness center. Mr. M was then discharged from PT.

In Summary

To reduce or eliminate bodily pain, a little bit of exercise will go a long way. The right comination of exercises will go even farther.

You do not have to live with pain. If you can make the commitment to do a few exercises everyday, you can reduce or eliminate your pain. You can reduce or eliminate the need for pain medicine. You can get back to your normal life. All that you have to do is a few exercises. Go for it!

About the Author

Brian is originally from Norfolk, Virginia and has lived in Charlottesville since graduating from Old Dominion University in 1983 with a Bachelor of Science in Physical Therapy. His work history includes five years at University of Virginia Hospital, six years at Martha Jefferson Hospital, and six years in private practices. From 2001 to the present, he has had his own practice in the Pantops area of Charlottesville. Brian's continuing education has included extensive training in osteopathic therapy techniques through the School of Osteopathy at Michigan State University, as well as through a multitude of inservices and other training programs.

Brian is married to Ann who is a medical technician at the University Medical Center. They have two boys. Will plays soccer at Longwood University and Kevin is a welder at a shipyard in the Tidewater area.

Brian's hobbies include windsurfing, softball, soccer, home improvement, and automotive restoration.

www.ingramcontent.com/pod-product-compliance
Lightning Source LLC
Chambersburg PA
CBHW080327270326
41927CB00014B/3126